W0043321

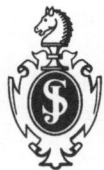

Dudley J. Pennell, Richard Underwood,
Durval C. Costa and Peter J. Ell

Thallium Myocardial Perfusion Tomography in Clinical Cardiology

With 157 Figures

Springer-Verlag
London Berlin Heidelberg New York
Paris Tokyo Hong Kong
Barcelona Budapest

Dudley J. Pennell, MA, MRCP
Amersham Research Fellow, Institute of Nuclear Medicine, University College and
Middlesex School of Medicine, Mortimer St, London W1N 8AA

S. Richard Underwood, MA, MRCP
Senior Lecturer in Cardiac Imaging, Royal Brompton National Heart and Lung
Institute, Dovehouse St, London SW3 6LY

Durval C. Costa, MD, MSc, PhD
Senior Lecturer in Nuclear Medicine, Institute of Nuclear Medicine, University
College and Middlesex School of Medicine, Mortimer St, London W1N 8AA

Peter J. Ell, MD, MSc, PD, FRCP, FRCR
Professor of Nuclear Medicine, Institute of Nuclear Medicine, University College and
Middlesex School of Medicine, Mortimer St, London W1N 8AA

The front cover illustration shows a normal myocardial perfusion image in the vertical long axis.

ISBN-13: 978-1-4471-1859-6   e-ISBN-13: 978-1-4471-1857-2
DOI: 10.1007/978-1-4471-1857-2

British Library Cataloguing-in-Publication Data
Thallium myocardial perfusion tomography in clinical cardiology.
    I. Pennell, Dudley J.
    I. Pennell, Dudley J.
    616.10754

Library of Congress Cataloging-in-Publication Data
Thallium myocardial perfusion tomography in clinical cardiology /
    Dudley J. Pennell . . . [et al.].
        p.   cm.

    1. Coronary heart disease—Tomography.   2. Heart—Radionuclide
imaging.   3. Thallium—Isotopes—Diagnostic use.   I. Pennell, Dudley J.,
1958–   .
    [DNLM: 1. Coronary Disease—radionuclide imaging.   2. Thallium
Radioisotopes—diagnosis use.   3. Tomography, Emission-Computed.
WG 300 T365]
RC685.C6T39   1991
616.1'2307575—dc20
DNLM/DLC   91–5007
for Library of Congress   CIP

Apart from any fair dealing for the purposes of research or private study, or criticism
or review, as permitted under the Copyright, Designs and Patents Act 1988, this
publication may only be reproduced, stored or transmitted, in any form or by any
means, with the prior permission in writing of the publishers, or in the case of
reprographic reproduction in accordance with the terms of licences issued by the
Copyright Licensing Agency. Enquiries concerning reproduction outside those terms
should be sent to the publishers.

© Springer-Verlag London Limited 1992

Softcover reprint of the hardcover 1st edition 1992

The use of registered names, trademarks etc. in this publication does not imply, even
in the absence of a specific statement, that such names are exempt from the relevant
laws and regulations and therefore free for general use.

Product liability: The publisher can give no guarantee for information about drug
dosage and application thereof contained in this book. In every individual case the
respective user must check its accuracy by consulting other pharmaceutical literature.

Typeset by Best-set Typesetter Ltd., Hong Kong

28/3830–543210   Printed on acid-free paper

Preface

Cardiologists have a tradition of performing their own imaging procedures. Only rarely are echocardiography and cardiac catheterisation delegated to others. This practice is efficient because the findings can be interpreted rapidly and accurately in the light of the clinical problem. In contrast, nuclear cardiology investigations are commonly performed by a third party. Both imager and cardiologist then need to be familiar with each other's practice if the patient is not to suffer. We are very fortunate to work in institutions where the importance of a close liaison is recognised. Indeed, the distinction between nuclear physician, nuclear cardiologist and cardiologist has become blurred. In this setting we are convinced that nuclear cardiology can improve the quality of patient management by providing the functional information to complement the anatomical information provided by, for instance, coronary arteriography.

The most important functional information in patients with coronary artery disease is myocardial perfusion, for it is abnormalities of perfusion that produce the symptoms that we treat with medication, angioplasty and bypass surgery. Despite the importance of myocardial perfusion, we have only one simple method with which it can be assessed. Thallium scintigraphy has been available for almost two decades but emission tomography is a more recent development that has made an important contribution. The high contrast resolution inherent to tomography means that the presence or absence of an abnormality can be determined with greater confidence than with planar imaging, particularly in borderline cases. The three-dimensional nature of tomograms means that the site and extent of the abnormality can be judged more accurately, and the images can be presented in planes familiar to cardiologists. Thallium tomography has a reputation, however, for being difficult to perform well. Certainly, the scope for artefact is greater with tomographic imaging than with planar imaging. We are eager, therefore, to offer our experience to others because, having conquered these problems, we can clearly recognise the importance of the technique. We hope that our experience will be helpful to cardiologists, nuclear physicians, radiologists and others involved in the assessment of the cardiac patient using radiopharmaceuticals. We intend it to act as a guide to normal and abnormal appearances and as an illustration of the way in which thallium emission tomography can contribute to patient management. Most of all, we hope that it will engender the same response from those unfamiliar with thallium tomography as it did from one of our colleagues who shall remain nameless:

"I didn't know you could do that. That could actually be useful."

London, April 1991

Dudley J. Pennell
Richard Underwood
Durval C. Costa
Peter J. Ell

Acknowledgements

We should like to thank the staff of the Institute of Nuclear Medicine for their assistance with the large number of scans that form the basis of our experience, and we are grateful to Amersham International PLC, CORDA and the Medical Research Council for financial assistance. DJP is an Amersham research fellow.

Abbreviations

BP	Blood pressure	PDA	Posterior descending artery
d	Diagonal branch of LAD	PET	Positron emission tomography
ECG	Electrocardiogram	RCA	Right coronary artery
HLA	Horizontal long axis	SA	Short axis
LAD	Left anterior descending	SPET	Single photon emission tomography
LCx	Left circumflex	VLA	Vertical long axis
LMS	Left main stem		

Notes

All exercise electrocardiograms reported in Chapter 6 were performed using the standard Bruce protocol. The description of findings at Coronary arteriography is limited to the abnormal findings only. The diagrams of coronary arteriograms show stenoses in red – one line, two lines or occlusion representing a mild or severe stenosis, or occlusion respectively. For reasons of clarity, only the most important stenoses are indicated and in cases with coronary bypass grafting only the native vessels are shown. The drawings that illustrate the site of thallium abnormalities are diagrammatic only and defects may not always be fully appreciated in the limited number of tomograms that can be displayed. White represents normal uptake, light grey, mid-grey and dark grey represent increasingly severe abnormalities.

Contents

1 Introduction 1

2 Radiopharmaceuticals 5
Myocardial Perfusion Tracers 5
Thallium-201 6
Technetium-99m 2-Methoxy-isobutyl-isonitrile 9
Technetium-99m Teboroxime 10

3 Stress Techniques 13
Drug Treatment 13
Dynamic Exercise 15
Pharmacological Stress 16
    Dipyridamole 16
    Adenosine 18
    Dobutamine 18
Choice of Stress Technique 19

4 Imaging Techniques 23
The Gamma Camera 23
Emission Tomography 23
Patient Preparation 25
Data Acquisition 26
Data Processing 27

5 Image Interpretation 31
Quality Control 31
Normal Appearances 31
Abnormal Appearances 33
Coronary Anatomy 36
Quantification 36
    Lung Uptake of Thallium 37
    Myocardial Distribution of Thallium 37
    Washout Analysis 41

6 Clinical Case Material 45
The Normal Heart 46
    Case 1   Normal Vertical Heart 46

CONTENTS

Case 2   Normal Horizontal Heart 48
Normal Variants.. 50
Case 3   Anterior Attenuation 50
Case 4   Inferior Attenuation........................... 52
Case 5   Apical Attenuation............................ 54
Case 6   Papillary Muscle 56
Single Vessel Reversible Ischaemia 58
Case 7   RCA 58
Case 8   LCx 60
Case 9   PDA 62
Case 10 Proximal LAD 64
Case 11 Diagonal LAD 66
Case 12 Distal LAD................................. 68
Single Vessel Myocardial Infarction 70
Case 13 RCA 70
Case 14 LCx 72
Case 15 PDA 74
Case 16 Proximal LAD 76
Case 17 Diagonal LAD 78
Case 18 Distal LAD................................. 80
Two Vessel Reversible Ischaemia 82
Case 19 RCA/LCx 82
Case 20 LAD/RCA 84
Case 21 LAD/LCx 86
Case 22 Left Main Coronary Artery 88
Two Vessel Myocardial Infarction 90
Case 23 RCA/LCx 90
Case 24 LAD/RCA 92
Case 25 LAD/LCx 94
Three Vessel Reversible Ischaemia....................... 96
Case 26 LAD/LCx/RCA 96
Three Vessel Myocardial Infarction 98
Case 27 LAD/LCx/RCA 98
Mixed Reversible Ischaemia and Infarction 100
Case 28 RCA Infarction/LAD Ischaemia..................... 100
Case 29 RCA Infarction/LCx Ischaemia 102
Case 30 LAD Infarction/LCx Ischaemia 104
Case 31 LAD Infarction/RCA Ischaemia................... 106
Case 32 LCx Infarction/RCA Ischaemia 108
Case 33 LCx Infarction/LAD Ischaemia 110
Prognosis Before Angiography 112
Case 34 No Chest Pain, Normal Scan 112
Case 35 Chest Pain, Normal Scan 114
Case 36 Controlled Chest Pain, Minor Ischaemia............ 116
Case 37 Controlled Chest Pain, Major Ischaemia 118
Prognosis After Angiography 120
Case 38 Controlled Chest Pain, Three Vessel Disease,
      Minor Ischaemia................................ 120
Case 39 Controlled Chest Pain, Three Vessel Disease,
      Major Ischaemia 122
Adverse Prognostic Signs............................... 124

CONTENTS

Case 40 Increased Lung Uptake............................ 124
Case 41 Dilated Left Ventricle on Exercise 126
Case 42 Dilated Left Ventricle After Infarction 128
Coronary Angioplasty 130
Case 43 Two Vessel Disease, Culprit Lesion 130
Case 44 Before Angioplasty Study.......................... 132
Case 45 After Angioplasty Study........................... 134
Case 46 Recurrence of Stenosis 136
Coronary Bypass Grafting 138
Case 47 Preoperative Study 138
Case 48 Postoperative Study............................... 140
Case 49 Recurrent Ischaemia 142
ECG Correlations.. 144
Case 50 Marked ECG Changes with No Ischaemia 144
Case 51 Marked ECG Changes with Minor Ischaemia 146
Case 52 Wolff–Parkinson–White Syndrome................. 146
Case 53 Left Bundle Branch Block 150
Case 54 Left Ventricular Hypertrophy 152
Coronary Angiogram Correlations............................ 154
Case 55 Normal Angiogram, Syndrome X 154
Case 56 Normal Angiogram, Left Bundle Branch Block 156
Case 57 Abnormal Angiogram, Normal Thallium Scan 158
Other Cardiology.. 160
Case 58 Dilated Cardiomyopathy 160
Case 59 Ischaemic Cardiomyopathy 162
Case 60 Hypertrophic Cardiomyopathy 164
Case 61 Coronary Muscle Bridge 166
Case 62 Orthotopic Cardiac Transplantation............... 168
Case 63 Reversible Right Ventricular Ischaemia 170
Case 64 Unusual Coronary Artery Anatomy................ 172
Case 65 Myocardial Damage Following Acute Anaphylaxis... 174
Case 66 Anomalous Origin of LAD......................... 176
Quantification.. 178
Case 67 Polar Mapping 178
Pharmacological Stress 180
Case 68 Dipyridamole 180
Case 69 Dobutamine 182
Case 70 Adenosine 184
Case 71 Dipyridamole with Exercise 186
Chest Pain and Ischaemia 188
Case 72 Chest Pain with No Ischaemia..................... 188
Case 73 No Chest Pain with Ischaemia..................... 190
Artefacts 192
Case 74 Motion 192
Case 75 Poor Count Rate 194
Case 76 Upward Creep 196
Case 77 Objects 198
Reperfusion... 200
Case 78 Reversed Redistribution 200
Case 79 24 Hour Imaging 202
Case 80 Reinjection....................................... 204

CONTENTS

7 Clinical Applications **207**

Detection of Coronary Artery Disease 207
Management of Established Coronary Artery Disease 209
    Stable Angina 209
    Myocardial Infarction 209
    Monitoring the Effects of Intervention 210
Prognosis in Coronary Artery Disease 211

8 The Future **215**

Instrumentation 215
Radiopharmaceuticals 216
Alternative Imaging Techniques 217

Subject Index **223**

Chapter 1

Introduction

Nuclear medicine has enjoyed a resurgence of interest in recent years as the value of the functional information that it provides is appreciated.[1] In almost every branch of medicine radiopharmaceuticals are used to measure organ function and, combined with the anatomical information provided by other imaging techniques such as ultrasound and radiology, this allows a more objective approach to patient management than when functional information is lacking. Cardiac patients in particular have benefitted from this information. Since Laennec invented the stethoscope a steady stream of technical developments has helped to measure cardiac function. By using radiopharmaceuticals it is now possible to quantify more elusive aspects of function such as global and regional ventricular function, valve function, and myocardial perfusion and metabolism.

Radioactive tracers are uniquely suited to this non-invasive assessment. They can almost be tailor made and can be administered in small volumes into a peripheral vein either at rest or during one of a number of forms of stress. Highly sensitive detectors are able to map the distribution of the emitted radiation and either projectional (planar) images or three-dimensional (tomographic) images can be recorded. Because the recording process is computer controlled, the digital data are amenable to further processing. Functional images can aid interpretation, and findings in any patient can automatically be compared with a normal database. Thallium has a unique place in non-invasive cardiac imaging. It is taken up by normal myocardium in proportion to myocardial perfusion and for many years it has provided the only simple method of assessing myocardial perfusion. A large body of experience has accumulated and it is now used in the diagnosis of disease, in its follow-up, and in the assessment of prognosis.

In contrast with the importance of nuclear medicine is its variable practice between different hospitals and countries. The relatively low use of thallium scintigraphy in Great Britain has been demonstrated in a recent survey.[2] The number of nuclear cardiological investigations performed in Great Britain in 1988 was 500 per million population. In the USA, the equivalent figure in 1985 was 3550.[3] Despite higher utilisation in the USA nuclear cardiology facilities are not evenly spread and the majority of studies are performed in a few active centres with other centres performing very few scans. These discrepancies highlight a number of problems with thallium as an imaging agent.

1

- Only 5% of the injected dose is concentrated in the myocardium and the remainder is taken up by skeletal muscle, stomach and gut.
- It has a relatively long half-life and only a small dose can be given without exposing the patient to unacceptable amounts of radiation.
- Its main emission is the 80 keV mercury X-ray which is of relatively low energy and is easily attenuated by body tissue.

The three factors combine to produce thallium scintigrams of low resolution with a low signal to noise ratio, and the nuclear physician requires considerable experience if the images are to be interpreted with confidence. Using traditional planar imaging the superimposition of normally and abnormally perfused areas reduces the contrast of the abnormal areas and this further complicates the interpretation of their severity and extent. Fortunately, a number of developments have greatly improved the position, most important of which has been the growth of emission tomographic imaging which is to planar imaging as X-ray tomography is to the plain X-ray.

Several studies have compared planar thallium imaging with tomography. The results vary but the general trend is that tomographic imaging provides a higher sensitivity for the detection of perfusion abnormalities without the loss of specificity. For instance, Fintel et al.[4] found the sensitivity and specificity using planar imaging to be 84% and 90% respectively, and using tomography to be 91% and 90%. Because these figures depend to a large extent on the characteristics of the population tested, they also used receiver operating characteristics curves (or ROC analysis) to compare techniques. Over the entire range of decision thresholds, tomography was superior to planar imaging for the territories of the left anterior descending and circumflex arteries, although there was no difference for the right coronary artery. Tomography was particularly helpful in males, those with mild or single vessel coronary disease and those without prior infarction. These simple numbers probably underestimate the value of tomography because the information in a thallium scan is much more than the binary result of disease present or disease absent. It is also possible to quantify the site, extent and severity of the perfusion abnormalities and in this respect tomography is helped by the avoidance of overlapping structures.

It must be acknowledged at the outset that not all nuclear physicians agree about the superiority of tomography over planar imaging. Whilst none can doubt the theoretical superiority of tomographic imaging, there are practical problems in acquiring good quality tomograms. If errors of technique and artefacts are not recognised, then tomograms certainly do have a greater potential than planar imaging to provide misleading results. Our own experience indicates that good quality tomography is an essential part of myocardial perfusion imaging and for this reason we document our experience in subsequent chapters.

References

1. McAfee JG, Kopecky RT, Frymoyer PA. Nuclear medicine comes of age: its present and future roles in diagnosis. Radiology 1990;174:609–20.
2. Underwood SR, Gibson CJ, Tweddel A, Flint J. A survey of nuclear cardiology practice in Great Britain. Br Heart J 1991 (in press).

3. Subcommittee of the Health and Environment Research Advisory Committee, Office of Energy Research, US Department of Energy. Review of the Office of Health and Environment Research Program, Nuclear Medicine, 1989. Washington DC: US Department of Energy, 1989.
4. Fintel DJ, Links JM, Brinker JA, Frank TL, Parker M, Becker LC. Improved diagnostic performance of exercise thallium-201 single photon emission computer tomography over planar imaging: a receiver operating characteristic analysis. J Am Coll Cardiol 1989;13: 600–12.

Chapter 2
Radiopharmaceuticals

The use of radiopharmaceuticals for the investigation of the cardiovascular system began in 1927 with the use of radium C to measure circulation time by Blumgart and Weiss.[1,2] Since then, there has been considerable development and the milestones are summarised in Table 2.1. The tracers can be divided into three groups. First, those that label the blood and hence allow the assessment of ventricular function and blood flow. Second, those that label the myocardium to provide information on myocardial perfusion or metabolism. Third, those that are localised in damaged endothelium or atheroma and so can be used to assess disease of the arterial wall directly. The following discussion is limited to the common tracers used to image myocardial perfusion.

Myocardial Perfusion Tracers

Early myocardial perfusion imaging used the monovalent cations caesium-131,[3] rubidium-81[4] and potassium-43[5,6] but did not gain widespread clinical acceptance because of the relatively poor imaging characteristics of the radiopharmaceuticals. The development of thallium-201[7] paved the way for routine myocardial perfusion imaging in the detection of reversible and irreversible ischaemia.

The ideal tracer for the assessment of myocardial perfusion possesses a number of properties. It should be distributed in the myocardium in proportion to blood flow over the range of values experienced in health and disease. It should be extracted efficiently from the blood by the myocardium on its first passage through the heart. It should remain within the myocardium for the period of data acquisition. After acquisition, rapid elimination from the body should allow repeat studies under different conditions. Other desirable properties are that it should have a high photon flux at an energy between 100 and 200 keV, a low radiation burden to the patient, it should be easily available, and it should be cheap. Needless to say, no tracer so far possesses all of these properties and compromises have to be made.

Unfortunately, none of the tracers in routine use allows measurement of myocardial perfusion in absolute terms (ml/min/g) and the best that can be achieved is a measure of the relative distribution throughout the myocardium.

5

Table 2.1 Milestones in the development of nuclear cardiology tracers

Year	Procedure	Tracer	Authors
1924–27	Circulation time	Radium C	Blumgart, Weiss
1948	Radiocardiography	^{24}Na	Prinzmetal
1955	Radiocardiography	^{131}I-albumin	McIntyre, Donato
1960/65	Myocardial perfusion	^{86}Rb, ^{131}Cs	Carr, Planiol
1964	Pulmonary perfusion	^{131}I-MAA	Taplin
1970/71	Radionuclide ventriculography	^{99m}Tc-erythrocytes	Adam, Bitter, Strauss, Pitt
1973	Myocardial infarct imaging	^{99m}Tc-pyrophosphate	Bonte
1973	Myocardial perfusion	^{201}Tl chloride	Lebowitz
1977	Myocardial metabolism	^{131}I fatty acids	Feinendegen, Stoecklin
1981	Myocardial innervation	^{123}I-MIBG	Kline
1984	Myocardial perfusion	^{99m}Tc-MIBI	Jones, Holman
1987	Myocardial perfusion	^{99m}Tc-teboroxime	Meerdink

Thallium-201

Thallium-201 is the most commonly used radionuclide for myocardial perfusion studies. Compared with the ideal tracer outlined above, it has a number of unfavourable properties but, because of the large experience with its use, it is the standard against which other tracers must be judged. Elemental thallium was discovered in 1861 by Crookes, who later invented the vacuum tube which is known by his name and with which Roentgen discovered X-rays in 1895. It is a metallic element in group IIIB of the periodic table under boron, aluminium, gallium and indium. Thallium-201 is a cyclotron-produced radioisotope. A generator is not available and it is therefore supplied in unit doses. It decays by electron capture to mercury-201 with a physical half-life of 72 h. Gamma photons of 135 and 167 keV are emitted (12% abundance) but the main emission is the mercury X-ray of 67–82 keV (88% abundance). There is no physical difference between γ-rays and X-rays but the former are the result of nuclear transitions and the latter of electron transitions.

$$^{201}_{81}\text{Tl} + e^- \xrightarrow{72h} {}^{201}_{80}\text{Hg} + X + \gamma$$

Thallium is administered intravenously as thallous chloride and the usual dose is 80 MBq. Higher doses have become popular in some countries although the high radiation burden associated with such doses is a problem. Uptake is rapid and the biological half-life in the blood is only 30 s.[8] Following intravenous injection, approximately 88%[9] is cleared from the blood after the first circulation but because the heart receives 5% of the cardiac output, only 4% of the total dose is taken up by the myocardium.[8,10] The hydrated thallous ion (Tl$^+$) is similar in size to the hydrated potassium ion (K$^+$) and the early literature suggested that uptake into cardiac and skeletal muscle cells is an active process involving the sodium–potassium ATPase enzyme system.[11,12] More recently this has been questioned because uptake is not reduced by cardiac glycosides[13,14] and the thallium may enter the cells passively along an electropotential gradient. Myocardial extraction exceeds that of other tissues which is helpful for cardiac imaging, and it is unaffected by beta-blockade.[15] The extraction efficiency is reduced by acidosis and hypoxaemia[14] although these are only small effects and may not reduce extraction significantly until close to cell death.[16-18] The commonly held belief that thallium uptake depends on both perfusion and ischaemia appears to be incorrect.[15] Distribution within the myocardium is therefore proportional to myocardial blood flow over a wide range of values although at high rates of flow, extraction may become rate limiting.[19,20] Although defects reflect impaired perfusion it has been suggested that in some cardio-myopathies, especially those associated with the muscular dystrophies, defects may arise from impaired extraction alone.

Once within the heart, the half-life of elimination of thallium is 7 h. The slow washout may either be explained by binding within the cell[21] or by the adverse electropotential gradient. The infusion of glucose and insulin in animals increases the clearance of thallium from the myocardium[22] and a carbohydrate meal between stress and redistribution imaging has been shown in humans to interfere with the diagnosis of reversible ischaemia. The redistribution thallium images should therefore be acquired under fasting conditions.[23]

Thallium is usually given at peak exercise which is then continued for two minutes in order to maintain stable conditions over the period of extraction of tracer by the myocardium. Imaging is begun within five minutes of injection and should be completed within 30 minutes. During this period the distribution of thallium within the myocardium is relatively fixed and, despite the cessation of exercise, the images reflect myocardial perfusion at peak stress. In fact, there is a slow equilibration between intracellular thallium and the very low level of intravascular thallium, so that the pattern of distribution slowly alters to reflect the changing conditions. Several hours after injection at stress, the thallium has redistributed and the images obtained at this time are similar to those that would have been obtained had the thallium been injected at rest. This redistribution is not entirely passive since the rate at which thallium washes out from ischaemic myocardium is lower than that from normal myocardium. This is shown in Fig. 2.1 in which the activity of three territories of myocardium have been plotted against time. The normal region shows the highest uptake but rapid and substantial washout. The ischaemic region shows depressed initial uptake and little washout with time, so that after 120 minutes the activity is similar to the normal region. In an infarcted region the initial activity is low and falls with time maintaining a clear difference with the other territories.[24]

The practical consequence of the slow redistribution of thallium is that the images acquired shortly after injection reflect myocardial perfusion during stress and those several hours later reflect resting perfusion. Non-viable myocardium such as in an area of infarction will show a fixed defect but myocardium that is affected by a haemodynamically significant coronary stenosis will show an initial defect of uptake that becomes normal in the redistribution images. This simple explanation is complicated by factors such as delayed redistribution and stunned or hibernating myocardium which are discussed in Chapter 5.

In normal volunteers, little thallium is taken up by the lungs although uptake is sometimes seen in heavy smokers. A high pulmonary capillary pressure leads to exudation of fluid and thallium into the extracellular and

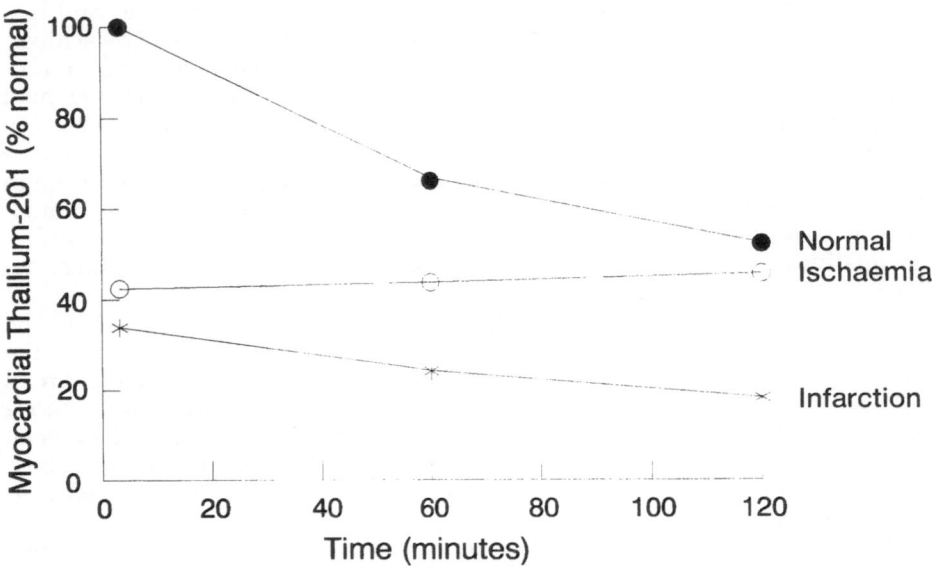

Fig. 2.1. Time–activity curves for three myocardial regions after [201]thallium injection at peak stress. See text for details. (Adapted from reference 24 with permission.)

alveolar spaces, and so patients with left ventricular dysfunction leading to a raised left ventricular end diastolic pressure and pulmonary oedema may have significant lung uptake at rest. Even in the absence of resting left ventricular dysfunction, stress-induced myocardial ischaemia may lead to similar changes. Such a finding, therefore, indicates a significantly jeopardised left ventricle and hence a poor prognosis.

Thallium has been used routinely as a tracer of myocardial perfusion for almost two decades and the experience collected over this time is considerable. Normal appearances of both planar and tomographic images are well established and the protocols for acquisition and image processing have been standardised. The radiopharmaceutical is widely available at short notice and its cost is low. It does, however, have some important limitations.

First, because of the relatively long half-life within the body, radiation exposure to the patient is high. Eighty megaBecquerel delivers an effective dose equivalent of 25 mSv which is considerably less than the normal exposure during coronary arteriography and is similar to that during X-ray transmission tomography or intravenous urography. On the principle that radiation exposure should be minimised it is difficult to justify frequent scans in an individual. Second, because of the desire to limit radiation exposure the injected dose is kept low and, to compound the problem, only 5% of the injected dose is taken up by the myocardium. The rest is widely distributed mainly to skeletal muscle and the gut. The count density of the myocardial images is therefore low with high background levels. Third, the low energy emission at 80 keV leads to low resolution images with significant attenuation by soft tissues. Technetium-99m compounds do not suffer the first and third of these problems and this has encouraged the development of such tracers.

Technetium-99m 2-Methoxy-isobutyl-isonitrile

Although thallium has provided excellent service since its introduction in 1975,[7] its physical limitations have led to the search for technetium-99m analogues. Two main classes of compounds have emerged: the isonitriles[25] and the substituted oximes. A number of early technetium-99m isonitriles suffered from high lung and liver uptake. 2-Methoxy-isobutyl-isonitrile (MIBI) has the best myocardium to background ratio and is now available commercially. Its advantages over thallium are its lower radiation burden to the patient and the higher resolution images that it provides, but it is expensive. In clinical practice it provides at least the same sensitivity and specificity for the detection of coronary artery disease.[26,27]

^{99m}Tc-MIBI is a cationic complex of 2-methoxy-isobutyl-isonitrile copper (1) tetrafluoroborate and formamidine sulphinic acid. It concentrates mainly in the cytosol of normally perfused myocardium by an active uptake mechanism that is impaired by ischaemia.[28] Its clearance from the blood is rapid with a half-life of less than two minutes, although first pass extraction is lower than thallium. Within the cytosol, it is bound to proteins with molecular weights between 5000 and 8000 daltons. In contrast to thallium, ^{99m}Tc-MIBI is taken up by the liver and this hinders imaging of the myocardium if only planar images are acquired.

The most important clinical difference between ^{99m}Tc-MIBI and thallium is that the technetium compound does not redistribute from its initial pattern of uptake. Thus, in order to compare stress and resting perfusion, two separate injections have to be given. The 6 h half-life of technetium-99m means that the two studies should be performed on separate days if activity from the first injection is not to confuse the images following the second injection. Alternatively, the two studies can be performed on the same day if a larger dose (three to five times) is given on the second occasion in order to swamp the activity remaining from the first injection. Same day protocols are, however, probably inferior to separate day protocols.[29]

Another consequence of the lack of redistribution of ^{99m}Tc-MIBI is that stress imaging can be delayed for some time after injection. Indeed, it is advisable to do so in order to allow the ratio of myocardial to liver and lung uptake to increase. Best contrast is obtained in images acquired 1–2 h after injection. There is no longer a need to perform exercise close to the gamma camera and injections can be made during normal treadmill exercise testing, in the catheter laboratory, or in the coronary care unit immediately before thrombolysis. Particularly promising studies involve giving the injection immediately before thrombolysis in patients with acute myocardial infarction. Later reinjection and imaging allow the amount of myocardium that has been salvaged by thrombolysis to be established.[30] Yet another consequence of the lack of redistribution is the ability to perform ventricular function studies either by following the first pass of the tracer through the heart or by electrocardiographically gated acquisition of the myocardial image.

Emission tomograms using ^{99m}Tc-MIBI have higher spatial resolution and higher count densities than when using thallium because of the higher energy photon produced by [99m]Tc (140 keV) and the shorter half-life (6 h) which allows larger doses to be given for the same radiation burden. For a total dose of 1370 MBq split into two parts for stress and rest imaging, the effective dose equivalent is 17 mSv.

Technetium-99m Teboroxime

Another group of compounds that has shown promise for myocardial perfusion imaging is that of boronic acid adducts with technetium dioxime.[31] Technetium-99m teboroxime is a neutral lipophilic molecule which is efficiently extracted by the myocardium from the blood but which has a very short residence time within the myocardium. Washout from the myocardium is biphasic, with 60% of the injected dose having a half-life within the myocardium of 5 min and the remaining 40% having a half-life of more than 70 min. Data acquisition, therefore, has to be very rapid although repeat studies can be performed rapidly. If emission tomography is to be performed, specialised equipment such as a multiple-headed gamma camera is probably necessary.

References

1. Blumgart HL, Yens OC. Studies on the velocity of blood flow. I. The method utilised. J Clin Invest 1927;4:1–13.
2. Blumgart HL, Weiss S. Studies on the velocity of blood flow. VII. The pulmonary circulation time in normal resting individuals. J Clin Invest 1928;4:399–425.
3. Carr EA. The direct diagnosis of myocardial infarction by photoscanning after administration of cesium-131. Am Heart J 1964;68:627–36.
4. Martin ND, Zaret BL, McGowan RL, Wells HP Jr, Flamm MD. Rubidium-81: a new myocardial scanning agent. Radiology 1974;111:651–6.
5. Hurley PH, Cooper M, Reba RC, Poggenburg KJ, Wagner HN. ^{43}KCl: a new radiopharmaceutical for imaging the heart. J Nucl Med 1971;12:516–19.
6. Zaret BL, Strauss HW, Martin ND, Wells HP, Flamm MD. Non-invasive regional myocardial perfusion with radioactive potassium. N Engl J Med 1973;288:809–12.
7. Lebowitz E, Greene MW, Fairchild R et al. Thallium-201 for medical use. J Nucl Med 1975;16:151–60.
8. Okada RD, Leppo JA, Strauss HW, Boucher CA, Pohost GM. Mechanisms and time course for the disappearance of thallium-201 defects at rest in dogs. Relation of time to peak activity to myocardial blood flow. Am J Cardiol 1982;49:699–706.
9. Grunwald AM, Watson DD, Holzgrefe HH et al. Myocardial thallium-201 kinetics in normal and ischaemic myocardium. Circulation 1981;64:610–18.
10. Svensson SE, Lomsky M, Olsson L, Persson S, Strauss HW, Westling H. Non-invasive determination of the distribution of cardiac output in man at rest and during exercise. Clin Physiol 1982;2:467–77.
11. Ku D, Akera T, Tobin T et al. Comparative species studies in the effect of monovalent cations on cardiac Na^+/K^+-adenosine triphosphatase and contractile force. J Pharmacol Exp Ther 1976;197:458–69.
12. Schelbert H, Ingwall J, Watson R et al. Factors influencing the myocardial uptake of thallium-201 (abstract). J Nucl Med 1977;18:598.
13. Krivokapich J, Shine KI. The effects of hyperkalaemia and glycoside on thallium-201 exchange in rabbit myocardium. Am J Physiol 1981;1981:H612–19.
14. Weich H, Strauss HW, Pitt B. The extraction of thallium-201 by the myocardium. Circulation 1977;56:188–91.
15. Melin JA, Becker LC. Quantitative relationship between global left ventricular thallium uptake and blood flow: effects of propranolol, ouabain, dipyridamole and coronary artery occlusion. J Nucl Med 1986;27:641–52.

16. Ingwall JS, Kramer M, Kloner NM et al. Thallium accumulation: differentiation between reversible and irreversible myocardial injury (abstract). Circulation 1979;59:678.
17. Goldhaber SZ, Newell JB, Ingwall JS et al. Effects of reduced coronary flow on thallium-201 accumulation and release in an in vitro rat heart preparation. Am J Cardiol 1983;51:891−6.
18. Pohost GM, Alpert NM, Ingwall JS, Strauss HW. Thallium redistribution: mechanisms and clinical utility. Semin Nucl Med 1980;10:70−93.
19. Neilson AP, Morris ML, Murdock R, Bruno FP, Cobb FR. Linear relationship between the distribution of thallium-201 and blood flow in ischaemic and non-ischaemic myocardium during exercise. Circulation 1980;61:797−801.
20. Mueller TM, Marcus ML, Ehrhardt JC, Chandhuri T, Abboud FM. Limitations of thallium-201 myocardial perfusion scintigrams. Circulation 1976;54:640−6.
21. Britten JS, Blank M. Thallium activation of the (Na^+-K^+)-activated ATPase of rabbit kidney. Biochim Biophys Acta 1968;159:160.
22. Wilson RA, Okada RA, Brown KA, Pohost GM, Strauss HW. The effect of glucose-insulin potassium on thallium-201 myocardial redistribution (abstract). J Am Coll Cardiol 1983; 1:590.
23. Wilson RA, Sullivan PJ, Okada RD, Boucher CA, Morris C, Pohost GM. The effect of eating on thallium myocardial imaging. Chest 1986;89:195−8.
24. Beller GA, Holzgrefe BS, Watson DD. Effects of dipyridamole induced vasodilation on myocardial uptake and clearance kinetics of thallium-201. Circulation 1983;68:1328−38.
25. Jones AG, Abrams MJ, Davison A. A new class of water soluble low valent technetium unipositive cations: hexakisisonitrile technetium (I) salts. J Nucl Med Allied Sci 1982;26:149.
26. Iskandrian AS, Heo J, Kong B, Lyons A, Marsch S. Use of technetium-99m isonitrile (RP30A) in assessing left ventricular perfusion and function at rest and during exercise in coronary artery disease, and comparison with coronary arteriography and exercise thallium-201 SPECT imaging. Am J Cardiol 1989;64:270−5.
27. Taillefer R, Lambert R, Dupras G et al. Clinical comparison between thallium-201 and Tc99m-methoxy isobutyl isonitrile (hexamibi) myocardial perfusion imaging for detection of coronary artery disease. Eur J Nucl Med 1989;15:280−6.
28. Sands H, Delano ML, Gallagher BM. Uptake of hexakis (t-butyl isonitrile) technetium (I) and hexakis (isopropyl-isonitrile) technetium (I) by neonatal rat myocytes and human erythrocytes. J Nucl Med 1986;27:404−8.
29. Whalley DR, Murphy JJ, Frier M, Wastie ML, Wilcox RG. A comparison of same day and separate day injection protocols for myocardial perfusion SPECT using 99mTc-MIBI. Nucl Med Commun 1991;12:99−104.
30. Wackers FJT, Gibbons RJ, Verani MS et al. Serial quantitative planar technetium-99m isonitrile imaging in acute myocardial infarction: efficacy for noninvasive assessment of thrombolytic therapy. J Am Coll Cardiol 1989;14:861−73.
31. Hendel RC, McSherry B, Karimeddini M, Leppo JA. Diagnostic value of a new myocardial perfusion agent, teboroxime (SQ 30,217), utilizing a rapid planar imaging protocol: preliminary results. J Am Coll Cardiol 1990;16:855−61.

Chapter 3
Stress Techniques

The response to stress is central to the assessment of most aspects of cardio-vascular function. It is particularly important for coronary artery disease because resting coronary flow is normal until the luminal cross-sectional area of a coronary artery is reduced by approximately 85%, and resting ischaemia only occurs when the artery is virtually occluded.[1] However, the maximal flow in the artery is impaired when a luminal stenosis of 50% is present.[1] Thus it is the failure of coronary flow to increase in response to stress that is the predominant functional impairment in coronary artery disease. The ratio of maximal to resting flow in an artery is defined as the coronary flow reserve[2] and this measure is useful because it assesses the overall haemodynamic significance of a lesion, without the difficult task of quantifying morphology.[3] Most investigative techniques use some form of cardiovascular stress to highlight differences in the coronary flow reserve between arteries (Table 3.1). Most of these induce myocardial ischaemia by the manipulation of myocardial oxygen demand but some, such as dipyri-damole, have a primary action on myocardial blood flow.

The most commonly used method of stressing the cardiovascular system is dynamic exercise. This has the advantage that it is physiological and mimics the stress that may provoke symptoms in patients with coronary artery disease. Particularly for myocardial perfusion imaging, other methods of challenging the cardiovascular system are possible, and it is important to be aware of the strengths and weaknesses of each technique so that they can be applied appropriately. Our own routine is to use maximal dynamic exercise combined with intravenous dipyridamole, but we use intravenous dobutamine if exercise is difficult, or if dipyridamole is contraindicated, and we anticipate that we shall use adenosine increasingly as a substitute for dipyridamole as more experience is gained.

Drug Treatment

A common question is what to do with the patient's medication before a stress test. Most cardiac drugs will affect the response to stress and beta-blockers in particular will blunt the heart rate response to exercise. It is important therefore to record the patient's medication and the time of the last dose. Whether to stop medication before the test depends on the in-

Table 3.1. Common forms of cardiovascular stress

	Advantages	Disadvantages
Dynamic exercise	• effective • familiar to all cardiologists • physiological and mimics everyday life	• often limited by non-cardiac symptoms
Isometric exercise	• easily performed • high specificity	• very poor sensitivity • uncomfortable for the patient
Cold pressor stress	• easily performed • high specificity	• very poor sensitivity • painful for the patient
Mental stress	• physiological	• very poor sensitivity
Atrial pacing	• level of stress easily controlled and reversed • easily coupled with invasive measurements	• non-physiological • invasive
Dipyridamole (oral)	• easily administered • avoids the need for dynamic exercise but can be coupled with it if desired • easily reversed by aminophylline	• non-physiological • unpredictable rate of absorption • frequent side effects • contraindicated with bronchospasm • increased splanchnic uptake of thallium • defects milder than produced by exercise
Dipyridamole (intravenous)	• as for oral • more predictable action • fewer side effects of shorter duration, especially if coupled with exercise	• as for oral, but see advantages (left) • not an ideal agent for electrophysiological or wall motion studies
Adenosine	• easily administered • rapid recovery	• non-physiological • relatively expensive
Dobutamine	• easily administered • rapid recovery • almost physiological action and maximum tolerated dose is related to exercise time • abnormalities of perfusion and wall motion more marked than with vasodilators • suitable for electrophysiological, wall motion, perfusion or metabolism studies	• antagonised by beta-blockade

formation that is required. If the clinical problem is the diagnosis of coronary artery disease then the test will be most sensitive in the absence of anti-anginal therapy. More commonly, the clinical question is whether there is evidence of reversible ischaemia in a patient with known coronary artery disease. Drugs need not then be stopped although the findings will have to be interpreted in the light of the current medication. If drugs are to be temporarily withdrawn, 24 h is sufficient for most short-acting drugs such as nitrates and calcium antagonists, but 48 h is required for beta-blockers because of their prolonged antianginal effect. Concern is sometimes expressed that withdrawal of beta-blockers may lead to a worsening of angina, rest pain or even infarction. This is uncommon, however, and temporary withdrawal is normally considered to be safe, provided that the patient is instructed to take glyceryl trinitrate as required and to contact a doctor or restart normal medication in case of intractable angina.

Dynamic Exercise

Dynamic exercise is performed on a treadmill or a bicycle ergometer. The increase in heart rate and blood pressure raises myocardial oxygen demand to the point where demand exceeds supply in territories served by diseased coronary vessels. During maximal dynamic exercise in humans, coronary flow has been shown to increase by a mean of 2.7 times the baseline value,[4] with limitation in diseased vessels. Dynamic exercise is safe in the cardiac patient, although there is a small morbidity and mortality and it should be performed under controlled conditions by personnel familiar with resuscitation.[5,6] Contraindications to dynamic exercise include unstable angina, previous adverse event during exercise, and obstruction to left ventricular outflow. Some physicians are also reluctant to exercise patients with recent infarction or with extensive ischaemia such as might be caused by left mainstem coronary disease. As with many contraindications these are only relative, and patients in the above categories may be exercised cautiously by experienced physicians.

There are both physiological and practical differences between exercise on a treadmill and on a bicycle. The most important practical difference is that all patients are familiar with walking but some are unable to coordinate sufficiently to pedal a bicycle. Heart rates achieved are usually less on a bicycle than on a treadmill because leg fatigue is often a limiting factor especially in the frail and elderly. It is difficult to compare levels of exercise achieved in stages on a treadmill with the number of watts achieved on a bicycle, because body weight affects the former but not the latter.

Despite the potential advantages of the treadmill over the bicycle, our own preference is for the bicycle because it is simpler to coordinate the injection of tracer or pharmacological stressor, and the incidence of hypotension caused by vasodilators such as dipyridamole is reduced and simpler to treat if the patient is already supine. To achieve high levels of exercise in the majority of patients is a skilled task that should not be delegated to the inexperienced. Exercise is begun at 25 W and increased each 2 min in 25 W increments until limited by symptoms, relative hypotension, or significant ventricular dysrhythmia such as ventricular tachycardia (Table 3.2). Exercise should not be stopped simply because a target heart rate is achieved, because of ST segment changes or because of benign dysrhythmias such as ventricular ectopic beats. It is useful to know the maximum predicted heart rate for the patient since the closer the heart rate to this level, the more complete

Table 3.2. Indications to terminate a dynamic exercise test

- patient fatigue, provided they have been suitably encouraged
- intolerable symptoms such as chest pain, dyspnoea, claudication. With encouragement, the patient may exercise beyond initially reporting the symptom
- fall of systolic blood pressure by more than 10 mmHg compared with the previous level of stress
- new ventricular dysrhythmia such as couplets, tachycardia or fibrillation. Isolated ectopic beats need not be a reason for termination
- new atrial dysrhythmia if poorly tolerated such as rapid tachycardia or fibrillation

ST segment depression alone or achievement of a target heart rate need not be a reason for stopping.

has been the stress. A rough guide to the maximum heart rate is 220 minus the age of the patient for men and 210 minus age for women.

During dynamic exercise the electrocardiogram should be monitored and pulse and blood pressure should be recorded at the end of each stage. Many departments only monitor a single bipolar lead such as CM5, which is recorded between a lead placed in the fifth intercostal space in the anterior axillary line and another on the right shoulder. Other departments record a full twelve lead electrocardiogram. This gives additional information but requires more complex equipment, more time, and greater attention to detail. The site of ST segment changes is not a good guide to the site of ischaemia.[7]

Thallium is injected at peak exercise and is best given into a cannula in an antecubital vein and flushed with normal saline. The patient should be encouraged to exercise for a further minute to maintain stress while the thallium is taken up by the myocardium but, if necessary, the level of stress can be reduced in this final minute. Although imaging should be begun within 5 min of tracer injection, it is sometimes necessary to allow a longer period of recovery before moving the patient to the camera and away from ECG monitoring.

Pharmacological Stress

Many patients with coronary artery disease are unable to exercise to their full potential because of vascular disease elsewhere or other physical or psychological problems. Pharmacological manipulation of myocardial blood flow and myocardial oxygen demand can overcome this problem and a number of approaches have been used.

Dipyridamole

Dipyridamole is familiar as an inhibitor of platelet aggregation but it is also a potent coronary arteriolar dilator. It is relatively specific for the myocardial arteriole, although it dilates arterioles in a number of other organs including the skin and gut. It was initially proposed as an antianginal agent, but its lack of efficacy was soon demonstrated.[8] Its action on the arteriolar smooth muscle cell arises from an increase in the interstitial level of adenosine caused by inhibition of the facilitated uptake of adenosine, and by inhibition of the breakdown of adenosine by adenosine deaminase. Activation of the myocyte membrane purinoceptors by adenosine leads to an increase of intracellular cyclic adenosine monophosphate and hence arteriolar vasodilation.[9] The increase in coronary arterial flow in humans using Gould's original regime of 0.56 mg/kg over 4 min[10] is variable but it is reported to be between 250%[11] and 600%.[12] The flow reserve is reduced in arteries with fixed stenoses,[13] and the differential flow between territories served by normal and by stenosed arteries may be sufficient to produce an apparent defect of thallium uptake even though flow may be increased in the abnormal area.[14]

It is also possible to produce ischaemia in the territory of a stenosed artery, and although the mechanisms of this ischaemia are complex there are three possible explanations. First, an increase of flow across a stenosis leads to a fall in distal perfusion pressure with preferential shunting to the subepicardium[14,15] which may be sufficient to cause subendocardial ischaemia.[10] Second, flow in high-resistance collateral vessels serving the area of a diseased artery may be reduced because of the generalised vasodilation and fall in perfusion pressure. This will be exacerbated by the small reduction in diastolic blood pressure caused by dipyridamole.[16] Third, dipyridamole causes a small increase in the rate pressure product, mainly because of the reflex tachycardia which raises myocardial oxygen demand.[16]

Dipyridamole can be given either orally or intravenously. It does not have a licence for intravenous administration in all countries, but this exists in the UK and was approved in 1991 for the USA. When given orally, the normal dose is 300 mg of crushed tablets and intravenously it is given as a 4 min infusion of 0.56 mg/kg. The perfusion tracer is either given 1 h after oral dipyridamole or 4 min after the end of the infusion. Because gastric absorption of dipyridamole is very variable, plasma levels after an oral dose are unpredictable[17] and the time of maximum coronary flow is unknown. This makes oral administration unreliable for the production of perfusion abnormalities and it leads to a high incidence of side effects. Intravenous administration is therefore preferred. In humans, peak coronary flow occurs approximately 4 min after the end of the infusion[12] and reaches an average of five times the baseline value.[12] The coronary flow remains elevated near peak levels for up to 10 min,[18] with a fall towards baseline values over 30 min.[19]

Following intravenous administration, chest pain occurs in roughly one-fifth of patients and non-cardiac side effects in one-third. Aminophylline is a specific antagonist of the action of adenosine on the purinoceptor and a slow intravenous injection (up to 250 mg) reverses the adverse effects. We normally only use aminophylline to counteract severe ischaemia caused by dipyridamole or the symptoms of peripheral vasodilation such as hypotension, but milder chest pain may also be helped by sublingual nitrates. Dipyridamole is contraindicated in patients with reversible airways disease, as it may also act on bronchial smooth muscle and provoke bronchospasm.[20] Because caffeine antagonises the action of dipyridamole, cocoa, tea, coffee or colas should not be taken for 12 h before the test.

Intravenous dipyridamole is as effective as dynamic exercise in the detection and assessment of coronary artery disease[21] and it has proved particularly useful in patients unable to exercise, such as those undergoing peripheral arterial surgery.[22] It also has a good safety record.[20,23] In the largest published study of 3911 patients, four (0.1%) suffered myocardial infarction within 24 h of infusion, but three of these had unstable angina.[20] Two of the patients died. In another study of 170 patients with known or suspected unstable angina, dipyridamole infusion was associated with two small infarctions (0.3%) but no deaths.[24] Because of the high risk of infarction in the natural history of patients with unstable angina, it is not possible to conclude that this was a specific effect of dipyridamole, but the use of dipyridamole stress in these patients has to be carefully balanced against the value of the result. Following dipyridamole, significant dysrhythmias are rare[25] but ventricular premature beats are common. Ventricular fibrillation has been described although this case was complicated by the use of high dose aminophylline.[26]

Adenosine

Dipyridamole acts as a vasodilator indirectly by increasing interstitial adenosine, but it is also possible to give adenosine intravenously for a direct effect. The main advantage of adenosine is its very short plasma half-life of less than 10 s which simplifies the control of plasma levels and leads to increased safety and a reduction in the duration of side effects. An intravenous infusion rate of 140 µg/kg/min causes maximal or near maximal hyperaemia in 92% of patients, with mean coronary flow increasing by 4.4 times the resting value.[27] During the infusion there is a marked increase in cardiac output and pulmonary capillary pressure. The heart rate increases with a fall in blood pressure and the epicardial coronary vessels dilate. For clinical imaging, this infusion rate can be given for 6 min with injection of thallium 2 min from the end. It should not be administered to patients with reversible airways disease.

At the time of writing, the published experience with adenosine in humans is limited. One study reported chest pain in 57% of patients,[28] although this does not necessarily imply myocardial ischaemia because adenosine may cause chest pain even in volunteers with normal coronary arteries and normal perfusion.[29] Headache and flushing were common and first degree atrioventricular block occurred in 10%. All these side effects were short lived. The predictive accuracy of adenosine stress was slightly higher than dynamic exercise stress (90% vs 80%),[30] and the combined sensitivity and specificity of these tomographic studies was 89% and 96% respectively. This compares favourably with the results obtained using dynamic exercise and it is likely therefore that the use of adenosine will increase.

Dobutamine

Both dipyridamole and adenosine are arteriolar dilators, but an alternative approach to pharmacological stress is to increase myocardial oxygen demand by increasing heart rate and blood pressure. This is more physiological than manipulation of coronary flow because it is more closely related to the cause of symptoms in everyday life. Myocardial oxygen demand can be increased using a β-agonist, the ideal properties of which should include: a short half-life, low arrhythmogenicity, peripheral vein administration, coronary vasodilation and familiarity of use. Dobutamine fulfils these criteria and dobutamine myocardial perfusion studies have been very successful[31-33] with a sensitivity of 94% and a specificity of 87% for the detection of coronary artery disease in tomographic studies. Dobutamine is infused into a peripheral vein starting at 5 µg/kg/min and increasing in increments of 5 µg/kg/min, usually to a maximum of 20 µg/kg/min, although some studies have used a maximum of 40 µg/kg/min. Each stage should last for 5 min to allow stabilisation of the haemodynamic effect (dobutamine has a plasma half-life of 90 s). In addition to the controlled increase in myocardial oxygen demand, dobutamine has some other important actions in the production of ischaemia.[34] The coronary perfusion pressure distal to a stenosis falls because of increased flow. This, combined with the increased wall tension, helps to explain the heterogeneity in coronary flow that occurs with dobutamine and the observed shunting of blood from the subendocardium to the subepicardium. Dynamic flow resistance may also increase at the site of a coronary stenosis. These effects mimic in part the actions of dipyridamole.

Dobutamine infusion is safe in patients with coronary artery disease and no serious complications have been reported, although experience is still accumulating. In our own study of 50 patients there were no serious side effects although 78% of patients experienced chest discomfort.[33] Arrhythmias occurred in 38% of patients but were never significant and consisted mainly of occasional ventricular premature beats. Non-cardiac side effects were reported by 64% of patients but were mild in nature, usually skin tingling, heart pounding or flushing. All side effects were relieved within a few minutes of stopping the infusion. Dobutamine increased systolic blood pressure and heart rate leading to a doubling of the double product at 20 µg/kg/min. The positive inotropic and chronotropic effects of dobutamine make it unsuitable for patients with contraindications to dynamic exercise, most importantly aortic stenosis and unstable angina. The action of dobutamine is antagonised by beta-blockers which must therefore be discontinued at least 48 h before the study. It is possible that higher doses of dobutamine will overcome the antagonism but the safety of such a policy has not been established.

Choice of Stress Technique

Dynamic exercise is the preferred technique for stressing patients during myocardial perfusion imaging because it is so familiar to cardiologists and because the level of exercise achieved is an important part of the objective assessment of symptoms. In patients unable to exercise, any of the pharmacological methods described above provide excellent alternatives. Dipyridamole myocardial perfusion imaging is well validated and produces results similar to dynamic exercise.[35,36] Experience with dobutamine is more limited but it should be used in patients with bronchospasm who are unable to exercise. Its advantages over dipyridamole are its short duration of action and the more profound perfusion defects that it produces. For imaging techniques that rely on abnormal wall motion for the detection of ischaemia, it is certainly superior.[37-39]

Our current routine practice is to combine maximal dynamic exercise with intravenous dipyridamole. This increases the sensitivity of the technique for the detection of perfusion defects and it increases the conspicuity of the defects.[40,41] The side effects of dipyridamole that are caused by peripheral vasodilation are reduced by exercise and the splanchnic vasoconstriction caused by exercise improves the ratio of myocardial to background counts when compared with dipyridamole alone. The combination has the added advantage that it is often difficult to predict in advance if exercise will be limited by non-cardiac symptoms. If it is, then the dipyridamole alone may be sufficient to provoke a defect.[42,43] Because the intravenous dipyridamole causes peak coronary flow 4 min after the end of infusion with an effect lasting up to 10 min, it is given at the beginning of exercise unless the patient has a poor exercise tolerance when it should be administered prior to exercise.

References

1. Gould KL, Lipscomb K. Effects of coronary stenoses on coronary flow reserve and resistance. Am J Cardiol 1974;34:48–55.
2. Kirkeeide RL, Gould KL, Parsel L. Assessment of coronary stenoses by myocardial perfusion imaging during pharmacological coronary vasodilation. VII. Validation of coronary flow reserve as a single integrated functional measure of stenosis severity reflecting all its geometrical dimensions. J Am Coll Cardiol 1986;7:103–13.
3. Fedele FA, Sharaf B, Most AS, Gewirtz H. Details of coronary stenosis morphology influence its haemodynamic severity and distal flow reserve. Circulation 1989;80:636–42.
4. Holmberg S, Serzysko W, Varnauskas E. Coronary circulation during heavy exercise in control subjects and patients with coronary heart disease. Acta Med Scand 1971;190:465–80.
5. Rochmis P, Blackburn H. Exercise tests. A survey of procedures, safety and litigation experience in approximately 170,000 tests. JAMA 1971;217:1061–6.
6. Gibbons L, Blair SN, Kohlk HW, Cooper K. The safety of maximal exercise testing. Circulation 1989;80:846–52.
7. Robertson D, Kostuk WJ, Ahuja SP. The localisation of coronary artery stenosis by 12 lead ECG response to graded exercise test: support for intercoronary steal. Am Heart J 1976;91:437–44.
8. Foulds T, Mackinnon J. Controlled double blind trial of Persantin in treatment of angina pectoris. Br Med J 1960;241:835–8.
9. Szegi J, Szentmiklosi AJ, Cseppento A. On the action of specific drugs influencing the adenosine induced activation of cardiac purinoceptors. In: Papp JG, ed, Cardiovascular pharmacology 1987: results, concepts and perspectives. Budapest: Akademiai Kiado, 1987; 591–9.
10. Gould KL. Noninvasive assessment of coronary stenoses by myocardial perfusion imaging during pharmacologic coronary vasodilatation. 1 Physiologic basis and experimental validation. Am J Cardiol 1978;41:267–78.
11. Brown G, Josephson MA, Petersen RD et al. Intravenous dipyridamole combined with isometric handgrip for near maximal coronary flow in patients with coronary artery disease. Am J Cardiol 1981;48:1077–85.
12. Wilson RF, Laughlin DE, Ackell PH et al. Transluminal, subselective measurement of coronary artery blood flow velocity and vasodilator reserve in man. Circulation 1985;72:82–92.
13. Feldman RL, Nichols WW, Pepine CJ, Conti CR. Acute effects of intravenous dipyridamole on regional coronary haemodynamics and metabolism. Circulation 1981;64:333–44.
14. Beller GA, Holzgrefe HH, Watson DD. Effects of dipyridamole induced vasodilation on myocardial uptake and clearance kinetics of thallium-201. Circulation 1983;68:1328–38.
15. Flameng W, Wusten B, Schaper W. On the distribution of myocardial blood flow II. Effects of arterial stenosis and vasodilatation. Basic Res Cardiol 1974;69:435–46.

16. Chambers CE, Brown KA. Dipyridamole induced ST segment depression during thallium-201 imaging in patients with coronary artery disease: angiographic and haemodynamic determinants. J Am Coll Cardiol 1988;12:37–41.

17. Segall GM, Davis MJ. Variability of serum drug level following a single oral dose of dipyridamole. J Nucl Med 1988;29:1662–7.

18. Harris DNF. The use of dipyridamole with myocardial imaging. MD Thesis, Bristol University, UK, 1982.

19. Brown BG, Josephson MA, Petersen RB et al. Intravenous dipyridamole combined with isometric handgrip for near maximal acute increase in coronary flow in patients with coronary artery disease. Am J Cardiol 1981;48:1077–85.

20. Ranhosky A, Rawson J. The safety of intravenous dipyridamole thallium myocardial perfusion imaging. Circulation 1990;81:1205–9.

21. Varma SK, Watson DD, Beller GA. Quantitative comparison of thallium-201 scintigraphy after exercise and dipyridamole in coronary artery disease. Am J Cardiol 1989;64:871–7.

22. Leppo J, Plaja J, Gionet M, Tumolo J, Paraskos JA, Cutler BS. Noninvasive evaluation of cardiac risk before elective vascular surgery. J Am Coll Cardiol 1987;9:269–76.

23. Homma S, Gilliland Y, Guiney TE, Strauss H, Boucher CA. Safety of intravenous dipyridamole for stress testing with thallium imaging. Am J Cardiol 1987;59:152–4.

24. Zhu YY, Chung WS, Botvinick EH et al. Dipyridamole infusion scintigraphy: the experience with its application in one hundred seventy patients with known or suspected unstable angina. Am Heart J 1991;121:33–43.

25. Pennell DJ, Underwood SR, Ell PJ. Symptomatic bradycardia complicating the use of intravenous dipyridamole for thallium-201 myocardial perfusion imaging. Int J Cardiol 1990; 27:272–4.

26. Bayliss J, Pearson M, Sutton GC. Ventricular dysrhythmias following intravenous dipyridamole during stress myocardial imaging. Br J Radiol 1983;56:686.

27. Wilson RF, Wyche K, Christensen BV, Zimmer S, Laxson DD. Effects of adenosine on human coronary arterial circulation. Circulation 1990;82:1595–606.

28. Verani MS, Mahmarian JJ, Hixson JB, Boyce TM, Staudacher RA. Diagnosis of coronary artery disease by controlled coronary vasodilation with adenosine and thallium-201 scintigraphy in patients unable to exercise. Circulation 1990;82:80–7.

29. Sylvén C, Beermann B, Jonzon B, Brandt R. Angina pectoris like pain provoked by intravenous adenosine in healthy volunteers. Br Med J 1986;293:227–30.

30. Nguyen T, Heo J, Ogilby D, Iskandrian AS. Single photon emission computed tomography with thallium-201 during adenosine induced coronary hyperaemia: correlation with coronary arteriography, exercise thallium imaging and two dimensional echocardiography. J Am Coll Cardiol 1990;16:1375–83.

31. Mason JR, Palac RT, Freeman ML et al. Thallium scintigraphy during dobutamine infusion: non-exercise dependent screening test for coronary artery disease. Am Heart J 1984;107: 481–5.

32. Pennell DJ, Underwood SR, Ell PJ. Thallium myocardial perfusion imaging using dobutamine: an alternative form of stress (Abstract). Eur J Nucl Med 1990;16:420.

33. Pennell DJ, Underwood SR, Swanton RH, Walker JM, Ell PJ. Dobutamine thallium-201 myocardial perfusion tomography. J Am Coll Cardiol 1991; (In press).

34. Warltier DC, Zyvoloski M, Gross GJ, Hardman HF, Brooks HL. Redistribution of myocardial blood flow distal to a dynamic coronary artery stenosis by sympathomimetic amines. Comparison of dopamine, dobutamine and isoproterenol. Am J Cardiol 1981;48:269–79.

35. Josephson MA, Brown BG, Hecht HS, Hopkins J, Pierce CD, Petersen RN. Noninvasive detection and localisation of coronary stenoses in patients: comparison of resting dipyridamole and exercise thallium-201 myocardial perfusion imaging. Am Heart J 1982;103: 1008–18.

36. Varma SK, Watson DD, Beller GC. Quantitative comparison of thallium-201 scintigraphy after exercise and dipyridamole in coronary artery disease. Am J Cardiol 1989;64:871–7.

37. Fung AY, Gallagher KP, Buda AJ. The physiological basis of dobutamine as compared with dipyridamole stress interventions in the assessment of critical coronary stenosis. Circulation 1987;76:943–51.

38. Pennell DJ, Underwood SR, Ell PJ, Swanton RH, Walker JM, Longmore DB. Dipyridamole magnetic resonance imaging: a comparison with thallium-201 emission tomography. Br Heart J 1990;64:362–9.

39. Pennell DJ, Underwood SR, Manzara CC et al. Magnetic resonance imaging of reversible myocardial ischaemia during dobutamine stress (abstract). Proceedings of the Society of Magnetic Resonance in Medicine 1990;116.

40. Walker PR, James MA, Wilde RPH, Wood CH, Russell RJ. Dipyridamole combined with exercise for thallium myocardial imaging. Br Heart J 1986;55:321–9.
41. Casale PN, Guiney TE, Strauss HW, Boucher CA. Simultaneous low level treadmill exercise and intravenous dipyridamole stress thallium imaging. Am J Cardiol 1988;62:799–802.
42. Iskandrian AS, Heo J, Kong B, Lyons E. Effect of exercise level on the ability of thallium-201 tomographic imaging in detecting coronary artery disease: analysis of 461 patients. J Am Coll Cardiol 1989;14:1477–86.
43. Young DZ, Guiney TE, McKusick A, Okada RD, Strauss HW, Boucher CA. Unmasking potential myocardial ischaemia with dipyridamole thallium imaging in patients with normal submaximal exercise thallium tests. Am J Noninvasive Cardiol 1987;1:11–14.

Chapter 4

Imaging Techniques

The Gamma Camera

Almost without exception, modern nuclear medicine images are acquired using a gamma camera based on the principles first suggested by Anger in 1957 (Fig. 4.1).[1] The camera consists of a scintillation detector made of a single sodium iodide crystal which is typically between 200 mm and 500 mm diameter and between 6 and 20 mm thick. Behind the crystal are a number of photomultiplier tubes (up to 90 or 100) which are optically coupled to the surface of the crystal and which sense the scintillations arising whenever a gamma ray is absorbed by the crystal. The areas of crystal seen by the tubes overlap, but the location of each scintillation can be computed from the relative responses in each tube. The energy of the photons can also be measured from the response of the tubes, and the electrical output from the camera head to the imaging computer consists of x and y coordinates and photon energy (z) for each scintillation that is detected. In front of the crystal is a collimator which consists of a disc of lead penetrated by a honeycomb of holes. The holes allow only gamma rays that are travelling perpendicularly to the crystal face to enter the crystal and in this way the gamma photons absorbed by the crystal form an image of the distribution of radionuclide in front of the camera.

In order to perform emission tomography, the camera must rotate around the patient. The mechanics of the rotation vary between manufacturers but an essential component is that the orbit must be precise, accurate and reproducible. Such mechanical stability does not always correspond with simplicity and elegance of design but good compromises have been achieved.

Emission Tomography

Emission tomography (from the Greek -τωμως, cutting) using radionuclides was first described in 1963 by Kuhl and Edwards,[2] 10 years before Hounsfield and Ambrose described X-ray transmission tomography,[3,4] but performance of the imaging hardware and reconstruction software was such that image quality was poor. Within the last ten years, improvements in both have led to the widespread use of emission tomography in nuclear

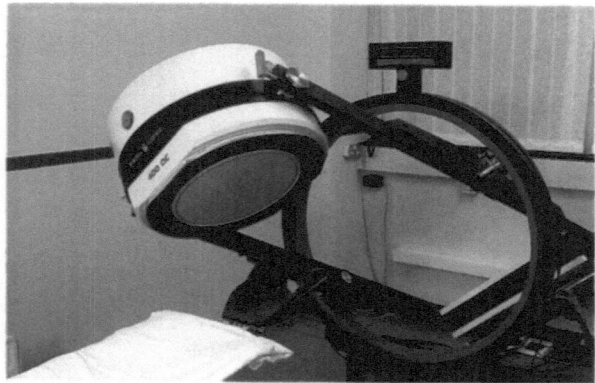

Fig. 4.1. A modern gamma camera.

medicine. Its use in nuclear cardiology has mainly been restricted to myocardial perfusion imaging and acute infarct imaging. Electrocardiogram gated blood pool emission tomography has not been widely developed, principally because appropriate computer software has not been available commercially, but there are some reports of its application.[5-8]

In general nuclear medicine, planar imaging is the normal method of image acquisition. Indeed, planar myocardial perfusion imaging using thallium has served cardiologists well for many years. Projectional imaging, however, suffers from the disadvantage that it is difficult to separate the activity from overlapping structures. The acquisition of multiple projections can ease this problem and it is usual to acquire anterior, left anterior oblique and left lateral images. With experience, the different areas of myocardium can be localised on these images and the site and extent of perfusion defects can be deduced.

Table 4.1. Guidelines to good quality thallium emission tomography

Technical aspects

- Regular checks of camera quality must be made, including weekly centre of rotation measurements and uniformity correction acquisitions of 3×10^7 counts.
- The camera orbit must be as close as possible to the chest wall.
- The patient must be comfortably positioned during acquisition in order to avoid motion artefact.

Clinical aspects

- The thallium must be injected at maximal or symptom limited exercise. The operator should be familiar with exercise testing and its potential complications and should not be afraid of stressing cardiac patients.
- The operator's clinical assessment at the time of exercise is invaluable. Clinical observations at peak exercise increase confidence in the assessment of the presence of ischaemia. The observations are an essential part of the report.
- There must be close liaison between the requesting clinician, the doctor performing the scan, and the reporter. Ideally, the three should be the same. Failing this, the clinical question must be clearly defined and the consequences of the findings must be understood by the reporting doctor.

Tomography is an extension of the multiprojection method of acquiring planar images. A number of equally spaced views (typically 32) is acquired as the camera rotates around the patient. The planar views are then reconstructed into tomograms using similar algorithms to those used in X-ray transmission tomography. The advantages of tomography over planar imaging include a true three-dimensional display of the distribution of the tracer within the heart which aids interpretation, improved image contrast because of the elimination of overlying structures, and the potential for quantification of the tracer uptake.

It is not our intention to provide a detailed description of the technique of emission tomography and the reader is referred to previous publications.[9,10] A number of points are vital for the acquisition of good quality thallium emission tomograms. These are summarised in Table 4.1, but the most important technical points are that the quality control of the acquisition system must be rigorous and the camera must be positioned as close as possible to the chest.

Patient Preparation

As already hinted, attention to detail is an important part of the acquisition of good quality tomograms. The thallium is injected at peak exercise (see Chapter 3), preferably through an intravenous cannula in an antecubital vein. The cannula should be flushed with normal saline after insertion although a dilute heparin flush may help to avoid clotting if a prolonged period between cannula insertion and thallium injection is anticipated. It is unwise to use an intravenous cannula that has been inserted for another purpose. If the injection is mistakenly given outside the vein no harm usually results, although there is the theoretical risk of localised radiation necrosis. A more important problem with an injection which is partly extravascular is that the quality of the images will suffer and the slow absorption of thallium from the injection site will complicate the analysis of washout rate from the myocardium. After the thallium injection it is sensible practice to flush the syringe with 10–20 ml of normal saline from a second syringe connected via a three-way tap to ensure that the full dose of thallium is administered.

For imaging, the patient lies supine on the couch with the left arm (for 180° rotation) or both arms (for 360° rotation) held above the head. This position is uncomfortable, particularly for elderly patients with cervical spine or shoulder problems but the majority of patients will tolerate the position for 15–20 min. A pillow placed under the knees gives some comfort and helps the patient to keep still. This is very important because motion artefact may not be easily identified after the acquisition (cases 33 and 74). The arm needs to be raised above the head so that it does not cause attenuation in the lateral projections and so that the camera can be as close as possible to the chest wall. For cameras which rotate in a circular orbit the positions which limit the proximity of the camera are usually the right shoulder and the left arm. For cameras which rotate in non-circular orbits, better approximation of the camera to the chest wall can be achieved at all parts of the orbit.

Artefacts will be caused by any attenuating structure which comes between the heart and the camera. Metallic objects in pockets (case 77) and metal buttons must be avoided but it is sometimes difficult to avoid the artefact from an implanted pacemaker. In ladies with large breasts, the site of artefact in the tomograms will depend on where the breast attenuates the planar images. It is recommended that the breasts are strapped against the chest so that the attenuation is as uniform as possible (case 3). Prone imaging is another possibility although the images tend to be of poorer quality. The left hemidiaphragm will also cause attenuation if it is elevated by, for instance, a large meal. For this reason, and because fasting increases insulin levels and hence myocardial uptake of thallium, the patient should fast for four hours before the study.

Data Acquisition

The ideal tomographic acquisition spans 360° and includes as many steps as possible but, in practice, a compromise has to be made. One way to reduce imaging time is to rotate the camera over only 180°. The heart is well suited for a 180° acquisition since it lies in the left anterior hemithorax and images acquired over the right posterior hemithorax are degraded by attenuation of between 16- and 64-fold. A 360° acquisition may therefore only add to the noise without adding any useful information. This has been established for thallium emission tomography[11] although there is some dispute.[12-14] Our own protocol is to acquire 32 images over 180° as the camera rotates anteriorly from the right anterior oblique position to the left posterior oblique projection. Table 4.2 summarises the other acquisition parameters.

The stress images are acquired as soon as possible after the end of exercise and should be completed within 30 min. Redistribution images are traditionally acquired 4 h after injection for planar imaging but redistribution tomographic imaging is sometimes performed earlier without loss of diagnostic accuracy, and this avoids excessive loss of thallium from the heart at the time of imaging. Much later imaging (12 or 24 h) is sometimes performed because of the increasing evidence that 4 h redistribution imaging can underestimate the extent of viable myocardium (case 79). Image quality with such a late acquisition is poor, however, and an alternative approach is to

Table 4.2. Acquisition parameters used for all images displayed in this book

Number of projections	32
Time per projection	30 s immediate, 40 s redistribution
Type of orbit	circular
Arc of rotation	180°
Collimator	low energy general purpose, parallel hole
Photopeaks	80 and 167 keV
Energy window, offset	20%, 0%
Image size	400 mm unzoomed, 64 × 64 pixels

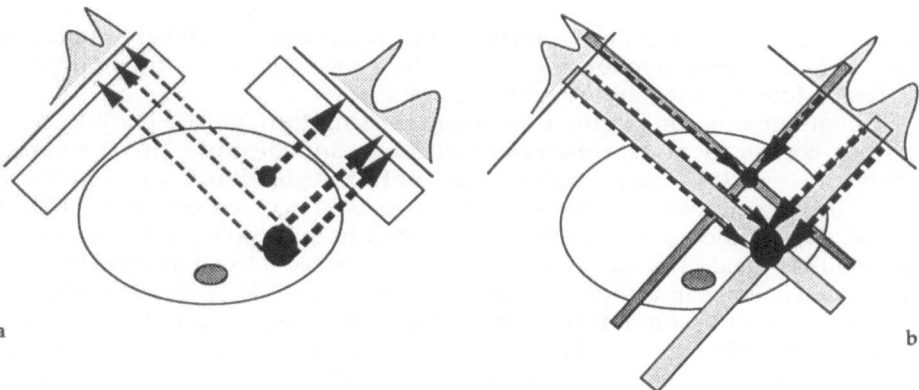

a   b

Fig. 4.2. Image reconstruction. **a** Each line of pixels in the planar image represents a profile of counts acquired from a tomographic plane perpendicular to the camera face. **b** Backprojection reverses this process but, because there is no depth information in the acquired counts, the values in the profile are laid down in columns projected back into the tomographic image. When this has been repeated for each of the projections there is reinforcement at the true position of a source of activity but no reinforcement at other positions.

image again after an additional resting injection of thallium. This improves the detection of viable myocardium but at the expense of an increased radiation burden to the patient (case 80).

Depending on clinical details and on local practice, normal stress images may avoid the need for redistribution imaging. There is no circumstance in which a study could be considered abnormal if the stress images are un-equivocally normal.

Data Processing

The set of planar images is reconstructed into a stack of transaxial tomo-grams by filtered backprojection. The technique is illustrated for a simple object in Fig. 4.2. Each line of pixels in the planar image represents a profile of counts acquired from a tomographic plane perpendicular to the camera face. Backprojection reverses this process but, because there is no depth information in the acquired counts, the values in the profile are laid down in columns projected back into the tomographic image. When this has been repeated for each of the projections there is reinforcement at the true posi-tion of a source of activity but no reinforcement at other positions. The result is a tomographic image showing the position of the source although, in the simple case illustrated, the image will have very poor resolution with a lot of surrounding reconstruction artefact. The artefact can be eliminated by backprojecting negative values alongside the original data, to interfere with and remove the unwanted positive values. The negative values are produced by filtering the data with an appropriately chosen filter before backprojection. The theory of these filters is beyond the scope of this book, but many different types have been developed. The principal difference between filters is whether they preserve or selectively attenuate the high spatial frequencies within the image. Both noise and fine detail are present in the high spatial frequencies and so the choice of filter is a compromise between loss of detail and removal of noise.

The attenuation of gamma photons in passing through the body leads to higher counts in more superficial structures and destroys the theoretical ability of emission tomography to quantify the distribution of uptake in megaBecquerel per gram of tissue. It is possible to correct for attenuation in three ways, although the mathematics involved is complex and none of the methods is ideal. The simplest approach is prereconstruction correction, in which each point in a projection profile is multiplied by a factor depending on the depth of tissue contributing to that point on the profile. No account is taken of the distribution of activity within the object, and so although this method may be suitable for uniform distributions (as in a liver scan), it is not suitable for cardiac work. Postreconstruction correction does take account of the distribution of activity within the body by considering the way in which a point source would be attenuated, and calculating a correction matrix to apply to the reconstructed image. This method performs reasonably well in clinical practice although it is not an exact solution to the problem and is not sufficiently accurate for reliable quantification. The third method is intrinsic correction in which an exponential attenuation within the body is assumed and taken into account during the filtering and backprojection. This is theoretically the most attractive method but its advantage over postprocessing methods remains to be demonstrated. None of the methods is suitable for a 180° acquisition and so it is normal to omit attenuation correction for thallium emission tomography.

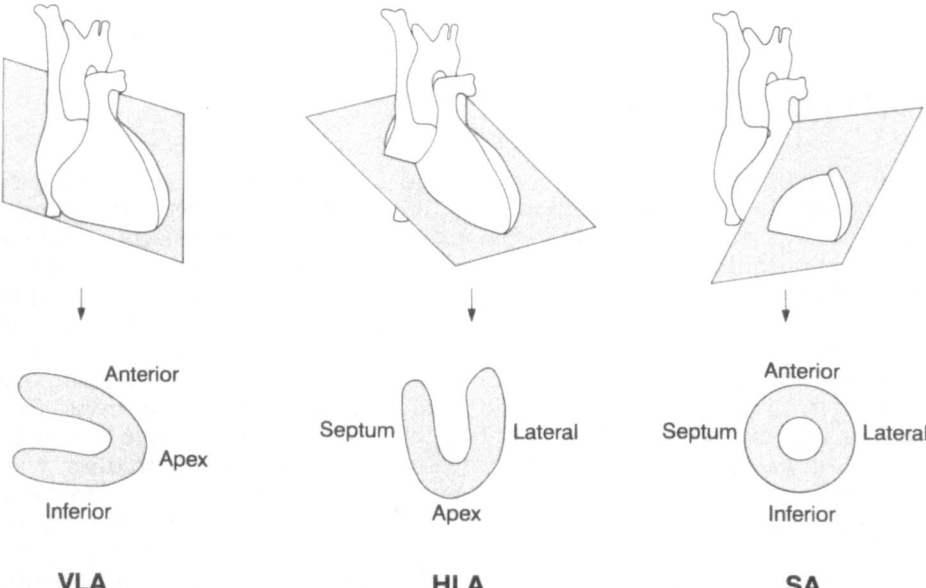

Fig. 4.3. The vertical long axis plane (VLA), horizontal long axis plane (HLA) and short axis plane (SA) with the segments of the myocardium which they cut. The diagram can be used as a key for the interpretation of the images in Chapter 6.

The stack of transaxial slices produced by filtered backprojection is a three-dimensional data set and it is a relatively simple computer task to reorientate the data into oblique slices. For the heart, the most useful oblique planes are the vertical and horizontal long axis (VLA and HLA) and the short axis planes (SA) (Fig. 4.3). These planes which pass perpendicularly through the major left ventricular walls are familiar to cardiologists from other imaging techniques. This enhances interpretation and acceptance by cardiologists without nuclear medicine training and allows a direct comparison of perfusion with functional or anatomical measures such as wall motion.[15] In order to define the angles of the planes, a central transaxial slice is displayed on the computer screen and the long axis is drawn on this image. Perpendicular to the transaxial plane and including the long axis as drawn, the vertical long axis slices are reconstructed. From the central vertical long axis slice, the caudal inclination of the true long axis can be seen and the horizontal long axis and short axis slices can be generated, both perpendicular to the vertical long axis slice.

References

1. Anger H. Scintillation camera. The review of scientific instruments 1958;29:27–33.
2. Kuhl DE, Edwards RQ. Image separation radioisotope scanning. Radiology 1963;80:653–61.
3. Hounsfield GN. Computerised transverse axial scanning (tomography). 1 Description of system. Br J Radiol 1973;46:1016–22.
4. Ambrose J. Computerised transverse axial scanning (tomography). 2 Clinical application. Br J Radiol 1973;46:1023–47.
5. Moore ML, Murphy PH, Burdine JA. ECG-gated emission computed tomography of the cardiac blood pool. Radiology 1980;134:233–5.
6. Maublant J, Bailly P, Mestas D et al. Feasibility of gated single-photon emission transaxial tomography of the cardiac blood pool. Radiology 1983;146:837–9.
7. Tamaki N, Mukai T, Ishii Y et al. Multiaxial tomography of heart chambers by gated blood-pool emission computed tomography using a rotating gamma camera. Radiology 1983;147:547–54.
8. Underwood SR, Walton S, Ell PJ, Jarritt PH, Emanuel RW, Swanton RH. Gated blood-pool emission tomography: a new technique for the investigation of cardiac structure and function. Eur J Nucl Med 1985;10:332–7.
9. Ell PJ, Holman BL. Computed emission tomography. Oxford: Oxford Medical Publications, 1982.
10. Ell PJ, Jarritt PH. Gamma camera emission tomography: quality control and clinical applications. London: Chapman and Hall, 1984.
11. Hoffman EJ. 180° compared with 360° sampling in SPECT. J Nucl Med 1982;23:745–7.
12. Coleman RE, Jaszczak RJ, Cobb FR. Comparison of 180 deg and 360 deg data collection in thallium-201 imaging using single photon emission computed tomography (SPECT). J Nucl Med 1982;23:655–60.
13. Go RT, McIntyre WJ, Houser TS et al. Clinical evaluation of 360° and 180° data sampling techniques for transaxial SPECT thallium-201 myocardial perfusion imaging. J Nucl Med 1985;26:695–706.
14. Knesaurek K. Image distortion in 180° SPECT studies. J Nucl Med 1986;27:1792.
15. Pennell DJ, Underwood SR, Ell PJ, Swanton RH, Walker JM, Longmore DB. Dipyridamole magnetic resonance imaging: a comparison with thallium-201 emission tomography. Br Heart J 1990;64:362–9.

Chapter 5

Image Interpretation

Quality Control

An essential prelude to image interpretation is to review the planar images which form the raw data of the tomograms. Although the planar images have few counts and only coarse detail can be seen, it is at this stage that potential artefacts are most easily detected. A cine display of the planar images gives the impression of the patient rotating and allows both clinical and technical details to be assessed. Excessive lung uptake, the prognostic importance of which is discussed later in this chapter, can easily be judged. Motion of the patient during the acquisition can be seen and upward creep may also be apparent (case 76).[1,2] The phenomenon of upward creep is sometimes seen in stress images following vigorous exercise. As the cardiovascular system returns to the resting state there are changes in heart rate, respiratory rate and redistribution of blood through the body. The mean position of the diaphragm rises and this pushes the heart up. This can lead to an apparent defect which will not be present in the redistribution images, thus simulating a reversible perfusion defect. If there is any doubt whether upward creep has occurred, then the planar images can be summed to show the outline of the heart moving cranially through the acquisition. Another artefact that is easily detected by reviewing the planar images is attenuation from the breast (case 3) or from metallic objects (case 77).

Normal Appearances

After review of the planar images, the tomograms themselves should be reviewed and this is also best performed on the computer screen. It is important to become familiar with the colour scale used because this provides semiquantitative information on count distribution throughout the myocardium (Fig. 5.1). Each image should be displayed with the top and bottom colours of the scale representing the maximum and minimum number of counts in any voxel of the complete study and should not be displayed to the maximum and minimum of the individual image. This ensures that different tomograms can be compared with each other. We find it most helpful to present the vertical and horizontal long axis, and short axis tomograms in three quadrants of the screen. The positions at which the

31

planes intersect can be superimposed, and the tomograms can be leafed through to provide a three-dimensional impression of tracer uptake. A display of the whole set of tomograms on a single screen is less helpful.

For clinical purposes, most of the information is present in the central slices of the two long axis planes and it is from these alone that the five major segments of the left ventricular myocardium can be judged: anterior wall, septum, inferior wall, lateral wall and apex. The four major walls can be divided into basal and apical portions yielding a total of nine segments. Further subdivision is unhelpful since only very rarely will a clinically significant perfusion defect involve less than one of these segments. If a defect is seen in the central long axis slices, then its exact position can be confirmed by reference to the short axis slices.

An important part of image interpretation is to become familiar with normal appearances. Although myocardial perfusion when seen with the resolution of thallium tomograms is homogeneous, there is a wide variety of normal appearances arising from variation in size and position of the heart

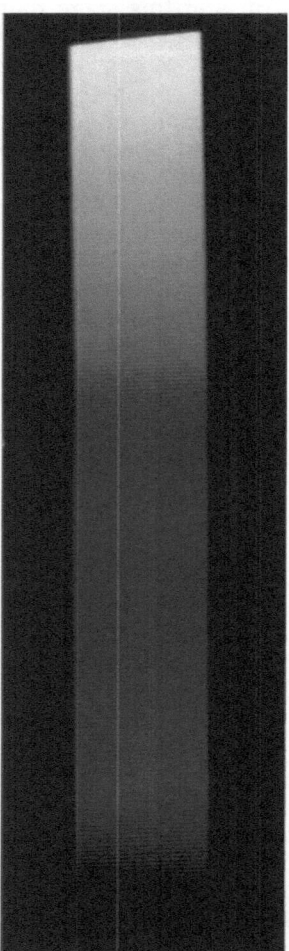

Fig. 5.1. The colour scale used to display all images in this book. Each pixel is displayed with a colour corresponding to the number of counts it contains. The top and bottom colours of the scale are assigned to the maximum number within the set of tomograms and to zero respectively.

Table 5.1. Common variations in normal thallium tomograms

Apical thinning	The apical myocardium is thinner than elsewhere and counts may be reduced to at least 50% of maximum
Short septum	The basal part of the septum is membranous and does not take up thallium
Inferior attenuation	The inferior myocardium is deeper than the rest of the heart leading to reduced counts, particularly in men. The basal part of the inferior wall may be reduced to 50% of maximum
Septal attenuation	It is normal for the septum to have lower counts than the lateral wall. This only rarely causes confusion
Anterior attenuation	This may be the result of breast artefact or upward creep
Lateral attenuation	Occasionally the basal part of the inferolateral wall is attenuated
Irregularity	Poor count statistics can lead to irregularity but this only rarely simulates the pattern of a perfusion defect
Wall thickening	Patient motion may lead to displacement of counts from one wall to another, smudging, or distortion of the normal anatomy

(cases 1 and 2), body habitus, and quality of the tomographic acquisition (case 75).[3] Common variations in tracer distribution are summarised in Table 5.1. It is sometimes difficult to distinguish between true perfusion defects and normal variation. If there is doubt, then repeat imaging in the prone position may help to identify inferior attenuation (case 4) and apical attenuation (case 5), and prone imaging or strapping of the breasts may help to identify attenuation from the breast (case 3). Another feature which aids interpretation is a knowledge of the normal distribution of coronary perfusion. If a defect involves a known coronary territory, such as the septum, anterior wall and apex (left anterior descending artery), then it is almost certainly a true perfusion defect, whereas if it does not fit with normal coronary anatomy it is more likely to be artefactual. If there is any doubt, then the clinical impression of whether myocardial ischaemia was present at the time of stress is very helpful. Some commentators believe that images should be interpreted in the absence of clinical information in order to avoid bias. We do not share that view. If the angiographic data pose the question whether a solitary lesion of the left anterior descending artery is haemodynamically significant, then there is little point worrying about how to interpret the inferior wall.

Abnormal Appearances

Chapter 6 provides a comprehensive illustration of abnormal appearances but it may be helpful to summarise some general rules. The size and shape of the ventricle are important. It is difficult to gauge the size of the ventricle in absolute terms but the best indicator is the relative size of the cavity and the myocardial wall. Of particular significance is dilatation which is present in the stess images but not in the redistribution images (case 41). This implies extensive reversible ischaemia and is associated with an adverse prognosis.[4] Thickening of the walls in patients with left ventricular hypertrophy (case 54) and hypertrophic cardiomyopathy (case 60) is sometimes apparent although, because the spatial resolution of thallium tomograms is not very good, it is difficult to draw reliable conclusions. The normal right ventricular myocardium is much thinner than the left ventricle but it is not unusual to see the right ventricle in tomograms. If the right ventricle is hypertrophied it may take up almost as much tracer as the left ventricle (case 63). Divergence of the anterior and inferior walls of the left ventricle is unusual and it implies apical aneurysm formation (cases 16 and 24). Again, such an interpretation can only be suggested and it should be confirmed by an alternative imaging technique such as radionuclide ventriculography or echocardiography.

Defects corresponding to areas of ischaemia are not normally subtle and it is preferable to err on the side of under-reporting than the opposite. It may be more harmful to suggest that a normal patient might be abnormal and hence to condemn him or her to further investigation, than to miss a mild abnormality which may not be of clinical significance. Allowing for the previous description of normal appearances, a defect that is less than 30% of maximum counts is unusual and areas of redistribution normally improve by at least 20% of maximum counts. When grading defects, both their extent and their depth should be reported. Dividing the myocardium into the nine segments described above, a defect can be described as mild if it involves one or two segments, moderate for three to five segments, and severe for six segments or more. Tracer uptake in each segment can be classified as normal, mildly, moderately or severely reduced, or absent, if uptake as a percentage of maximum in the whole set of tomograms is 100%–70%, 70%–50%, 50%–30%, 30%–10%, or 10%–0 respectively.

Abnormalities are normally classified as either fixed or reversible and are said to indicate infarcted and reversibly ischaemic myocardium respectively. Whilst this is a good guideline, we now know that it is simplistic. Redistribution is often incomplete if imaging is performed at 3–4 hours, but failure to return to normal does not necessarily imply that there is partial infarction since later redistribution imaging (case 79) or reinjection imaging (case 80) will often show further improvement.[5,6] It has been demonstrated that redistribution may be incomplete at 4 h in as many as 22% of segments[7] and even later images may be required if the extent of non-viable myocardium is not to be overestimated. This is not always practical and an alternative approach if delayed redistribution is suspected is to inject a second dose of thallium at rest. Although this involves an additional radiation burden it can be justified in some circumstances. Another method of avoiding 24 h imaging might be to follow stress thallium imaging with resting technetium isonitrile imaging since the 140 keV gamma ray of technetium-99m can be successfully imaged in the presence of thallium-201. Further experimentation is required before an alternative protocol could be recommended for routine use, but in the meantime it is reasonable to continue unchanged, bearing in mind the possibility of delayed redistribution when planning and reporting studies. The prognostic significance of delayed redistribution appears to be the same as that of early redistribution and it does not necessarily represent more profound ischaemia.[8]

Partial redistribution does not often present a practical problem. More difficult is failure of a potentially viable area to show any redistribution at all. Reinjection of thallium leads to an improvement in approximately 30% of such areas,[9–12] suggesting that the presence of viable myocardium is seriously underestimated by conventional thallium imaging.[13] Whilst reinjection may be a small price to pay if it provides information on the viability of myocardium,[14] it is difficult to believe that a complete assessment can be made without separate studies of perfusion and metabolism as are provided by positron emission tomography. Positron emission tomography reveals viable myocardium by virtue of its preserved uptake of [18F]-fluorodeoxyglucose, indicating a switch from the normal fatty acid metabolism to anaerobic glucose metabolism.

An important clinical problem which has been solved by positron emission tomography is the detection of "hibernating" myocardium. This is myocardium which is chronically ischaemic and has reduced its contractile function in order to make best use of what oxygen is available, but which has the potential for normal function when normal perfusion is restored. It has been suggested that thallium injected at rest will be taken up by hibernating myocardium and that a comparison of resting thallium uptake and ventricular function should reveal the hibernating myocardium. Whilst this may be so with mild resting ischaemia, profoundly ischaemic myocardium is unlikely to be detected in this way. Further studies comparing thallium scintigraphy with positron emission tomography are expected to resolve the issue.

Just as hibernating myocardium is the result of chronic ischaemia, stunned myocardium is the result of acute ischaemia. Following myocardial infarction and reperfusion by thrombolysis, mechanical function may be temporarily depressed despite the preservation of metabolic function. This is another occasion when a defect of thallium uptake at rest does not necessarily imply irretrievable infarction.

Reverse redistribution is a term that is applied to the unusual occurrence of normal uptake in the stress images with reduced uptake on redistribution (case 78). The appearance is the result of an area from which there is faster washout than surrounding myocardium, but there is uncertainty over its cause. It has been variously suggested that it has the same significance as reversible ischaemia or that it is the result of partial infarction with a patent coronary vessel.[15] Although not denying that such phenomena may occur, our own experience is that reverse redistribution is often the result of image artefact.

Defects of tracer uptake indicate inequalities of tracer delivery to the myocardium or of its active uptake by the myocytes, but this need not always be the result of atheromatous coronary artery disease. Other forms of pathology that may cause focal defects are coronary artery spasm,[16] anomolous coronary arteries or arteries constricted by muscle bridges (case 61),[17] small vessel disease as may occur in diabetes or syndrome X (case 55),[18,19] the dilated (case 58) and hypertrophic cardiomyopathies (case 60),[20,21] hypertrophy caused by outflow obstruction or hypertension (case 54), infiltrative disorders such as sarcoidosis[22] and amyloidosis (case 40), connective tissue disorders,[23] and conduction defects such as left bundle branch block (cases 53 and 56).[24] These defects are often fixed but reversible defects may also occur. The mechanism of such reversible defects is obscure. One theory that is appropriate in left bundle branch block is that the duration of diastolic coronary flow is shortened in the septum by delayed relaxation and so diastolic coronary flow may be inadequate at high heart rates.[25] The defects reduce the specificity of thallium scintigraphy for the detection of coronary artery disease and this has in the past been cited as a major limitation of the technique. In fact, it only rarely leads to a diagnostic problem and conventional epicardial coronary artery disease remains the commonest cause of thallium defects in patients with diabetes and left bundle branch block.[26]

There is insufficient experience of thallium imaging in patients following orthotopic heart transplantation to be confident of the significance of abnormalities. Accelerated atherosclerosis may occur in the donor coronary arteries and reversible defects would be expected to reflect this obstructive disease. Episodes of rejection may also lead to myocardial disease which would be expected to produce fixed defects. Because of these fixed defects, however, it may be difficult to diagnose accelerated coronary disease from the thallium scan alone. Myocardial hypertrophy has also been reported (case 62).

Coronary Anatomy

When interpreting thallium tomograms, it is important to remember that the distribution of the major coronary arteries varies greatly between individuals. The most constant vessel is the left anterior descending artery which supplies the distal anterior wall and apex, with septal and diagonal branches supplying the septum and proximal anterior wall (cases 10–12, 16–18). Depending on the arrangement of vessels, a proximal left anterior descending lesion may involve the whole of the anterior wall, apex and septum, or it may spare the septum. It is less usual to involve the septum without the anterior wall. A very large artery may extend around the apex to perfuse the distal inferior wall and, conversely, the inferior portion of the septum may be supplied by the posterior descending artery arising from the right or circumflex arteries.

In 85% of people the right coronary artery is dominant, meaning that it gives rise to the posterior descending artery which supplies the inferior wall (cases 7, 9, 13, 15). In the other 15%, the posterior descending artery arises from the distal circumflex artery. In a right dominant circulation, the circumflex artery normally supplies only the basal portions of the lateral and inferior walls and possibly the basal septum, and the lateral wall is supplied by the marginal branches of the circumflex artery (cases 8 and 14). Because of this variation, it can be difficult to assign areas to these two arteries unless the anatomy is known. It is nearly always safe to assign the anterior wall and septum to the left anterior descending artery and the lateral wall to the circumflex artery, but the inferior wall may be supplied either by the right coronary artery or by the left circumflex artery.

Quantification

Our description of normal and abnormal appearances assumes a certain familiarity with thallium tomograms and begs the question; "When is reduced tracer uptake abnormal?" There is no simple answer to this question because a number of factors unrelated to myocardial perfusion will alter the apparent uptake of tracer. Visual analysis of the images is normally adequate to assess all of these factors and to decide on the information content of the image, but there are two important reasons for wanting a more objective assessment. First, clinical experience does not come easily and it is hopefully based on some attempt at objective analysis. Second, objective analysis is more likely to be consistent both for the same observer and between observers.

The nuclear medicine computer can be used at three levels to aid image interpretation. At the simplest level, it can manipulate the display of the image by background subtraction, alteration of contrast, and the use of a colour scale to simplify visual quantification. At the next level, it can be used to analyse the counts within any region of the image, to compare these counts with established normal ranges and hence to identify abnormalities. On the highest level, artificial intelligence can be used to suggest a clinical interpretation of the images.[27] The first of these is trivial and does not require expansion. The third is beyond the scope of this book. We shall, therefore, concentrate on methods by which the computer can be used to quantify counts within the image.

Lung Uptake of Thallium

In 1987 it was reported that a high uptake of thallium in the lungs was the most important variable provided by thallium imaging for the prediction of future cardiac events (case 40).[28] Lung uptake is related to other prognostic variables including the extent and severity of coronary artery disease, the degree of impairment of left ventricular function, and the increase in pulmonary capillary pressure during exercise. The factors which affect uptake are complex but they include pulmonary transit time, extraction efficiency by the lungs, and pulmonary capillary pressure. All of these are related to left ventricular function and so a high uptake simply reflects poor function, either at rest or induced by ischaemia during exercise.[29]

Absolute lung uptake cannot be measured easily and so it is expressed as a ratio between uptake in the lungs and the heart. Despite variable cardiac uptake the ratio has proved helpful.[30] It can be measured either from an initial anterior planar image or from the appropriate image of the tomographic acquisition. Counts within regions placed over the whole of the right lung field and the whole of the heart are compared, although the exact positioning of the cardiac region of interest does affect the ratio. The upper limit in patients without coronary artery disease varies between 0.78 and 0.86[31] and values above this are associated with a high risk of future cardiac events.

Myocardial Distribution of Thallium

A number of methods have been used to quantify the distribution of thallium within the myocardium, including linear profiles, circumferential profiles[32] and analysis of count histograms. All of these are applicable to both planar and tomographic images but an additional method that has been used to simplify the display and quantification of tomographic images is the polar map (or "bullseye" image, case 67).[33-35] It must be emphasised that there is not a simple relationship between the amount of tracer uptake

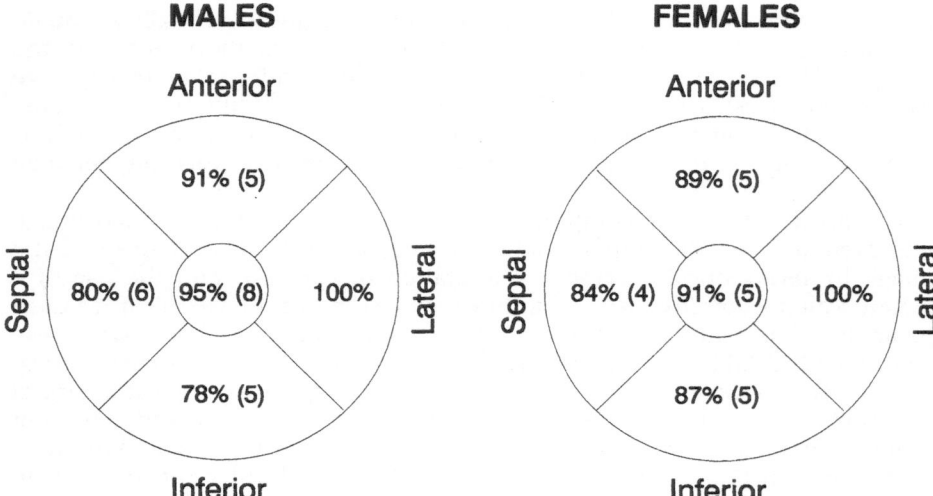

Fig. 5.2. Polar maps showing the mean distribution of thallium after exercise in normal subjects. The lateral wall normally contains the highest activity and is scaled to 100% to allow a comparison with other territories. (Adapted from reference 36 with permission.)

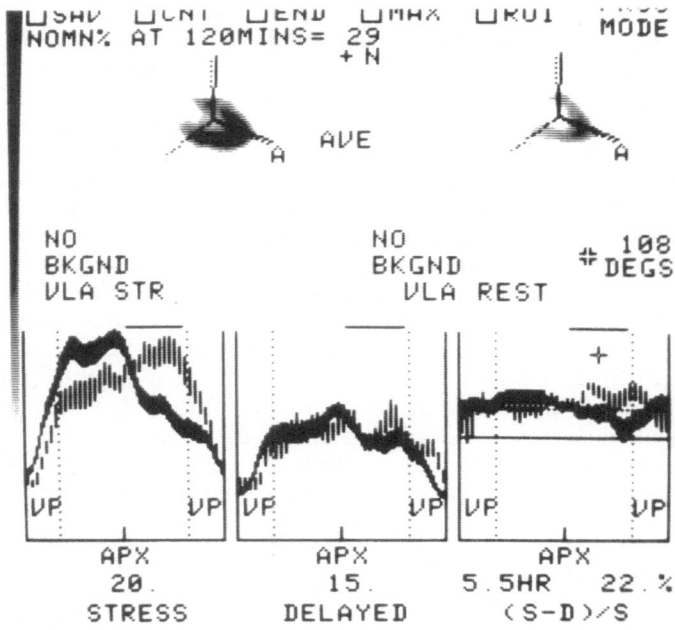

Fig. 5.3. Circumferential profile analysis of vertical long axis tomograms (stress, top left; redistribution, top right). A radius is swept around the image and a profile is plotted of the maximum counts at each point, excluding the valve plane (VP). The stress profile appears bottom left, the redistribution profile bottom centre, and the washout profile bottom right. This is calculated as (stress − redistribution) / stress. The profile from the patient (black) is compared with an established normal range (hatched). There is a reversible perfusion defect of the anterior wall with reduced washout in this region.

38

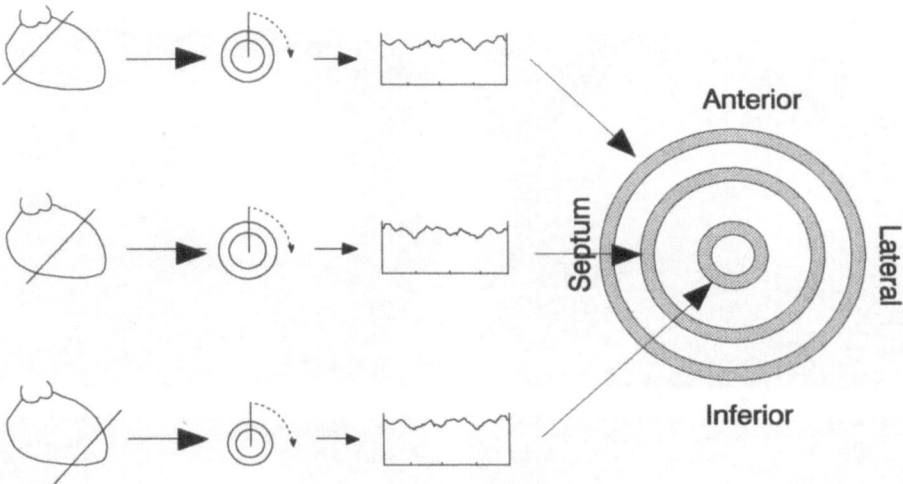

Fig. 5.4 Reconstruction of the polar plot or "bullseye" image. The apical short axis tomogram is laid down in the centre of a circular image with more basal slices appearing outside it. The resulting image has the effect of transforming the conical myocardium into a disk.

within the myocardium and the number of counts in each voxel, and quantification is normally relative to the maximum counts in any part of the myocardium. Thallium imaging is sometimes criticised because global depression of uptake might mask relative defects but in practice, this situation never occurs. Fig. 5.2 shows the distribution of myocardial counts in polar maps derived from normal males and females. The lateral wall normally contains the highest counts and the images are therefore scaled to 100% in this territory. The regional variation and the difference between the sexes is clearly shown. The largest variations occur in the septum and inferior wall.[36]

Fig. 5.3 shows an example of circumferential profile analysis of vertical long axis tomograms. The profiles of each tomogram are compared with normal ranges constructed from a bank of patients without cardiac abnormality. In this example, the profile through the anterior wall is abnormally low in the stress tomogram but normal in the redistribution tomogram. The washout profile also shows abnormally low washout in this region. The reversible ischaemia is mild and it is more easily seen from the profiles than from the images alone.

Fig. 5.4 shows the reconstruction of the polar map. This form of display has the advantage that all areas of the myocardium are represented in a single image, although it has the disadvantage that the image is less familiar to cardiologists and it is less easy to appreciate the relationship between the site of a defect and coronary arterial territories. Another problem is that equal areas of myocardium are not mapped to equal areas of the polar plot and so the size of a defect becomes distorted. Furthermore, if stress and redistribution polar plots are to be compared, the mapping of both studies must be identical. This may be difficult if there are count changes at the apex. Our own practice is only to refer to such a display in cases of doubt. Fig. 5.5 shows an example of a patient with reversible inferolateral ischaemia.

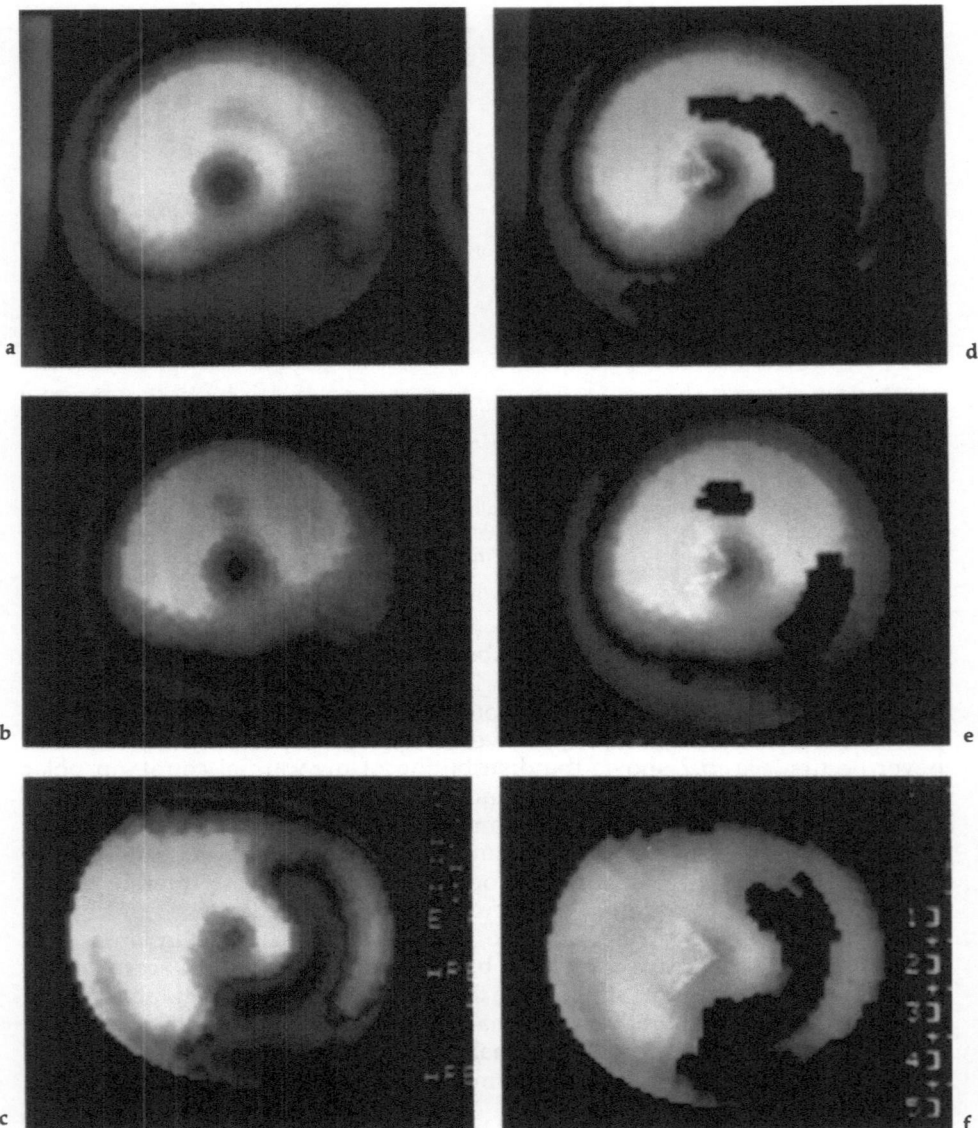

Fig. 5.5. Polar plots of a patient with reversible inferolateral ischaemia. **a** Stress, **b** redistribution, **c** washout. **d, e, f** The same images as **a, b** and **c** with areas that are more than two standard deviations from the mean of a normal population blacked out. This shows the extent of the abnormalities more clearly.

Table 5.2 summarises data from a number of studies to allow a comparison of qualitative and quantitative analyses of thallium scintigrams.[37] Although there is variation between the studies, the general trend is that quantification allows an increase in sensitivity for the detection of disease without a reduction in specificity. The differences between studies are related

Table 5.2. Sensitivity and specificity for the detection of coronary artery disease arranged to demonstrate the effects of quantitative analysis

Reference	Number of patients	Qualitative analysis		Quantitative analysis	
		Sensitivity (%)	Specificity (%)	Sensitivity (%)	Specificity (%)
Planar studies					
Maddahi et al.[39]	118	91	86	93	91
Tomographic studies					
Francisco et al.[40]	86	76	67	90	96
Tamaki et al.[41]	104	80	93	91	92
Niemeyer et al.[42]	131	74	68	69	86

to differences in technique and to differences in patient populations (patients with and without infarction, single or triple vessel disease, etc.).

Washout Analysis

Slow washout of thallium from the myocardium is an indicator of ischaemia, although there is considerable confusion over the interpretation of this phenomenon.[38] Following initial uptake of thallium there is a dynamic equilibrium between the intracellular, extracellular and intravascular compartments. As the thallium is slowly excreted by the kidneys and gut, so it washes out from the myocardium. In an area of reduced intracellular uptake caused by ischaemia at the time of injection, the rate of washout from the cell is reduced because of the lower intracellular concentration, and the rate of uptake into the cell is increased as normal cellular metabolism returns. Both of these conspire to increase intracellular thallium when compared with normal myocardium and estimates of the rate of washout from the ischaemic area will show it to be reduced. A diagnosis of abnormality based on washout only is suspect, because redistribution should be apparent in the images from which the washout is measured.

References

1. Friedman J, Van Train K, Maddahi J et al. "Upward creep" of the heart: a frequent source of false-positive reversible defects during thallium-201 stress-redistribution SPECT. J Nucl Med 1989;30:1718–22.
2. Mester J, Welle R, Claussen M et al. Upward creep of the heart in exercise thallium 201 single photon emission tomography: clinical relevance and a simple correction method. Eur J Nucl Med 1991 (in press).
3. DePuey EG, Garcia EV. Optimal specificity of thallium-201 SPECT through recognition of imaging artefacts. J Nucl Med 1989;30:441–9.
4. Weiss AT, Berman DS, Lew AS et al. Transient ischaemic dilatation of the left ventricle on stress thallium-201 scintigraphy: a marker of severe and extensive coronary artery disease. J Am Coll Cardiol 1987;9:752–9.
5. Cloninger KG, DePuey EG, Garcia EV et al. Incomplete redistribution in delayed thallium-201 single photon emission computed tomographic (SPECT) images: an overestimation of myocardial scarring. J Am Coll Cardiol 1988;12:955–63.

6. Ziessman HA, Keyes JW, Fox LM, Green CE, Fox SM. Delayed redistribution in thallium 201 SPECT myocardial perfusion studies. Chest 1989;96:1031–5.
7. Yang LD, Berman DS, Kiat H et al. The frequency of late reversibility in SPECT thallium-201 stress–redistribution studies. J Am Coll Cardiol 1990;15:334–40.
8. Botvinick EH. Late reversibility: a viability issue. J Am Coll Cardiol 1990;15:341–4.
9. Ohtani H, Tamaki N, Yonekura Y et al. Value of thallium-201 reinjection after delayed SPECT imaging for predicting reversible ischemia after coronary artery bypass grafting. Am J Cardiol 1990;66:394–9.
10. Dilsizian V, Rocco TP, Freedman NMT, Leon MB, Bonow RO. Enhanced detection of ischaemic but viable myocardium by the reinjection of thallium after stress–redistribution imaging. N Engl J Med 1990;323:141–6.
11. Rocco TP, Dilsizian V, McKusick KA, Fischman AJ, Boucher CA, Strauss HW. Comparison of thallium redistribution with rest "reinjection" imaging for the detection of viable myocardium. Am J Cardiol 1990;66:158–63.
12. Tamaki N, Ohtani H, Yonekura Y et al. Significance of fill-in after thallium-201 reinjection following delayed imaging: comparison with regional wall motion and angiographic findings. J Nucl Med 1990;31:1617–23.
13. Brunken RC, Kottou S, Nienaber CA et al. PET detection of viable tissue in myocardial segments with persistent defects at Tl-201 SPECT. Radiology 1989;172:65–73.
14. Bonow RO, Dilsizian V, Cuocolo A, Bacharach SL. Identification of viable myocardium in patients with chronic coronary artery disease and left ventricular dysfunction. Comparison of thallium scintigraphy with reinjection and PET imaging with 18F-fluorodeoxyglucose. Circulation 1991;83:26–37.
15. Weiss AT, Maddahi J, Lew AS et al. Reverse redistribution of thallium-201: a sign of nontransmural myocardial infarction with patency of the infarct-related coronary artery. J Am Coll Cardiol 1986;7:61–7.
16. Ricci DR, Orlick AE, Doherty PW, Cipriano PR, Harrison DC. Reduction of coronary blood flow during coronary artery spasm occurring spontaneously and after provocation by ergonovine maleate. Circulation 1978;57:392–5.
17. Bennett JM, Blomerus P. Thallium-201 scintigraphy perfusion defect with dipyridamole in a patient with a myocardial bridge. Clin Cardiol 1988;11:268–70.
18. Meller J, Goldsmith SJ, Rudin A et al. Spectrum of exercise thallium-201 myocardial perfusion imaging in patients with chest pain and normal coronary angiograms. Am J Cardiol 1979;43:717–23.
19. Berger BC, Abramowitz R, Park CH et al. Abnormal thallium-201 scans in patients with chest pain and angiographically normal çoronary arteries. Am J Cardiol 1983;52:365–70.
20. O'Gara PT, Bonow RO, Maron BJ et al. Myocardial perfusion abnormalities in patients with hypertrophic cardiomyopathy: assessment with thallium-201 emission computed tomography. Circulation 1987;76:1214–23.
21. von Dohlen TW, Prisant LM, Frank MJ. Significance of positive or negative thallium-201 scintigraphy in hypertrophic cardiomyopathy. Am J Cardiol 1989;64:498–503.
22. Bulkley BH, Rouleau JR, Whitaker JQ, Strauss HW, Pitt B. The use of thallium-201 for myocardial perfusion imaging in sarcoid heart disease. Chest 1977;72:27–32.
23. Follansbee WP, Curtiss EI, Medsger TA et al. Physiologic abnormalities of cardiac function in progressive systemic sclerosis with diffuse scleroderma. N Engl J Med 1984;310:142–8.
24. Braat SH, Brugada P, Bar FW, Gorgels APN, Wellens HJJ. Thallium-201 exercise scintigraphy and left bundle branch block. Am J Cardiol 1985;55:224–6.
25. Hirzel HO, Senn M, Nuesch K et al. Thallium-201 scintigraphy in complete left bundle branch block. Am J Cardiol 1984;53:764–9.
26. Jazmati B, Sadaniantz A, Emaus SP, Heller GV. Exercise thallium-201 imaging in complete left bundle branch block and the prevalence of septal perfusion defects. Am J Cardiol 1991;67:46–9.
27. DePuey EG, Garcia EV, Ezquerra NF. Three-dimensional techniques and artificial intelligence in thallium-201 cardiac imaging. AJR 1989;152:1161–8.
28. Gill JB, Ruddy TD, Newell JB et al. Prognostic importance of thallium uptake by the lungs during exercise in coronary artery disease. N Engl J Med 1987;317:1485–9.
29. Mannting F. Pulmonary thallium uptake: correlation with systolic and diastolic left ventricular function at rest and during exercise. Am Heart J 1990;119:1137–46.
30. Kurata C, Tawarahara K, Taguchi T, Sakata K, Yamazaki N, Naitoh Y. Lung thallium-201 uptake during exercise emission computed tomography. J Nucl Med 1991;32:417–23.
31. Mannting F. A new method for quantification of pulmonary thallium uptake in myocardial SPECT studies. Eur J Nucl Med 1990;16:213–22.

32. Burow RD, Pond M, Schafer AW, Becker L. Circumferential profiles: a new method for computer analysis of thallium-201 myocardial perfusion images. J Nucl Med 1979;20:771–7.
33. Garcia EV, Van Train K, Maddahi J et al. Quantitation of rotational thallium-201 myocardial perfusion tomography. J Nucl Med 1985;26:17–26.
34. DePasquale EE, Nody AC, DePuey EG et al. Quantitative rotational thallium-201 tomography for identifying and localising coronary artery disease. Circulation 1988;77:316–27.
35. Mahmarian JJ, Boyce TM, Goldberg RK, Cocanougher MK, Roberts R, Verani MS. Quantitative exercise thallium-201 single photon emission computed tomography for the enhanced diagnosis of ischaemic heart disease. J Am Coll Cardiol 1990;15:318–29.
36. DePasquale EE, Nody AC, DePuey EG et al. Quantitative rotational thallium-201 tomography for identifying and localising coronary artery disease. Circulation 1988;77:316–27.
37. Hör G. Myocardial scintigraphy – 25 years after start. Eur J Nucl Med 1988;13:619–36.
38. Leppo J. Thallium washout analysis: fact or fiction? J Nucl Med 1987;28:1058–60.
39. Maddahi J, Garcia EV, Berman DS, Waxman A, Swan HJC, Forrester J. Improved non-invasive assessment of coronary artery disease by quantitative analysis of regional stress myocardial distribution and washout of thallium-201. Circulation 1981;64:924–35.
40. Francisco DA, Collins SM, Go RT, Ehrhardt JC, Van Kirk OC, Marcus ML. Tomographic thallium-201 myocardial perfusion scintigrams after maximal coronary artery vasodilation with intravenous dipyridamole. Circulation 1982;66:370–9.
41. Tamaki NY, Yonekura T, Imkai T et al. Segmental analysis of stress thallium myocardial emission tomography for localisation of coronary artery disease. Eur J Nucl Med 1984;9:99–105.
42. Niemeyer MG, Laarman GJ, Lelbach S et al. Quantitative thallium-201 myocardial exercise scintigraphy in normal subjects and patients with normal coronary arteries. Eur J Radiol 1990;10:19–27.

Chapter 6
Clinical Case Material

THE NORMAL HEART

Case 1 – Normal Vertical Heart

History

A 48-year-old lady was referred for thallium imaging following coronary angiography which was performed because of atypical chest pain.

Thallium Myocardial Perfusion Tomography

Stress Technique Dipyridamole was infused during bicycle exercise to 100 W. Stress was limited by fatigue with lateral chest wall discomfort. The peak blood pressure and heart rate were 140/85 mmHg and 124/min.

Stress Images The pattern of uptake of tracer is normal.

Rest Images There is no change.

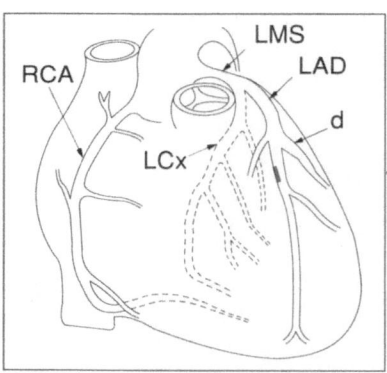

Coronary Angiography

There was a mild mid-segment left anterior descending artery stenosis of uncertain haemodynamic significance. Left ventricular wall motion was normal.

Conclusion

Normal myocardial perfusion during stress and rest. There is no ischaemia associated with the minor left anterior descending artery stenosis. Angioplasty to the stenosis was not performed.

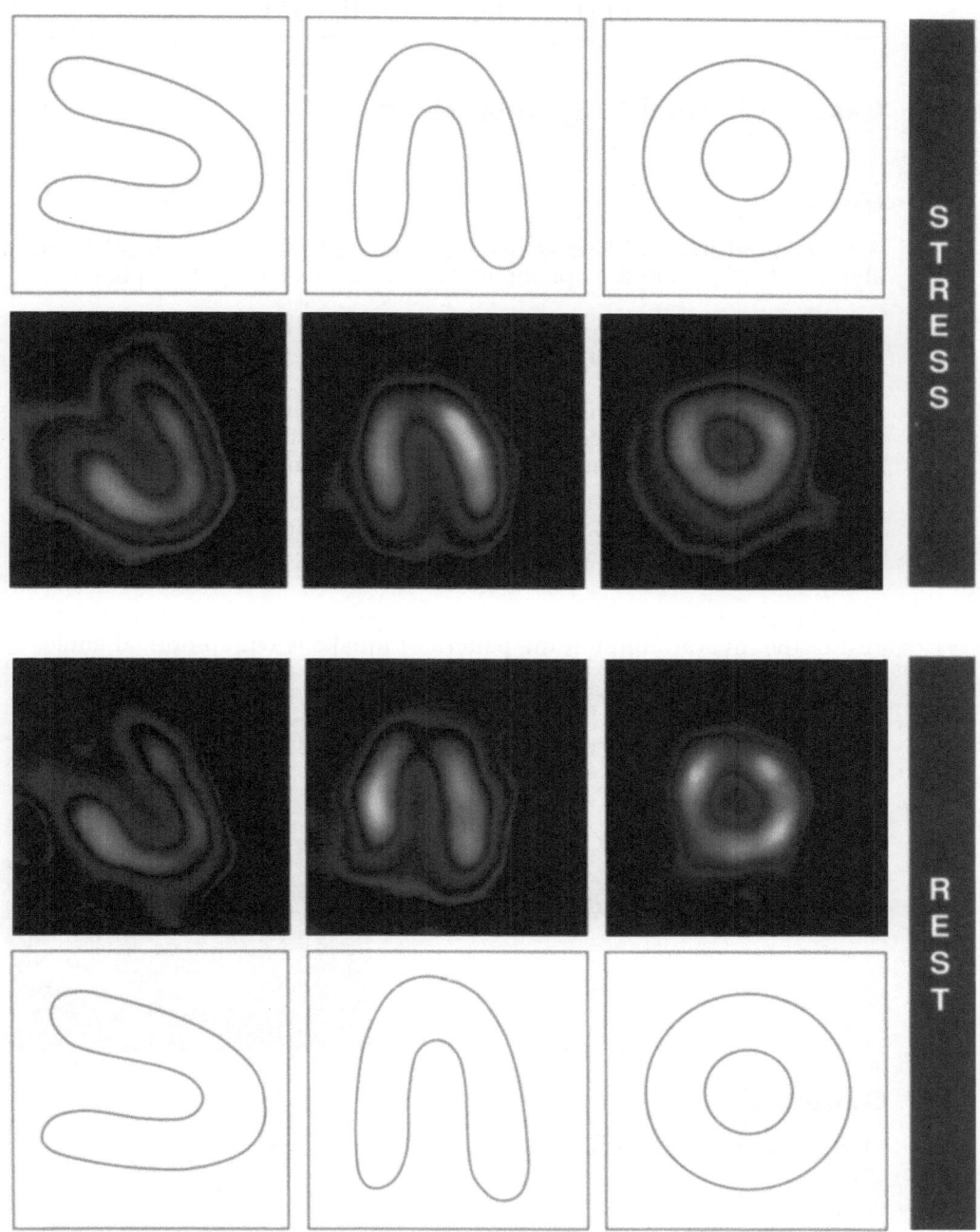

Normal myocardial perfusion in a vertically positioned heart. Minor variations in the distribution of tracer are normal and the right ventricle is not normally seen.

Case 2 – Normal Horizontal Heart

History

A 63-year-old hypertensive woman was referred for thallium imaging with atypical chest pain and palpitations. Her exercise tolerance was poor.

Thallium Myocardial Perfusion Tomography

Stress Technique Dipyridamole was infused during bicycle exercise to 50 W. Exercise was limited by fatigue without chest pain. At peak stress the blood pressure and the heart rate were 190/110 mmHg and 115/min.

Stress Images The pattern of uptake of tracer within the heart is normal. An anterior planar image is also shown below to illustrate low lung uptake (contrast with case 40), and high splanchnic uptake caused by dipyridamole-induced vasodilation.

Rest Images Washout of tracer from the apex is more rapid than from the rest of the myocardium but the pattern of uptake is within normal limits.

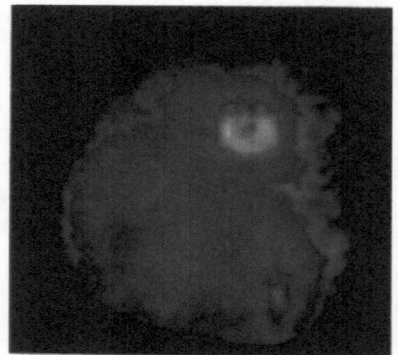

Coronary Angiography

The coronary arteries were normal. Left ventricular wall motion was normal.

Conclusion

Myocardial perfusion is normal.

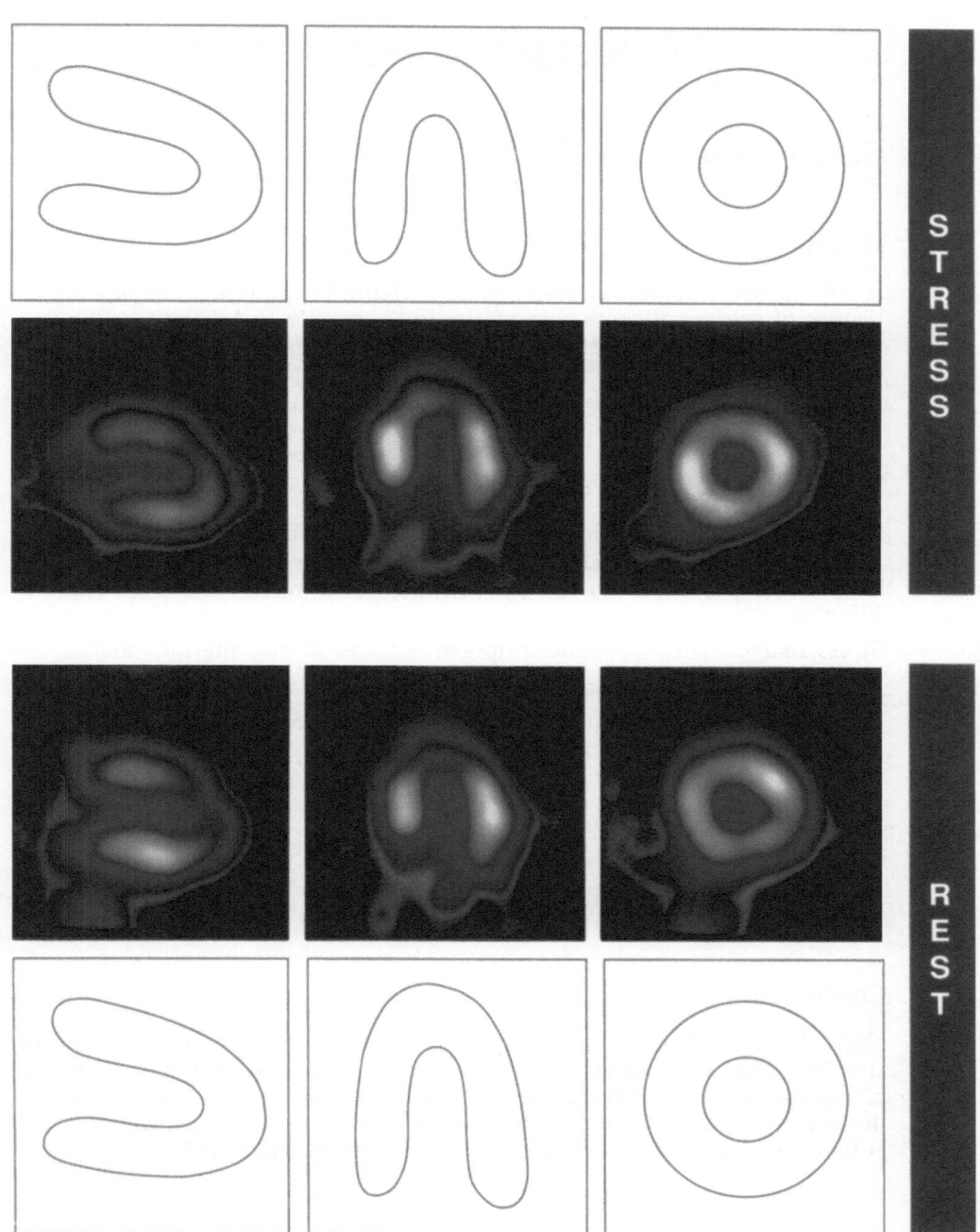

The heart is in a horizontal position in the chest but it is a normal size without dilatation during stress. The horizontal heart is a normal variant and commonly occurs in obese people because of elevation of the diaphragm.

Case 3 – Anterior Attenuation

History

A 50-year-old woman was referred for thallium imaging because of a 5-year history of exertional chest pain of atypical character and duration. She was hypertensive and obese. Her resting ECG was normal and her exercise ECG was limited at 5 minutes by fatigue with atypical pain at which time equivocal ST changes were present.

Thallium Myocardial Perfusion Tomography

Stress Technique Dipyridamole was infused during bicycle exercise to 100 W. Stress was limited by leg fatigue and chest pain beneath the left breast. The peak blood pressure and heart rate were 230/120 mmHg and 125/min.

Stress Images There is reduced uptake of tracer in the anterior wall.

Rest Images There is no change.

Prone Images Anterior wall uptake is now normal. Tracer within the stomach is seen in the short axis view because of elevation of the diaphragm in the prone position.

Coronary Angiography

The coronary arteries were normal. Left ventricular wall motion was normal.

Conclusion

Normal myocardial perfusion during stress and rest. There is significant anterior wall attenuation from large breasts which was apparent in the planar images. Prone imaging evens out the attenuation and helps to avoid the artefact. Radionuclide ventriculography during stress showed normal anterior wall motion and normal left ventricular ejection fraction.

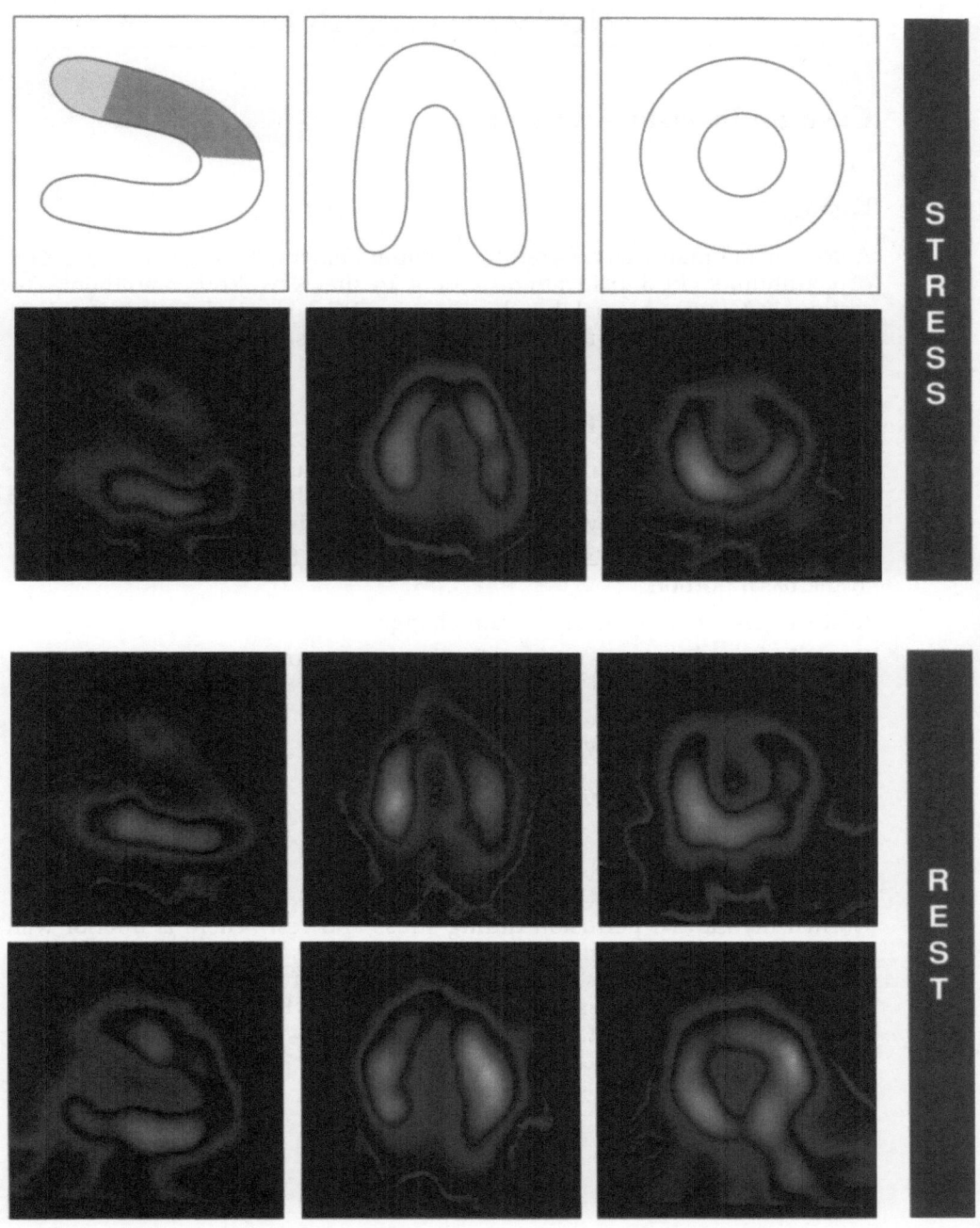

STRESS

REST

Breast attenuation can produce apparent perfusion abnormality. Patient positioning must be appropriately chosen.

NORMAL VARIANTS

Case 4 – Inferior Attenuation

History

A 44-year-old man was referred for thallium imaging having suffered 2 days of continuous chest pain after running in the New York marathon. The resting ECG was normal but his exercise ECG showed 2 mm lateral ST depression after 12 min although there was no associated chest pain.

Thallium Myocardial Perfusion Tomography

Stress Technique Dipyridamole was infused during bicycle exercise to 200 W. Stress was limited by leg fatigue without chest pain. The peak blood pressure and heart rate were 180/110 mmHg and 140/min.

Stress Images There is reduced uptake of tracer in the inferior wall especially in the basal portion.

Rest Images There is no significant change.

Prone Images The pattern of uptake of tracer is now normal.

Coronary Angiography

Coronary angiography was not performed.

Conclusion

Normal myocardial perfusion during stress and rest. There is inferior wall attenuation particularly affecting the basal inferior segment. This is common, especially in men, and is thought to be a result of increased attenuation of photons from the deeper posterior myocardium. Prone imaging alters the position of the heart and reduces this attenuation.

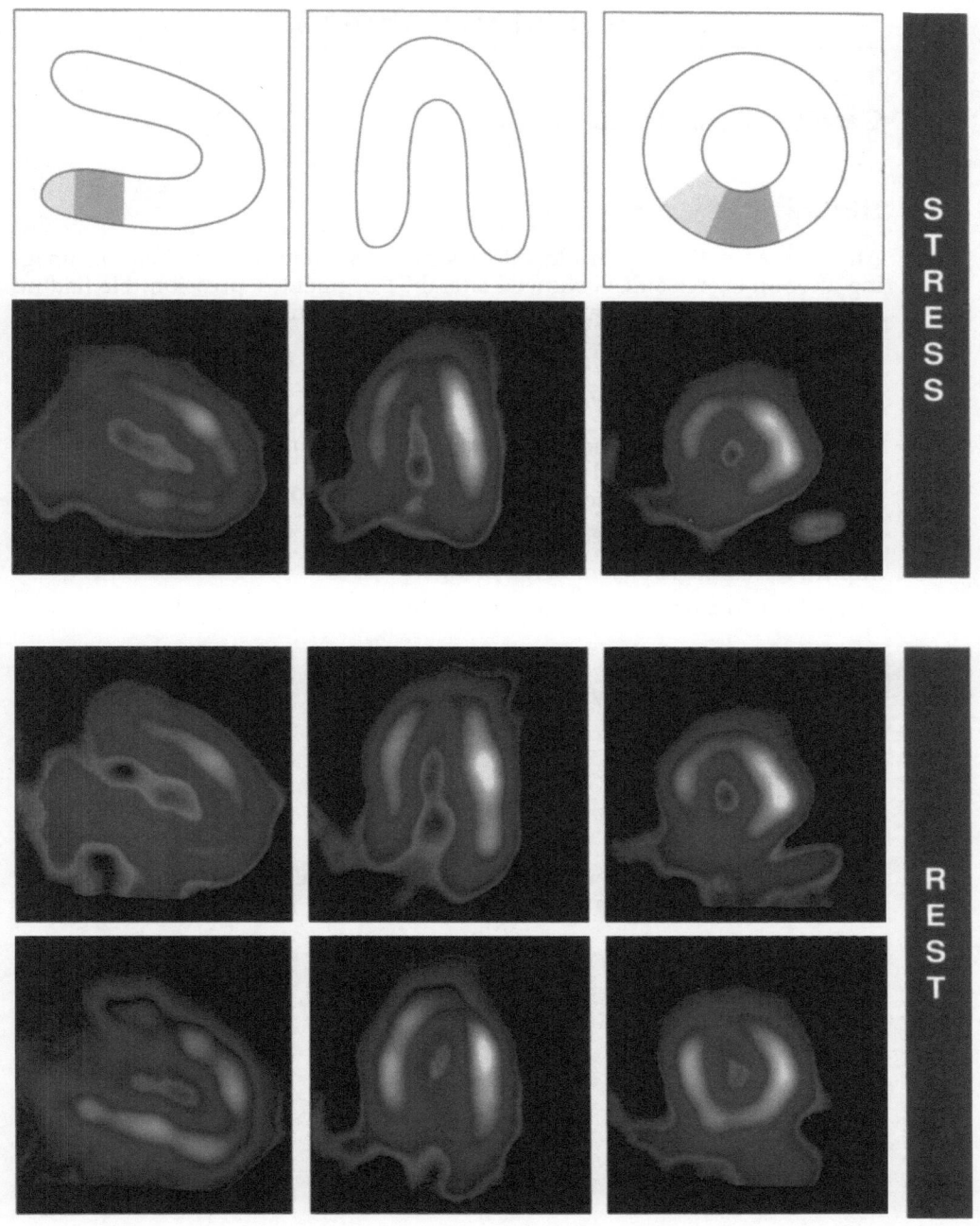

Inferior wall attenuation is common. Care should be taken that it is not interpreted as abnormal, especially if there is no other reason to suspect disease. In case of doubt, prone imaging may be helpful.

Case 5 – Apical Attenuation

History

An asymptomatic 56-year-old businessman was referred for thallium imaging after an exercise ECG showed lateral ST segment depression. He had no risk factors for coronary artery disease and the resting ECG was normal.

Thallium Myocardial Perfusion Tomography

Stress Technique Dipyridamole was infused during bicycle exercise to 100 W. Stress was limited by fatigue without chest pain. At peak stress the blood pressure and the heart rate were 180/110 mmHg and 145/min.

Stress Images There is reduced uptake of tracer in the apex.

Supine Rest Images There is no change.

Prone Rest Images The appearance of the apex has improved.

Coronary Angiography

This was not performed.

Conclusion

Reduced uptake of tracer in the apex is a normal variant and may result from anatomical thinning of the myocardium.

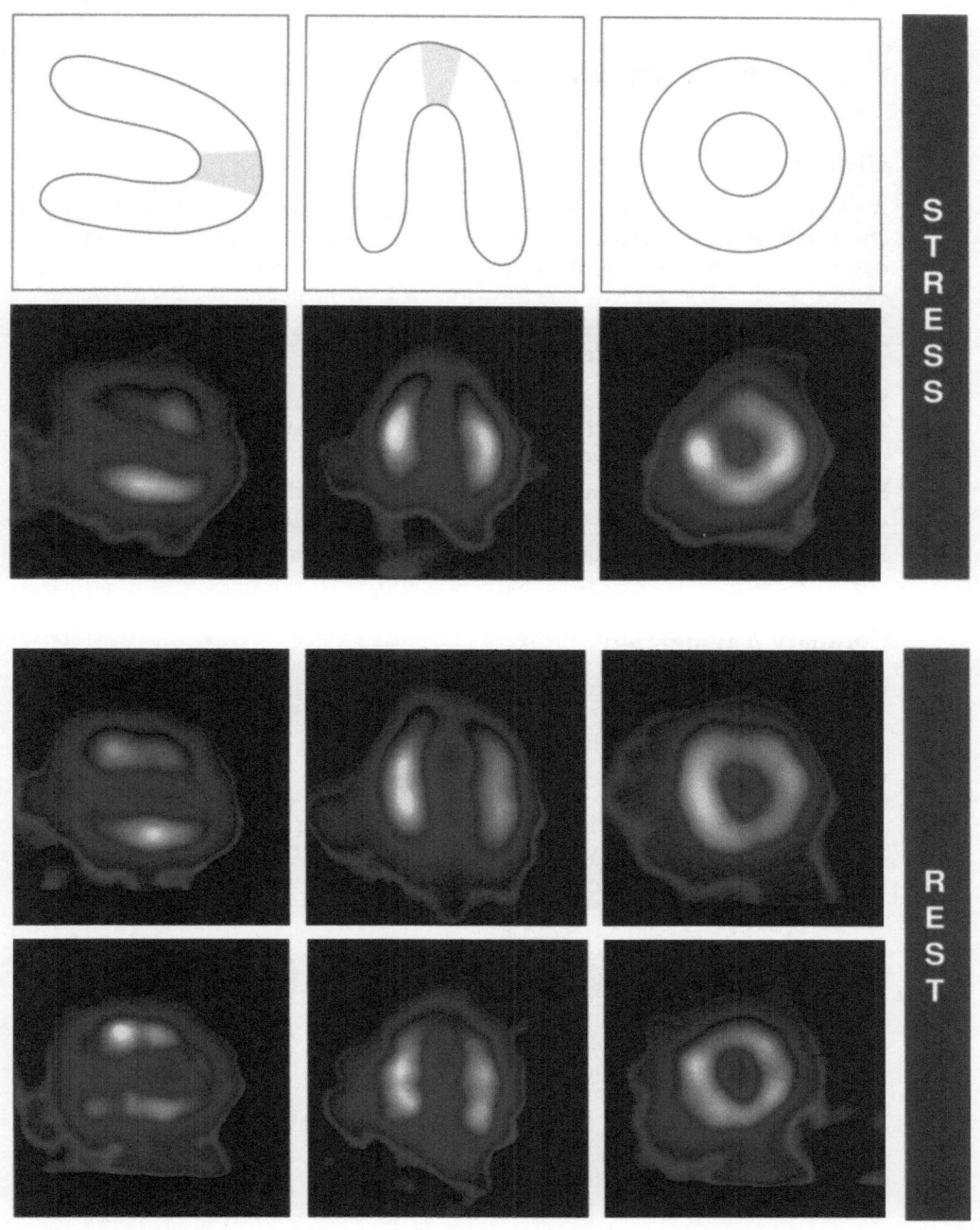

STRESS

REST

Apex attenuation is a normal variant and may show improvement with prone imaging.

Case 6 – Papillary Muscle

History

A 55-year-old woman was referred for thallium imaging because of atypical chest pain and an exercise ECG showing lateral ST segment depression. She had no risk factors for coronary artery disease. Her resting ECG was normal.

Thallium Myocardial Perfusion Tomography

Stress Technique Dipyridamole was infused during bicycle exercise to 100 W. Stress was limited by fatigue without chest pain. The peak blood pressure and heart rate were 170/90 mmHg and 140/min.

Stress Images The pattern of uptake of tracer is within normal limits but an area of increased uptake is seen in the inferior and the lateral walls (*arrows*).

Rest Images Redistribution imaging was not performed.

Coronary Angiography

Coronary angiography was not performed.

Conclusion

The bulges in the inferior and lateral walls are the papillary muscles. Because the pain was atypical and myocardial perfusion was normal, the patient was reassured.

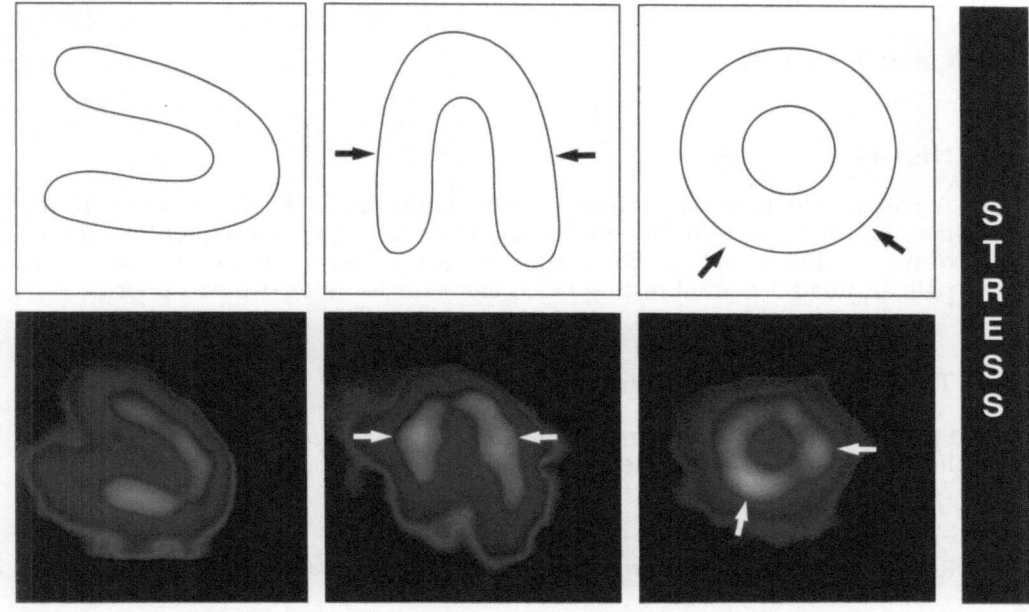

Prominent papillary muscles may give the appearance of a defect in neighbouring areas. Redistribution imaging can occasionally be avoided if the stress images are normal.

SINGLE VESSEL REVERSIBLE ISCHAEMIA

Case 7 – RCA

History

A 65-year-old lady was referred for thallium imaging after a hospital admission for chest pain thought to be cardiac in origin, but without evidence of myocardial infarction. She continued to experience mild exertional chest pain and had a normal resting ECG. Her exercise tolerance was poor.

Thallium Myocardial Perfusion Tomography

Stress Technique Dobutamine was infused to 20 µg/kg/min. Stress was limited by chest pain. The peak blood pressure and heart rate were 158/74 mmHg and 138/min.

Stress Images There is decreased uptake of tracer in the inferior wall.

Rest Images There is improvement in the inferior wall.

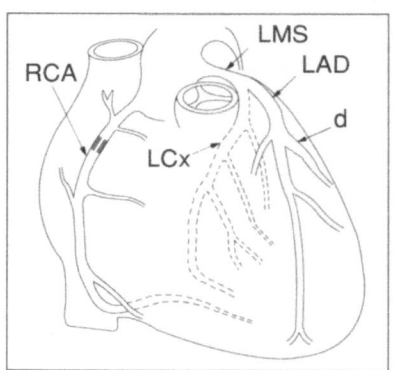

Coronary Angiography

There was a stenosis of the proximal right coronary artery. Left ventricular wall motion was normal.

Conclusion

Reversible inferior myocardial ischaemia. This is normally the territory of the right coronary artery although it may sometimes be supplied by the left circumflex artery.

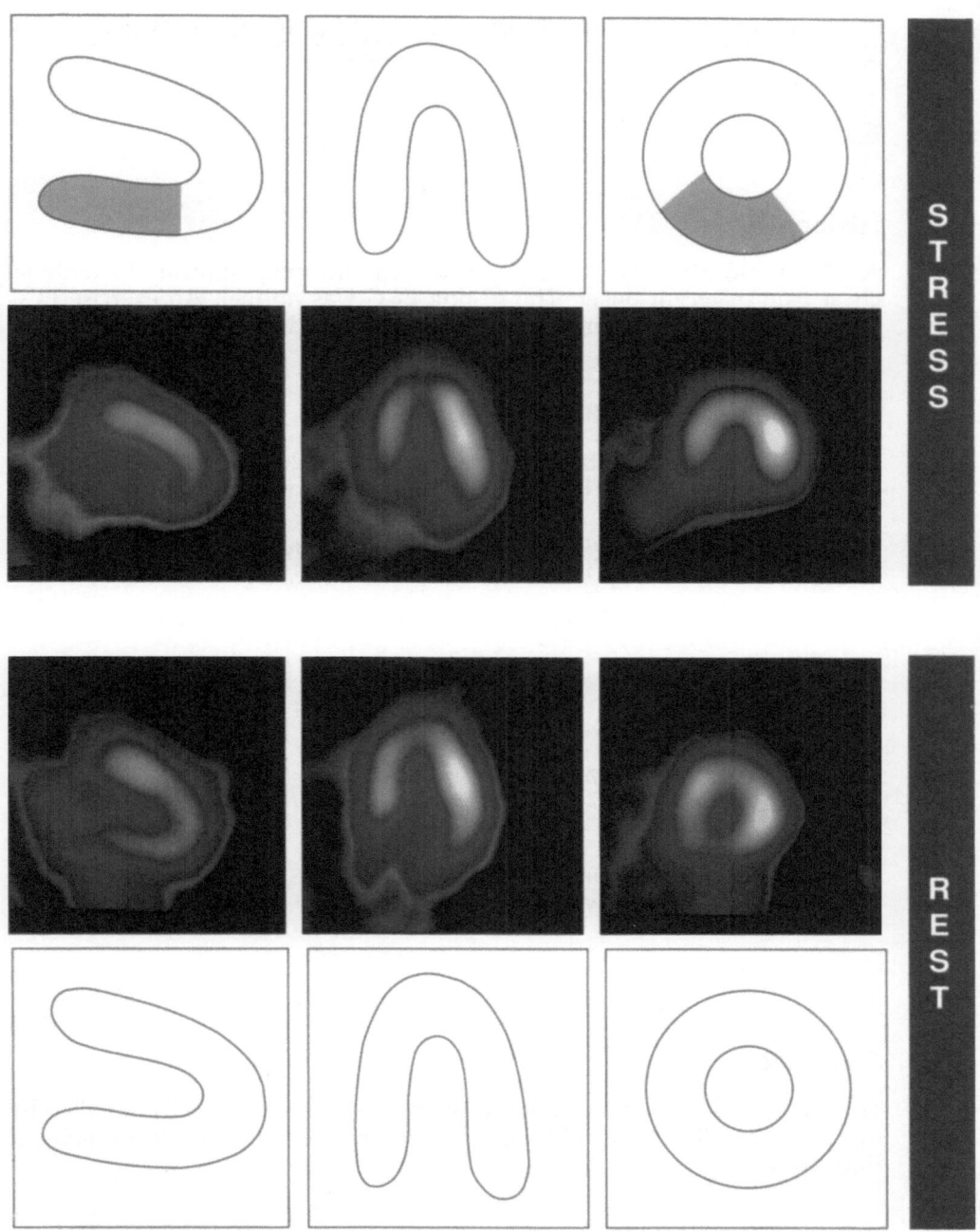

The site of coronary artery disease cannot be decided with certainty from the site of ischaemia, but disease of the right coronary artery commonly causes reversible ischaemia of the inferior myocardium.

Case 8 – LCx

History

A 53-year-old man was referred for thallium imaging because of exertional chest pain of recent onset. The resting ECG was normal. An exercise ECG was abnormal after 12 min with 1 mm anterior ST depression.

Thallium Myocardial Perfusion Tomography

Stress Technique Dobutamine was infused to 20 µg/kg/min. Stress was limited by chest pain. The peak blood pressure and heart rate were 140/84 mmHg and 124/min.

Stress Images Uptake of tracer in the lateral wall is reduced with extension of the defect into the apex and the basal inferior wall.

Rest Images The abnormal area is improved.

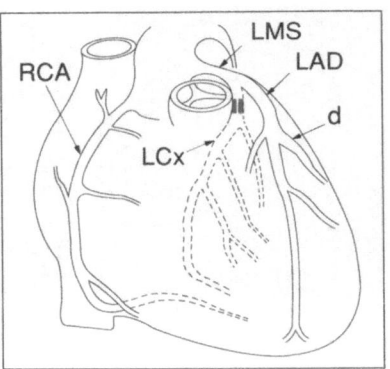

Coronary Angiography

There was a proximal stenosis of a dominant left circumflex artery and the right coronary artery was normal. Left ventricular wall motion was normal.

Conclusion

There is reversible ischaemia of the lateral wall. This is typically supplied by the left circumflex artery although it may also be supplied by a dominant right coronary artery.

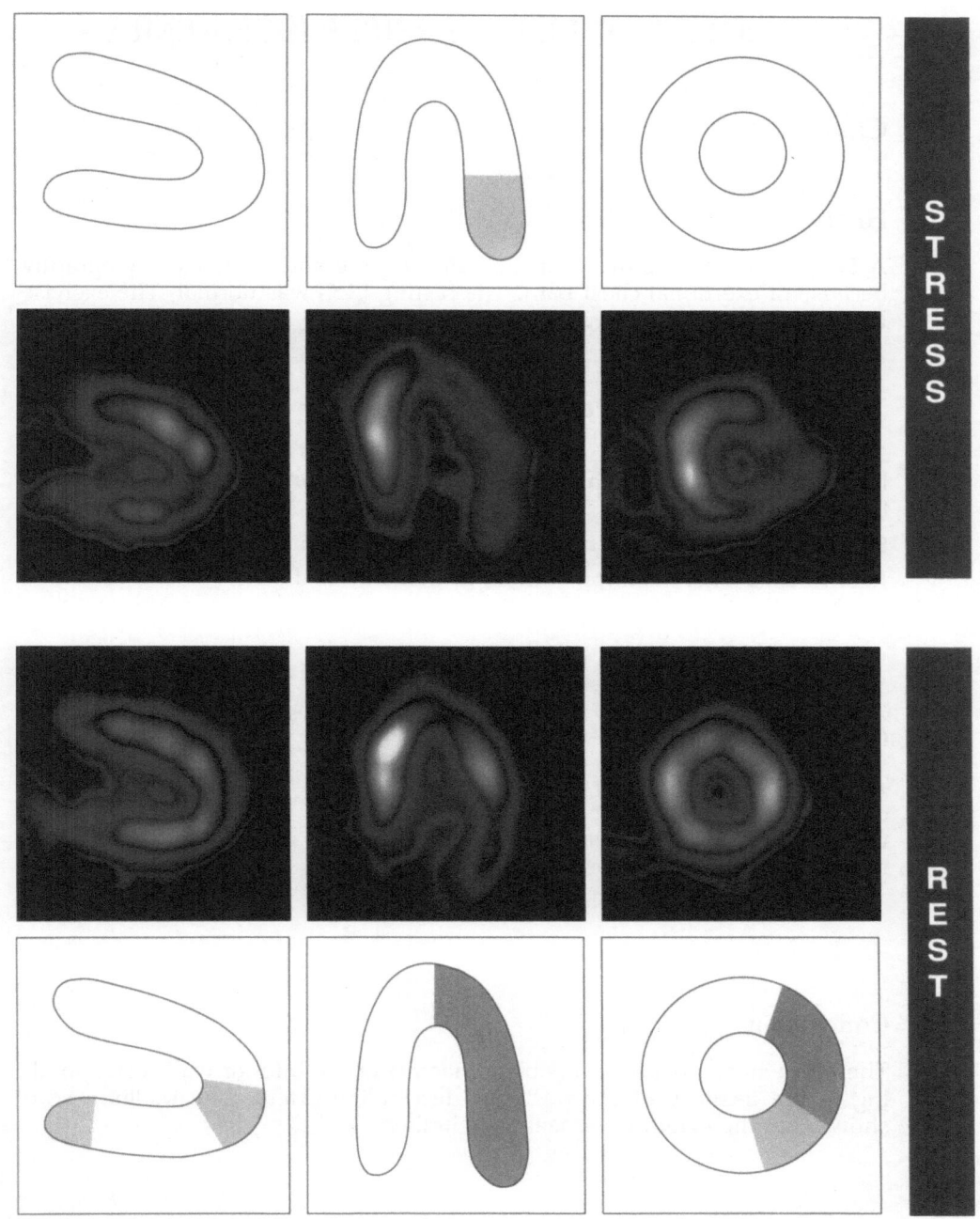

STRESS

REST

Reversible ischaemia of the lateral wall may be caused by disease of the left circumflex artery. As with the inferior wall, the corresponding coronary artery cannot be identified with certainty.

Case 9 – PDA

History

A 57-year-old man underwent thallium imaging and coronary angiography because of exertional chest pain. The resting ECG was normal. The exercise ECG showed 2 mm ST depression after 5 min.

Thallium Myocardial Perfusion Tomography

Stress Technique Dobutamine was infused to 15 µg/kg/min. Stress was limited by chest pain. The peak blood pressure and heart rate were 140/84 mmHg and 124/mim.

Stress Images Uptake of tracer in the basal inferolateral wall is reduced.

Rest Images There is improvement in the abnormal area.

Coronary Angiography

There was a stenosis of the posterior descending artery arising from a dominant right artery. Left ventricular wall motion was normal.

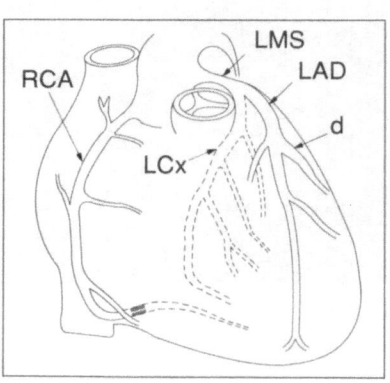

Conclusion

There is a small area of reversible ischaemia of the inferior wall corresponding to the territory of the posterior descending artery. The thallium scan shows that the extent of ischaemia is limited.

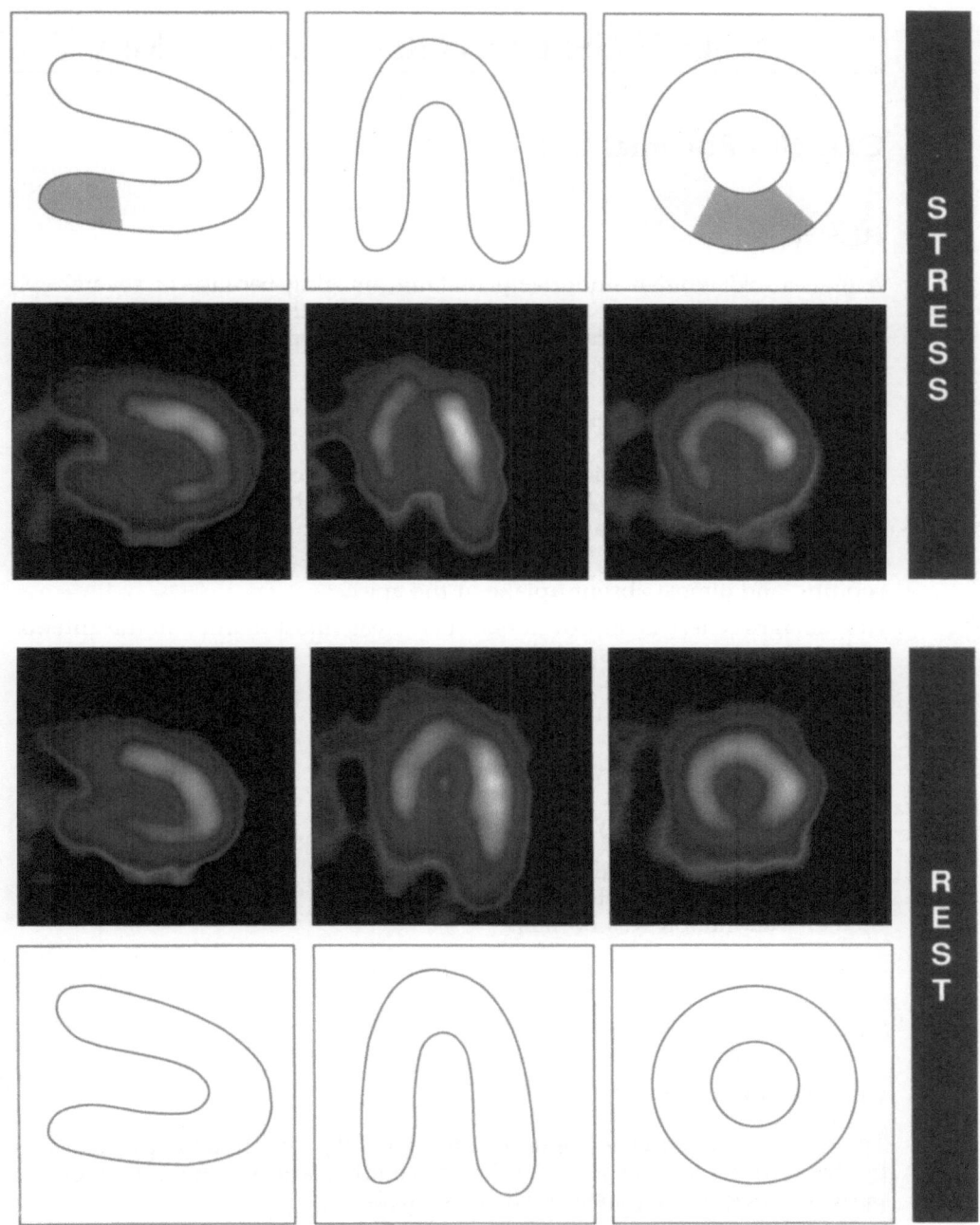

The posterior descending artery arises from the right coronary artery in 85% of people and from the left circumflex artery in the remainder. The site of ischaemia cannot help decide which artery is dominant.

SINGLE VESSEL REVERSIBLE ISCHAEMIA

Case 10 – Proximal LAD

History

A 69-year-old woman underwent thallium imaging because of several epi-sodes of exertional chest pain relieved by nitrate therapy. The resting ECG was normal and the exercise ECG showed equivocal ST segment changes.

Thallium Myocardial Perfusion Tomography

Stress Technique Dipyridamole was infused prior to bicycle exercise to 50 W. Stress was limited by chest pain. The peak blood pressure and heart rate were 120/80 mmHg and 100/min.

Stress Images There is reduced uptake of tracer in the anterior wall and septum, and almost absent uptake in the apex.

Rest Images There is improvement in all areas, most marked in the anterior wall and septum, but also at the apex.

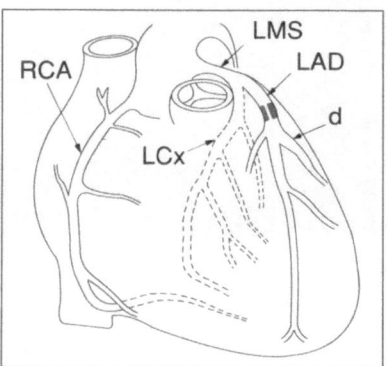

Coronary Angiography

There was a stenosis in the proximal left anterior descending artery. Left ven-tricular wall motion was normal.

Conclusion

There is reversible ischaemia of the anterior wall, septum and apex which is in the territory of the left anterior descending artery. The extent of the perfusion defect suggests a proximal stenosis.

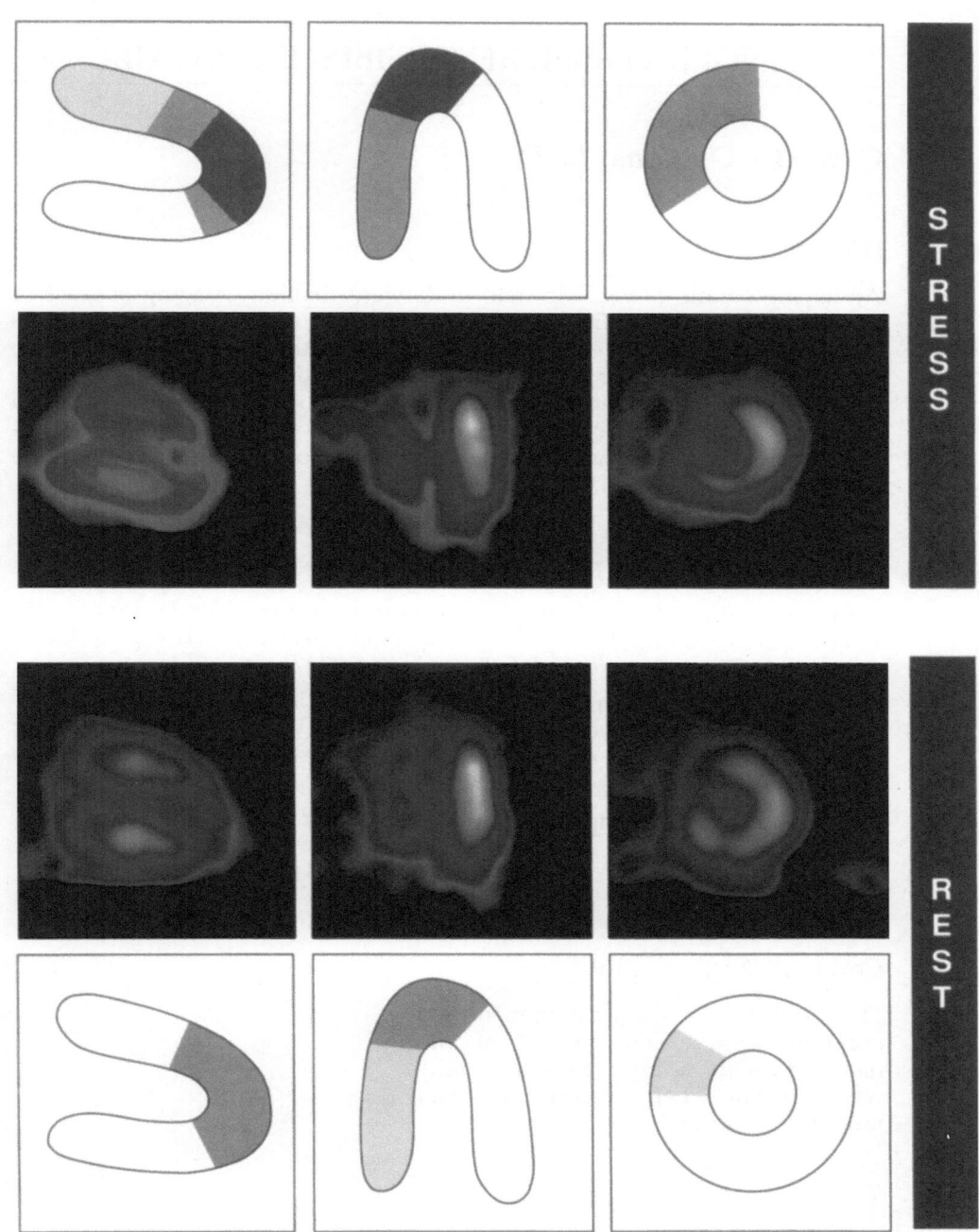

Reversible ischaemia of the anterior wall together with the septum is almost invariably caused by disease of the left anterior descending artery. The extent of ischaemia (five of nine segments) indicates a moderate risk of future cardiac events.

SINGLE VESSEL REVERSIBLE ISCHAEMIA

Case 11 – Diagonal LAD

History

An asymptomatic 43-year-old man underwent thallium imaging because of an abnormal exercise ECG performed routinely following triple bypass surgery to the diagonal branch of the left anterior descending artery, the marginal branch of the circumflex artery and the right coronary artery 6 years before. The referring physician wanted to assess the presence and extent of myocardial ischaemia before deciding whether coronary angiography was required. There was no history of myocardial infarction and the resting ECG was normal.

Thallium Myocardial Perfusion Tomography

Stress Technique Dipyridamole was infused during bicycle exercise to 125 W. Stress was limited by fatigue without chest pain. The peak blood pressure and heart rate were 160/90 mmHg and 117/min.

Stress Images There is reduced uptake of tracer in the mid-portion of the anterior wall. The apparent defect of the inferior wall which is seen in the short axis image is not significant because it was only seen in this single slice.

Rest Images There is improvement in the anterior wall.

Coronary Angiography

The graft to the diagonal branch was occluded with distal disease of the native coronary artery. The other grafts were patent. Left ventricular wall motion was normal.

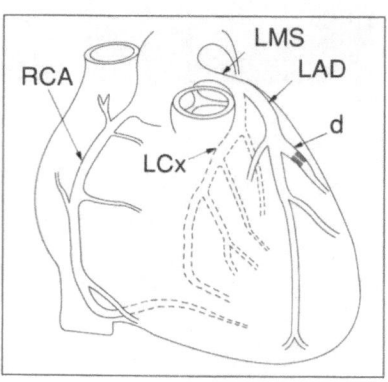

Conclusion

There is reversible ischaemia affecting a small portion of the anterior wall. Both the extent and the severity of the ischaemia is mild and the distribution is typical of a diagonal stenosis. Although the diagonal saphenous vein graft was occluded, no further action was taken because of the lack of symptoms and good prognosis implied by the thallium scan.

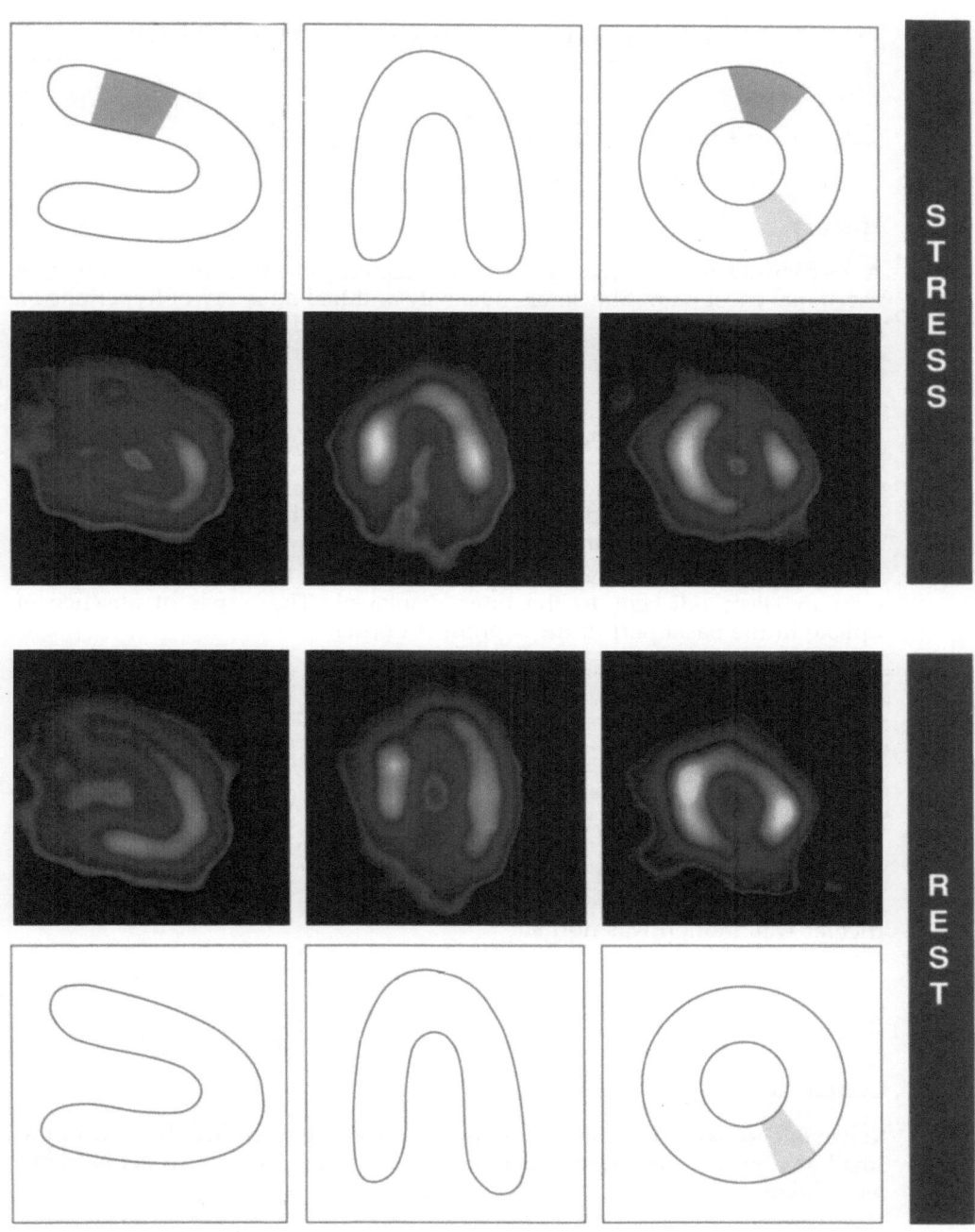

The diagonal branch of the left anterior descending coronary artery supplies the anterior wall of the left ventricle. Thallium tomography is a valuable method of assessing myocardial perfusion after coronary bypass grafting.

SINGLE VESSEL REVERSIBLE ISCHAEMIA

Case 12 – Distal LAD

History

A 77-year-old woman was referred for thallium imaging after the onset of exertional chest pain. She smoked heavily and had a history of hypertension and reflux oesophagitis. The resting ECG showed evidence of left ventricular hypertrophy but an exercise ECG was not performed.

Thallium Myocardial Perfusion Tomography

Stress Technique Dipyridamole was infused prior to bicycle exercise to 50 W. Exercise was limited by chest pain. The peak blood pressure and heart rate were 140/80 mmHg and 96/min.

Stress Images There is reduced uptake of tracer in the apex which was also seen in slices adjacent to the ones displayed. The apparent absence of uptake in the basal part of the septum is normal.

Rest Images The abnormal area improves.

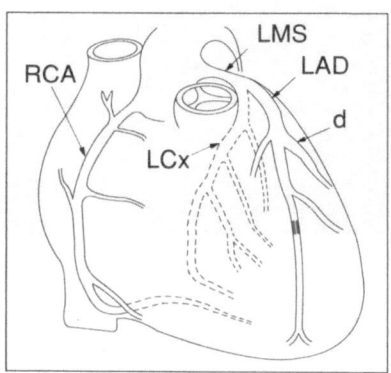

Coronary Angiography

There was a stenosis of the distal left anterior descending artery. Left ventricular wall motion was normal.

Conclusion

Reversible ischaemia of the apex with poor exercise tolerance. In view of the small area at risk the patient was reassured and her symptoms settled with medication.

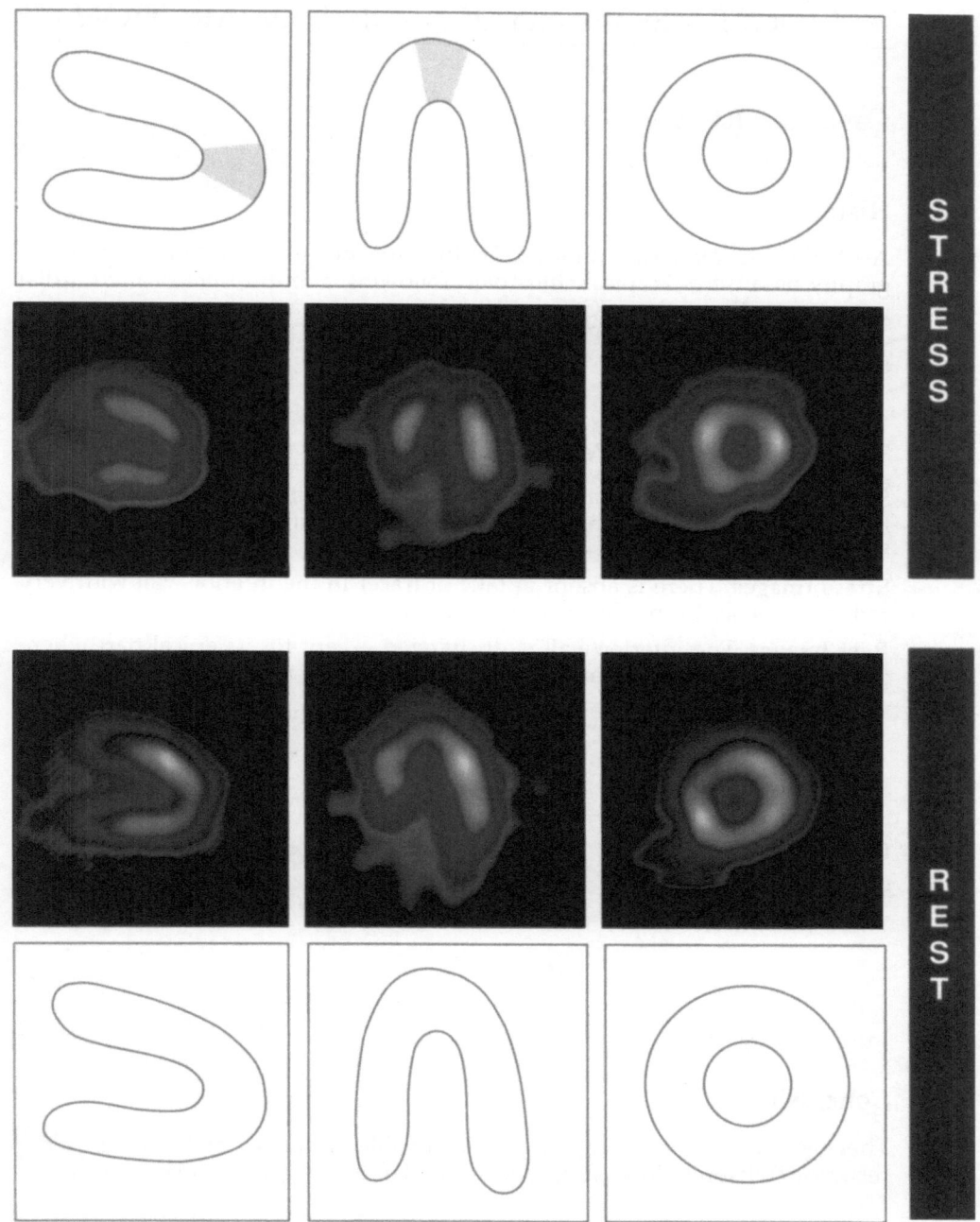

The distal left anterior descending artery usually supplies the apex, although it may also be supplied by a large posterior descending artery. The septum normally appears shorter than the lateral wall because of absent uptake in its membranous portion.

SINGLE VESSEL MYOCARDIAL INFARCTION

Case 13 – RCA

History

A 61-year-old man was referred for thallium imaging and coronary angio-graphy because of atypical chest pain following a recent inferior myocardial infarction. His resting ECG showed inferior Q-waves with repolarisation changes and his exercise ECG was abnormal after 8 min with 2 mm of lateral ST segment depression.

Thallium Myocardial Perfusion Tomography

Stress Technique Dobutamine was infused to 20 µg/kg/min. Stress was limited by chest pain. The peak blood pressure and heart rate were 180/84 mmHg and 129/min.

Stress Images There is absent uptake of tracer in the inferior wall with very reduced uptake in the distal portion and apex.

Rest Images The inferior wall is unchanged except for its apical part where there is minor improvement.

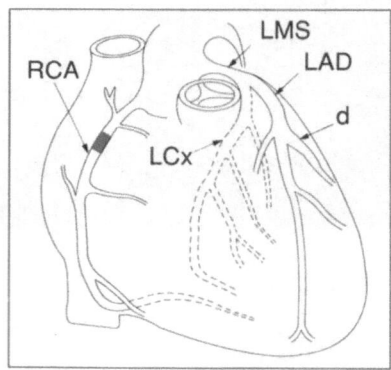

Coronary Angiography

The right coronary artery was occluded. There was inferior hypokinesis.

Conclusion

There is an inferior infarction. The reversible ischaemia at the apex is the result of collateral blood supply from the left anterior descending artery.

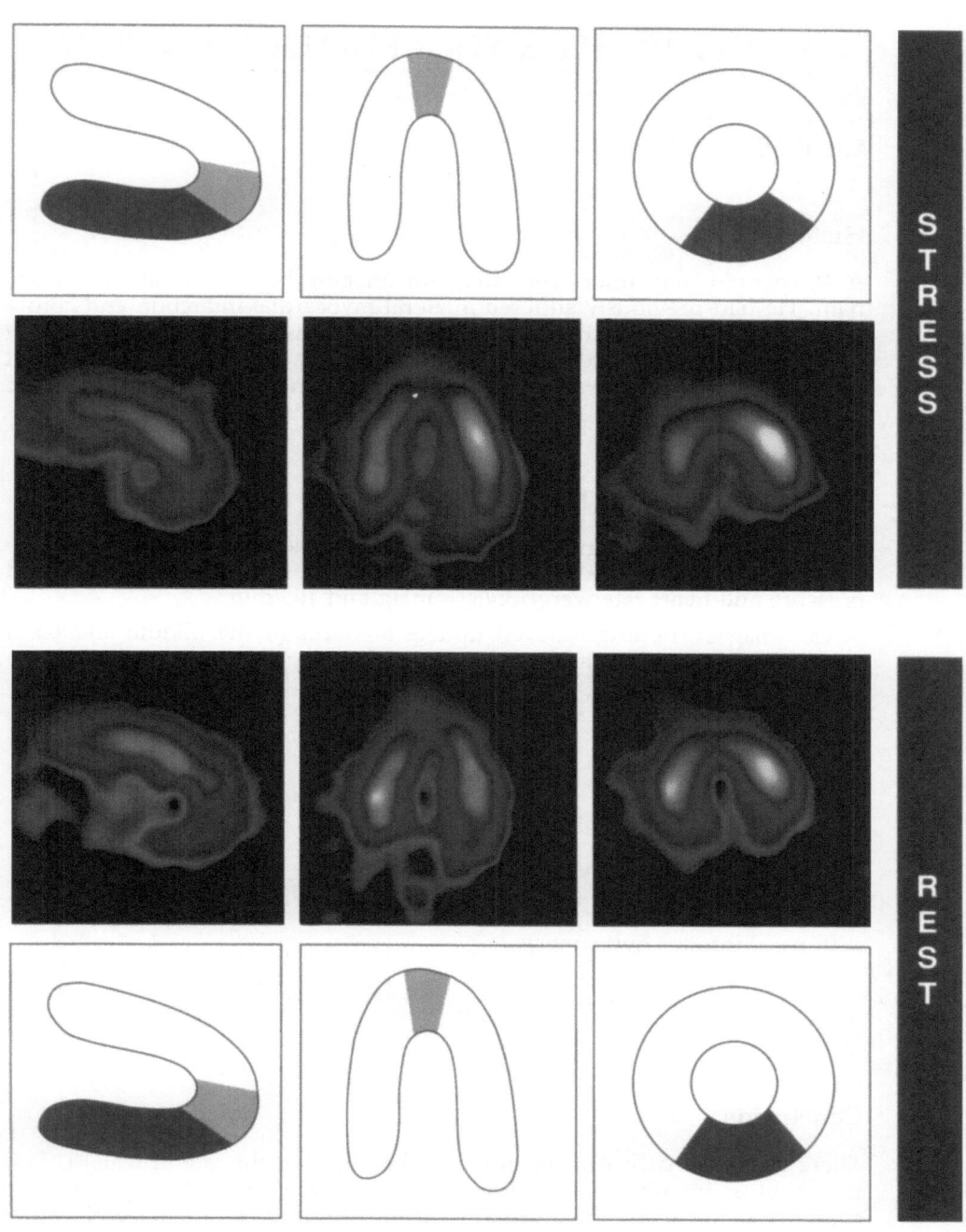

A fixed perfusion defect represents myocardial infarction, in this case, of the inferior wall. Myocardial perfusion imaging is indicated following myocardial infarction in order to assess the presence of residual myocardial ischaemia.

SINGLE VESSEL MYOCARDIAL INFARCTION

Case 14 – LCx

History

A 46-year-old man underwent thallium imaging because of atypical chest pain. He had previously suffered a lateral myocardial infarction and coronary angiography had shown single vessel disease with an occluded left circumflex artery. An exercise ECG was abnormal. The referring cardiologist wanted to know if there was evidence of continuing ischaemia which would have been an indication for angioplasty.

Thallium Myocardial Perfusion Tomography

Stress Technique Dipyridamole was infused prior to bicycle exercise to 50 W. Stress was limited by fatigue without chest pain. The peak blood pressure and heart rate were 135/80 mmHg and 105/min.

Stress Images There is reduced uptake of tracer in the middle and basal portions of the lateral wall and the basal inferior wall.

Rest Images There is no change.

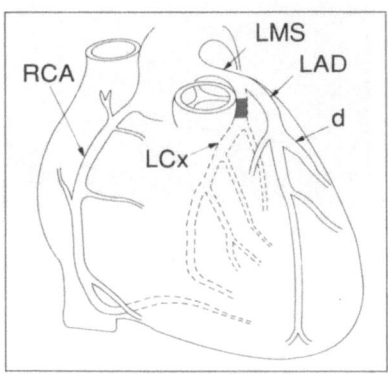

Coronary Angiography

The left circumflex artery was occluded with basal inferior hypokinesis.

Conclusion

There is a fixed defect of thallium uptake affecting the lateral wall. This is typical of an infarct in the territory of the left circumflex artery. There is no evidence of reversible myocardial ischaemia around the infarct or in other territories. No further intervention was performed.

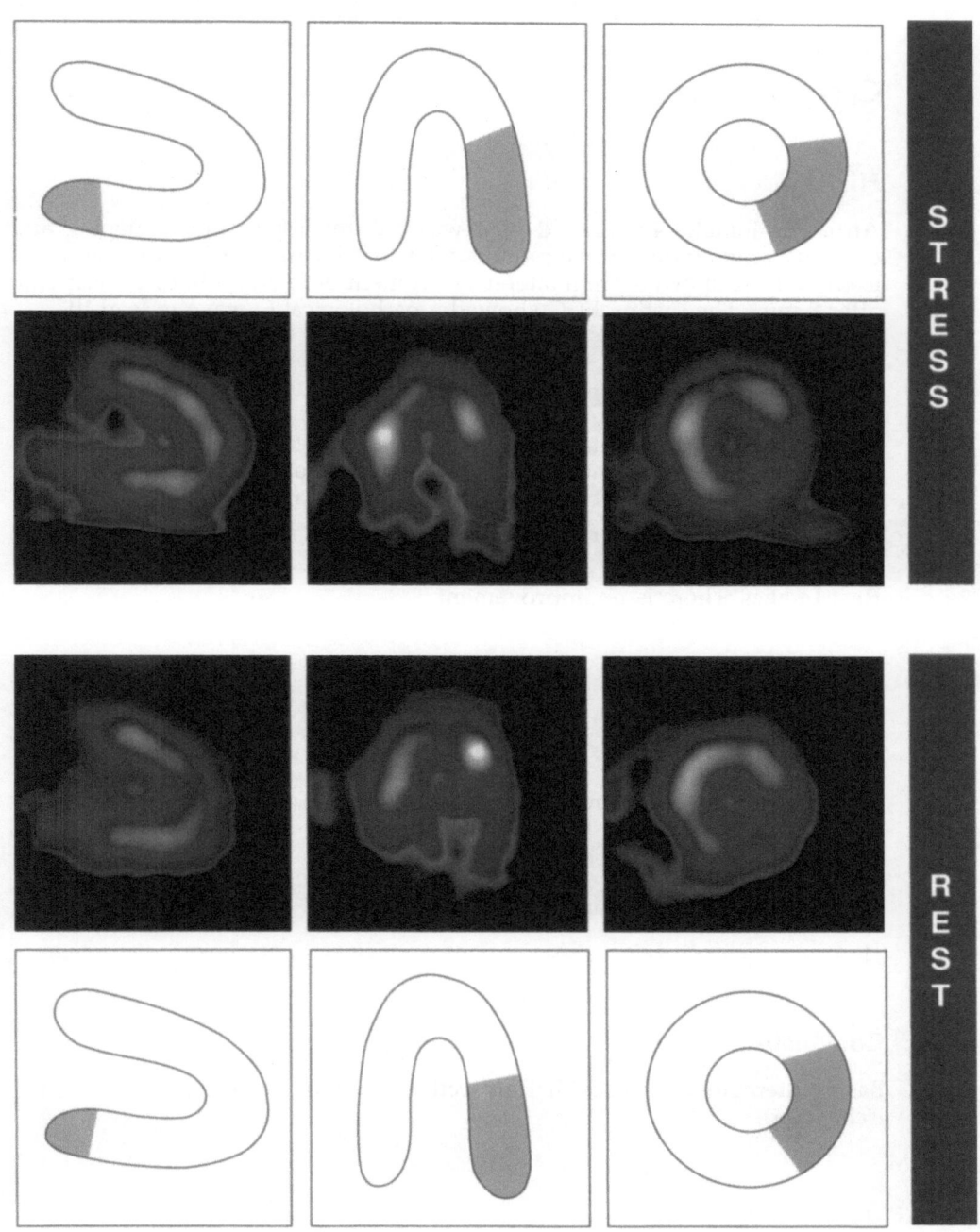

STRESS

REST

Occlusion of the left circumflex artery may cause infarction of the lateral wall. In the absence of reversible ischaemia, medical treatment is preferred.

SINGLE VESSEL MYOCARDIAL INFARCTION

Case 15 – PDA

History

An asymptomatic 42-year-old man was referred for thallium imaging and coronary angiography three months after inferior myocardial infarction. An exercise ECG showed 3 mm lateral ST segment depression but no chest pain after 8 min. The resting ECG showed a pathological Q-wave in lead III.

Thallium Myocardial Perfusion Tomography

Stress Technique Dobutamine was infused to 20 µg/kg/min. Stress was limited by the end of the infusion protocol without chest pain. The peak blood pressure and heart rate were 182/92 mmHg and 137/min.

Stress Images There is reduced uptake of tracer in the basal inferior and basal lateral walls.

Rest Images There is no improvement.

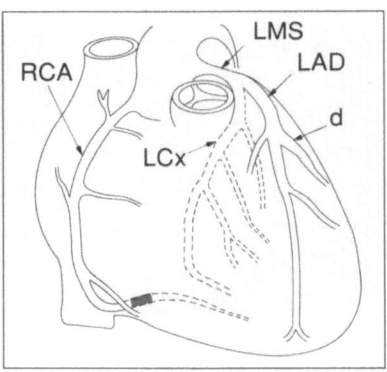

Coronary Angiography

An occlusion was present in the posterior descending branch of a dominant right coronary artery. There was basal inferior hypokinesis.

Conclusion

Basal inferolateral myocardial infarction without evidence of reversible ischaemia.

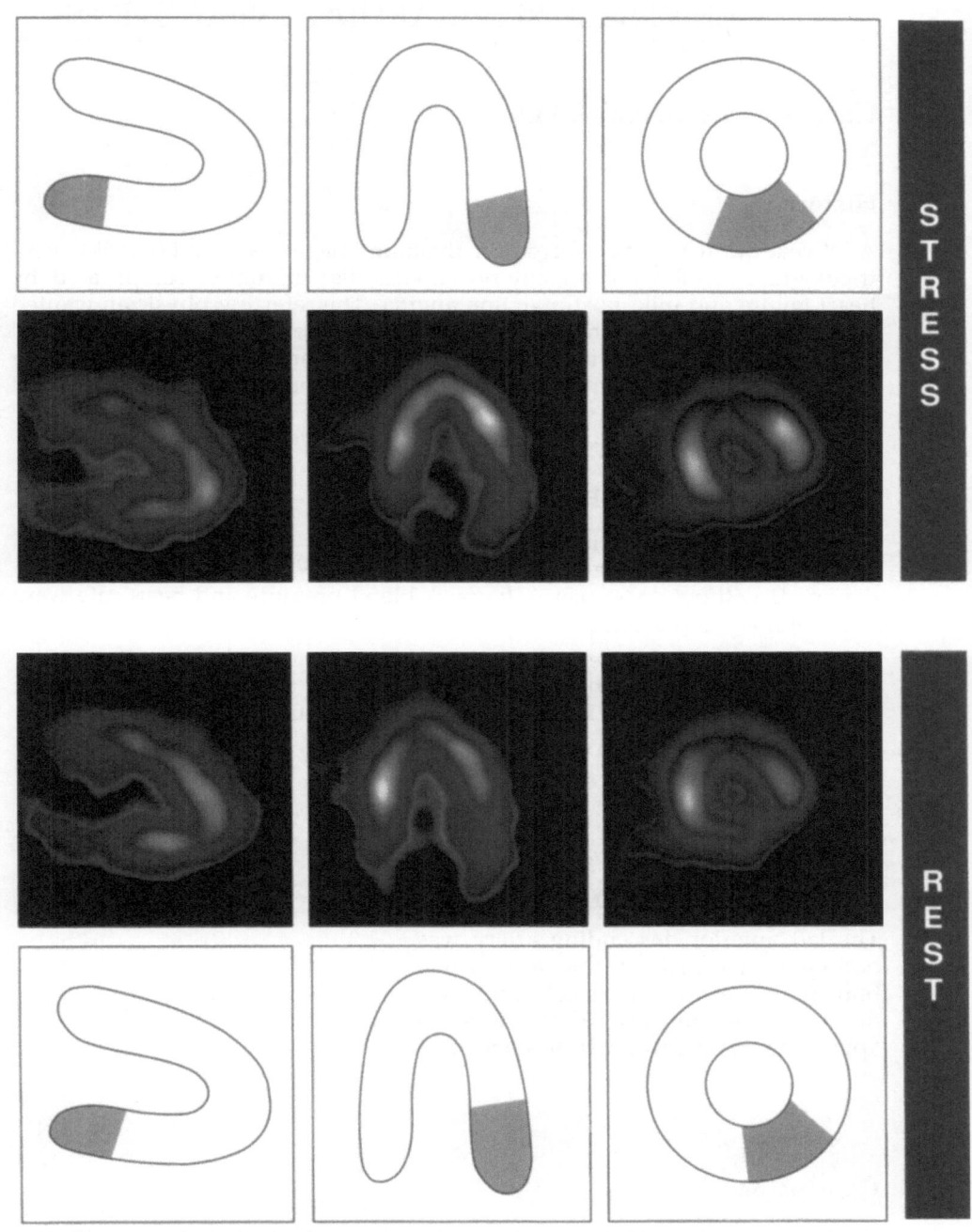

Occlusion of the posterior descending artery may lead to basal infero-lateral infarction.

SINGLE VESSEL MYOCARDIAL INFARCTION

Case 16 – Proximal LAD

History

A 78-year-old man was referred for thallium imaging and radionuclide ventriculography following an anterior myocardial infarction complicated by heart failure and mild postinfarction angina. The referring physician wanted to assess the extent of the infarction, the presence of reversible myocardial ischaemia, and the resting ejection fraction in order to plan any further management. The resting ECG showed right bundle branch block and anterior Q-waves.

Thallium Myocardial Perfusion Tomography

Stress Technique Dipyridamole was not infused because of a history of asthma. Bicycle exercise was performed to 50 W. Stress was limited by dyspnoea without chest pain. The peak blood pressure and heart rate were 140/70 mmHg and 105/min.

Stress Images The left ventricle is dilated and there was increased uptake of thallium in the lungs. There is reduced uptake of tracer in the inferior and distal anterior walls and absent uptake in the septum and apex.

Rest Images There is no change.

Coronary Angiography

The left anterior descending artery was occluded proximal to the first septal branch. There was a distal right coronary artery stenosis. There was an apical aneurysm and anterior akinesia.

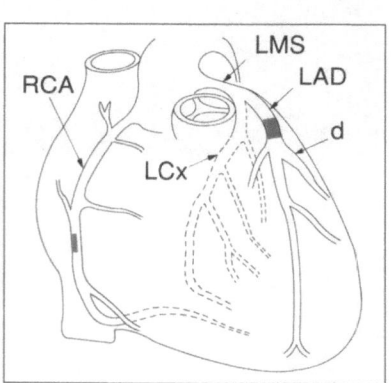

Conclusion

There is extensive anteroseptal and apical infarction with no evidence of reversible ischaemia. The dilatation of the left ventricle and the increased lung uptake imply impaired left ventricular function. Radionuclide ventriculography showed a resting ejection fraction of 12% with amplitude and phase abnormalities characteristic of an apical aneurysm.

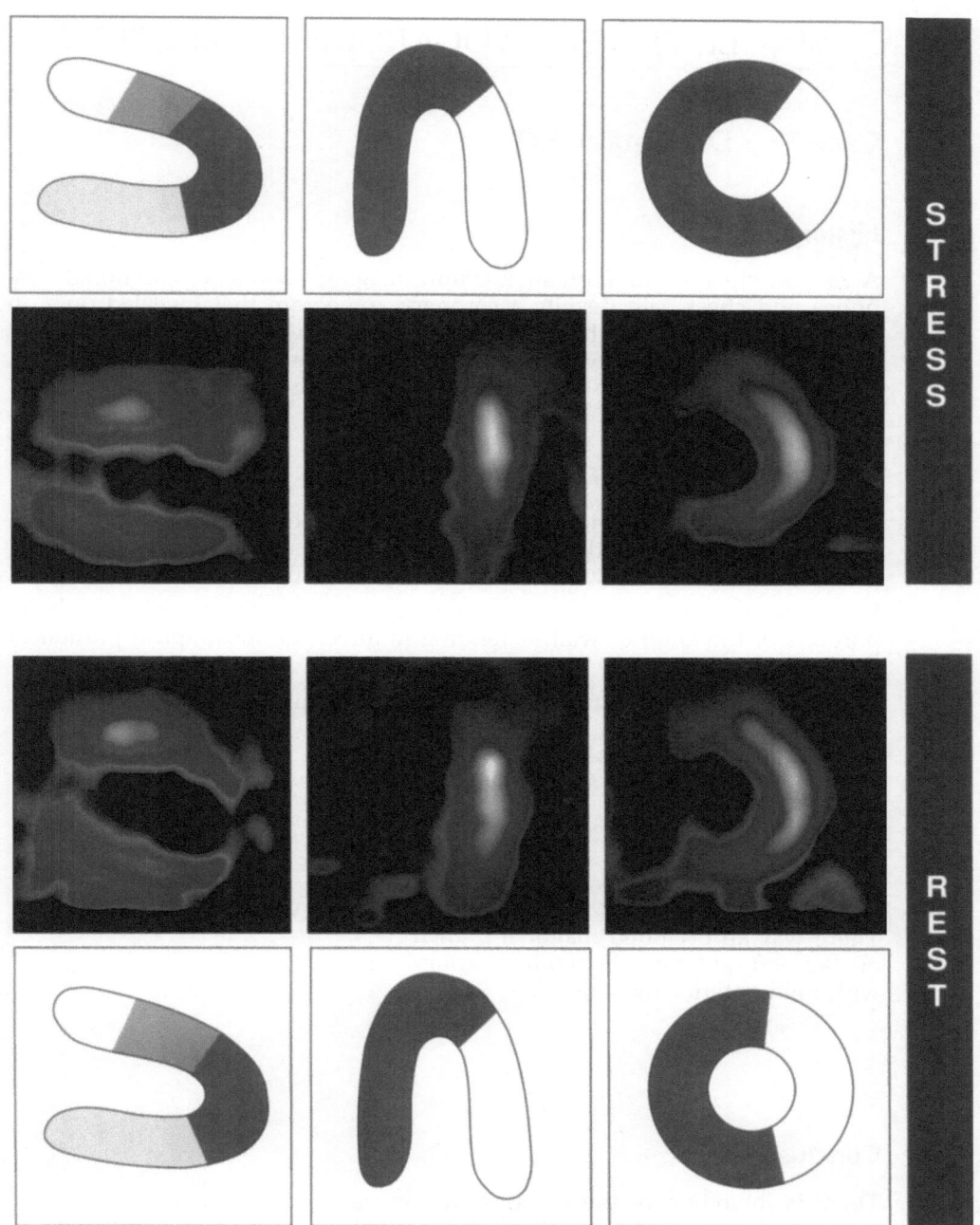

Proximal occlusion of the left anterior descending artery may cause extensive infarction. Divergence of the anterior and inferior walls suggests aneurysm formation. In extensive anterior infarction, inferior wall attenuation may be accentuated. Dipyridamole is contraindicated if there is a history of bronchospasm.

SINGLE VESSEL MYOCARDIAL INFARCTION

Case 17 – Diagonal LAD

History

A 75-year-old man underwent thallium imaging because of exertional dyspnoea and chest pain despite a coronary angiogram that revealed only an
occluded diagonal branch of the left anterior descending artery. Whilst it is
well recognised tht symptoms and extent of ischaemia are poorly correlated,
the request was made to establish the severity of ischaemia.

Thallium Myocardial Perfusion Tomography

Stress Technique Dipyridamole was infused prior to bicycle exercise to
50 W. Stress was limited by fatigue without chest pain. The peak blood
pressure and heart rate were 150/80 mmHg and 120/min.

Stress Images There is reduced uptake of tracer in the middle and basal
portions of the anterior wall, extending to affect the most apical portion of
the lateral wall.

Rest Images There is little change, except for minor improvement in the
basal anterior wall.

Coronary Angiography

There was an occluded diagonal branch
of the left anterior descending artery
with mild anterior hypokinesis.

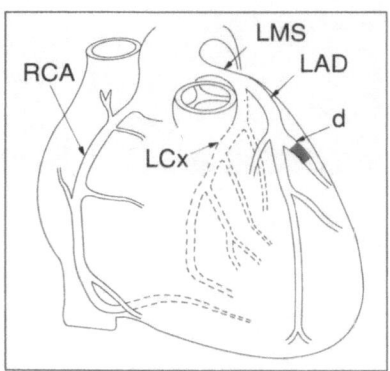

Conclusion

There is infarction of the anterior wall in its middle portion with a small
amount of associated reversible ischaemia. This area is typical of the distribution of the diagonal artery although there is considerable variation. The
scan reflects a low risk of future cardiac events and reinforces the fact that
symptoms are no guide to the extent of ischaemia.

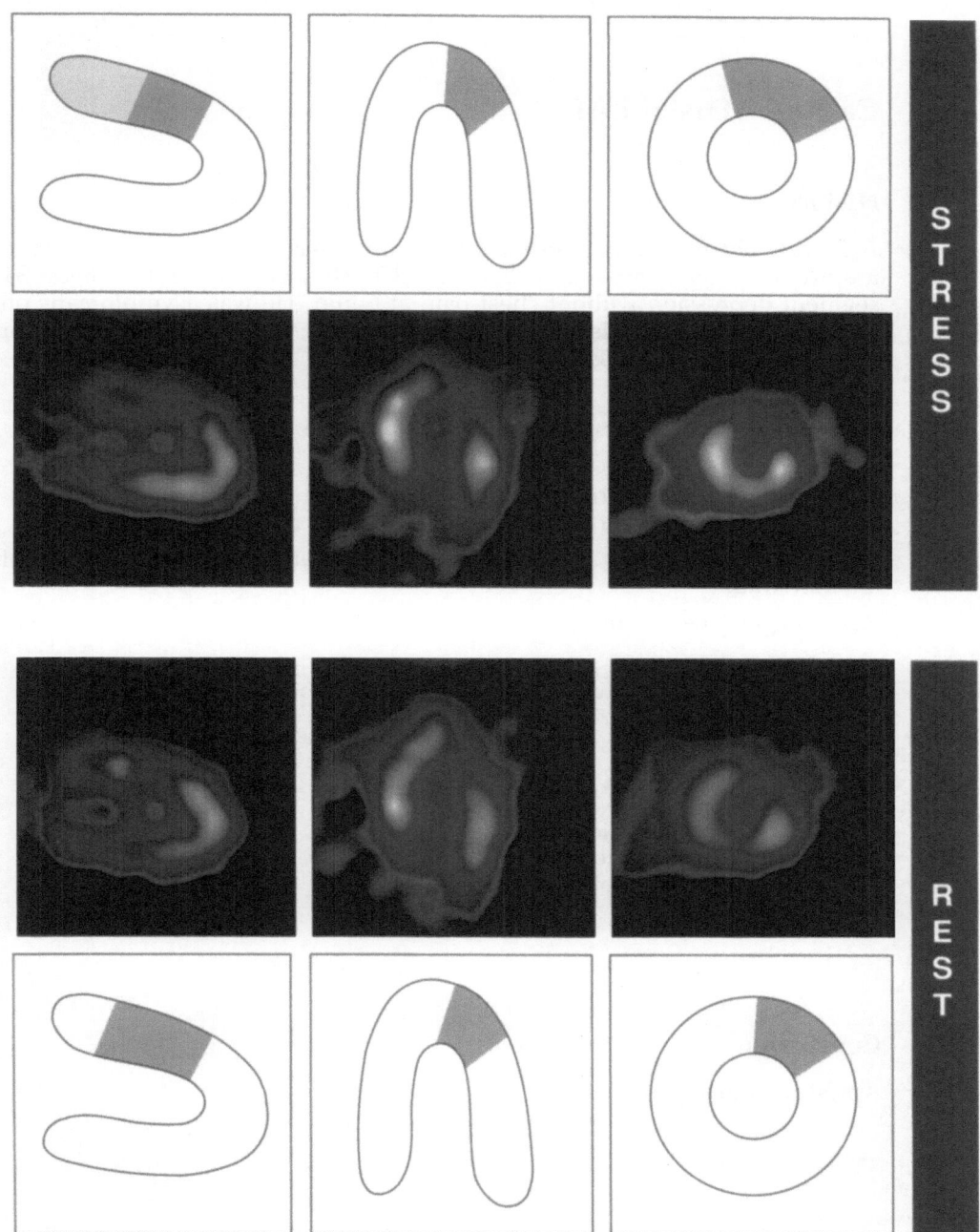

Occlusion of the diagonal branch of the left anterior descending artery may result in infarction of the anterolateral wall. In one-quarter of cases, myocardial infarction occurs without symptoms.

SINGLE VESSEL MYOCARDIAL INFARCTION

Case 18 – Distal LAD

History

A 51-year-old man was referred for thallium imaging and coronary angiography after apical infarction. Exercise ECG showed 2 mm inferolateral ST segment depression without chest pain at 6 min. He was asymptomatic on antianginal therapy. His resting ECG showed a Q-wave in aVl and poor anterior R-wave progression.

Thallium Myocardial Perfusion Tomography

Stress Technique Dipyridamole was infused without symptoms. The peak blood pressure and heart rate were 125/78 mmHg and 84/min.

Stress Images There is reduced uptake of tracer in the apex and apical anterior wall.

Rest Images There is no improvement.

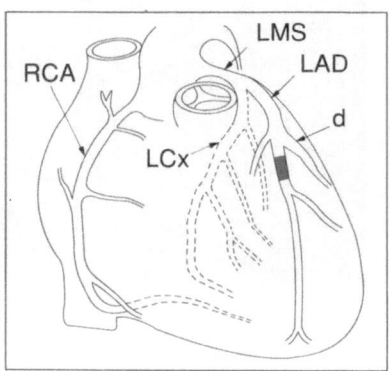

Coronary Angiography

There was an occlusion of the left anterior descending artery after a large diagonal branch with apical akinesis.

Conclusion

Apical myocardial infarction.

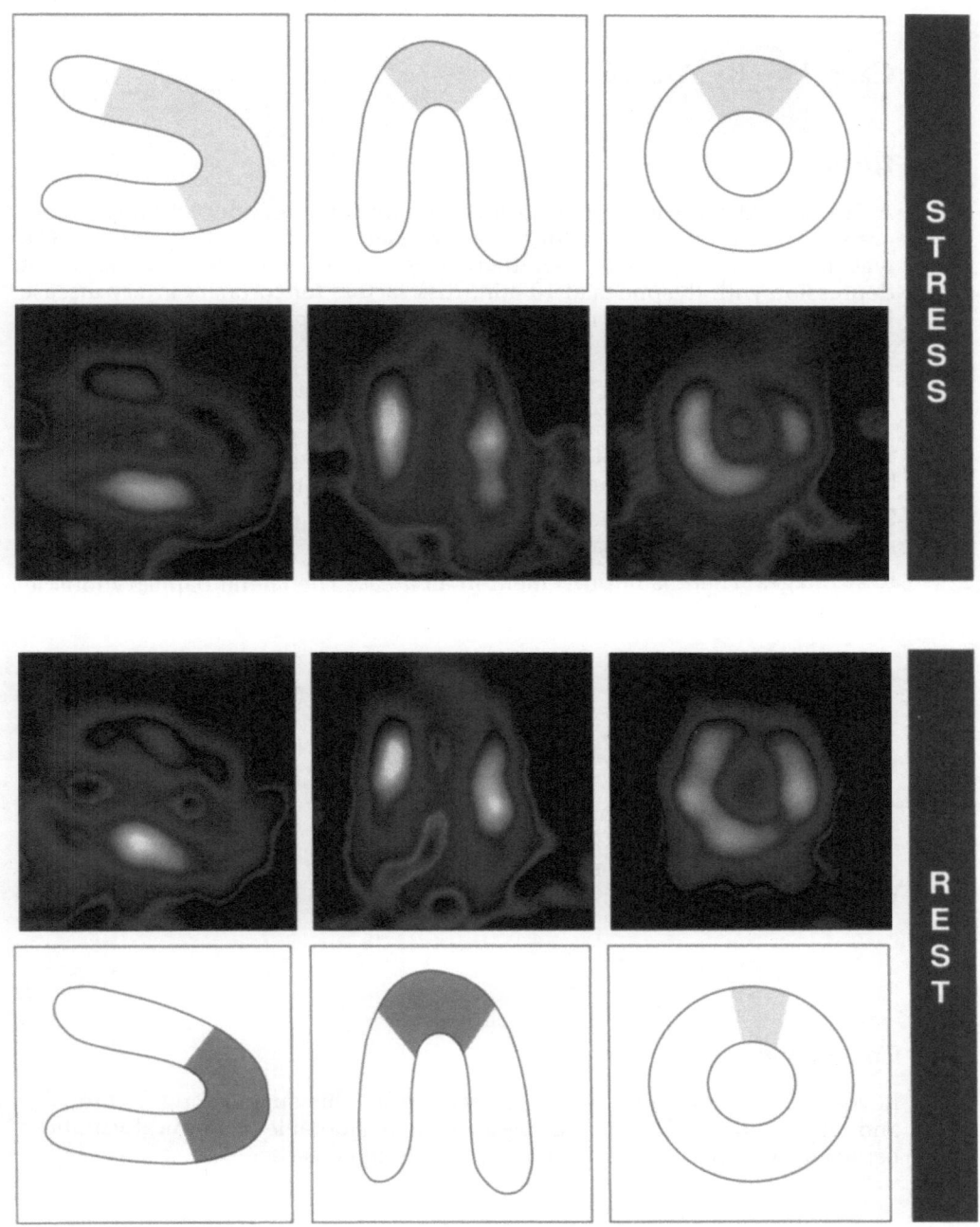

STRESS

REST

Occlusion of the left anterior descending artery after the septal and diagonal branches may cause apical infarction.

TWO VESSEL REVERSIBLE ISCHAEMIA

Case 19 – RCA/LCx

History

A 36-year-old man was referred for thallium imaging and coronary angiography with a one-year history of exertional chest pain. The resting ECG was normal but, on exercise, there was 3 mm inferolateral ST segment depression with dyspnoea at 10 min. Risk factors for coronary artery disease included hypertension, a raised cholesterol, and a positive family history.

Thallium Myocardial Perfusion Tomography

Stress Technique Dipyridamole was infused causing chest pain. The peak blood pressure and heart rate were 150/60 mmHg and 84/min.

Stress Images There is reduced uptake of tracer in the inferior wall extending into the apex and basal lateral wall.

Rest Images There is improvement in all areas. The lateral papillary muscle is prominent.

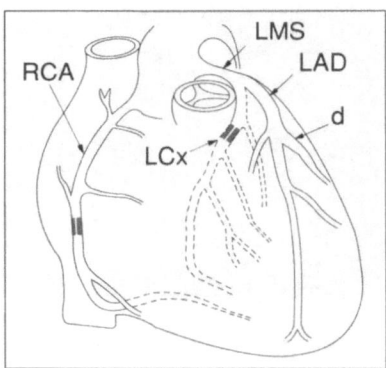

Coronary Angiography

There were stenoses of the proximal left circumflex artery and of the mid-right coronary artery. Left ventricular wall motion was normal.

Conclusion

Reversible inferior and lateral wall ischaemia. This suggests right coronary and left circumflex disease, but because of considerable anatomical variation between these two arteries it is not possible to be certain.

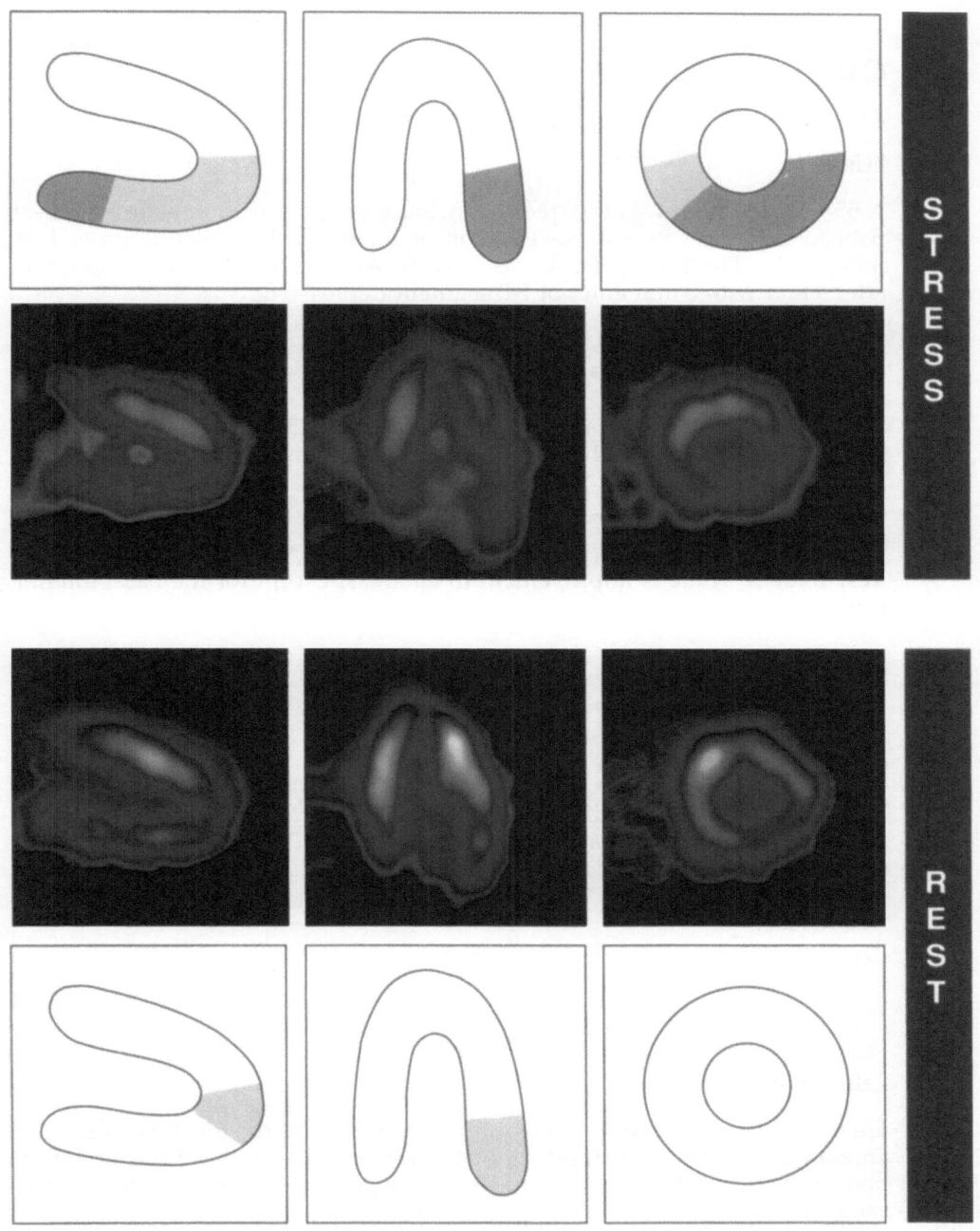

Lateral and inferior wall ischaemia suggest left circumflex and right coronary artery disease.

Case 20 – LAD/RCA

History

A 55-year-old man was referred for thallium imaging with a history of chest pain for 15 years. Recent exacerbation of symptoms had been improved by β-blockade. The resting ECG was normal. An exercise ECG was abnormal after 4 min with 3 mm anterior ST segment depression.

Thallium Myocardial Perfusion Tomography

Stress Technique Dobutamine was infused to 15 µg/kg/min. Stress was limited by chest pain. The peak blood pressure and heart rate were 166/76 mmHg and 125/min.

Stress Images There is reduced uptake of tracer in the anterior and inferior walls, the septum, and the apex.

Rest Images There is improvement in all areas, except for the basal inferior wall.

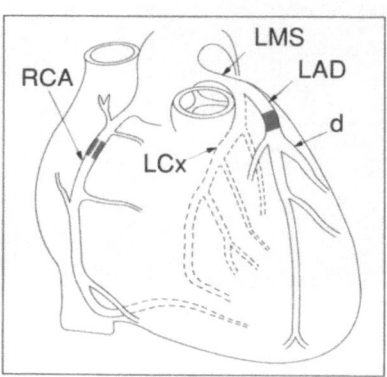

Coronary Angiography

The left anterior descending artery was occluded and there was a proximal stenosis in a dominant right coronary artery. Left ventricular wall motion was normal.

Conclusion

There is extensive reversible myocardial ischaemia in the territory of the left anterior descending and right coronary arteries. The extent of this implies a poor prognosis. The patient underwent coronary bypass grafting in the same admission.

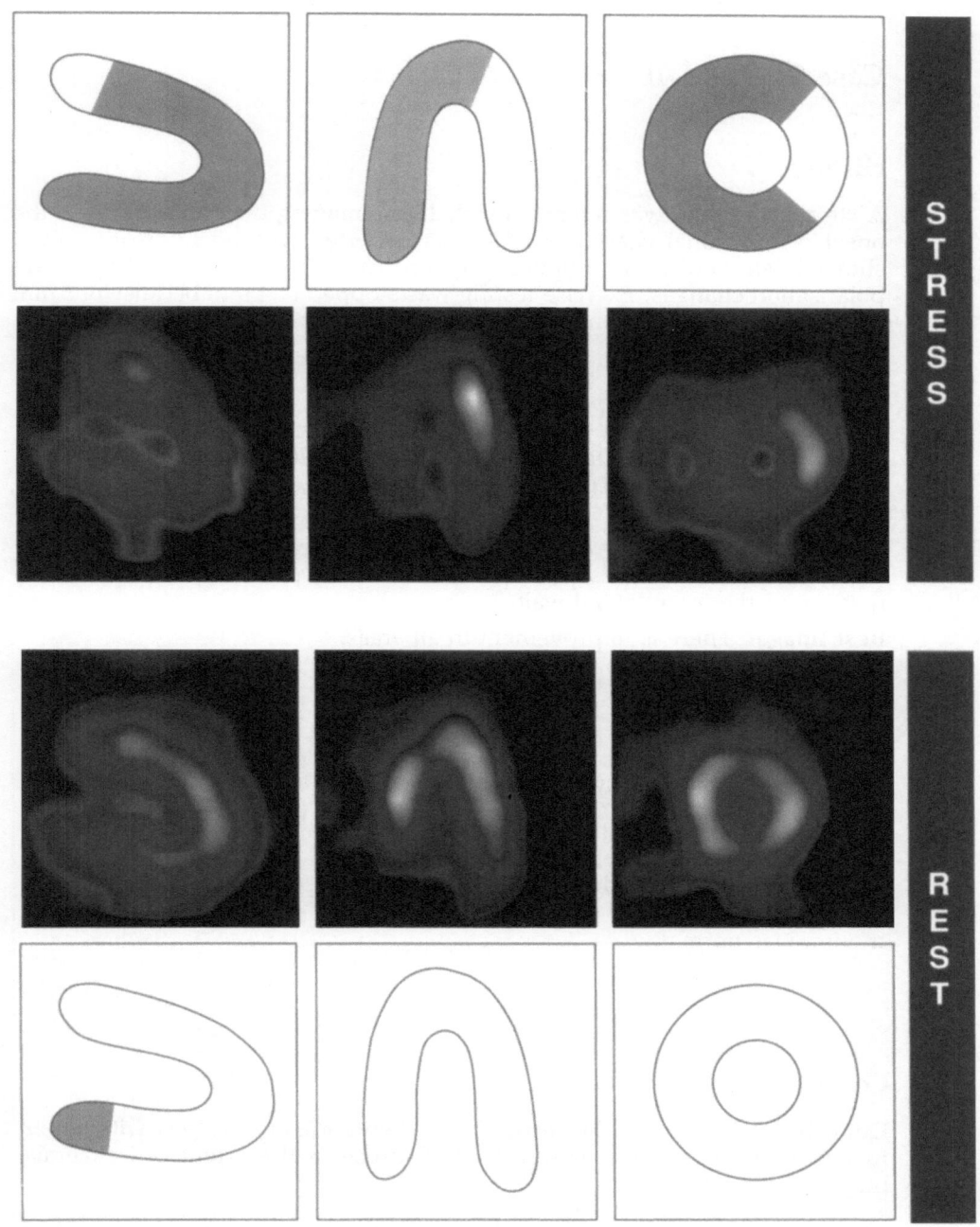

STRESS

REST

Extensive reversible ischaemia implies a poor prognosis and warrants urgent revascularisation.

Case 21 – LAD/LCx

History

A 60-year-old man was referred for thallium imaging three months after the onset of exertional chest pain. He was hypertensive and his resting ECG showed left ventricular hypertrophy on voltage criteria but without re-polarisation changes. Exercise testing was stopped at 4 min because of 5 mm of ST segment depression without chest pain.

Thallium Myocardial Perfusion Tomography

Stress Technique Dobutamine was infused to 20 µg/kg/min. Stress was limited by chest pain. The peak blood pressure and heart rate were 164/86 mmHg and 126/min.

Stress Images There is greatly reduced uptake of tracer in the entire anterior wall and apex, although septal uptake is relatively preserved. Uptake is also reduced in the inferolateral wall.

Rest Images There is improvement in all areas.

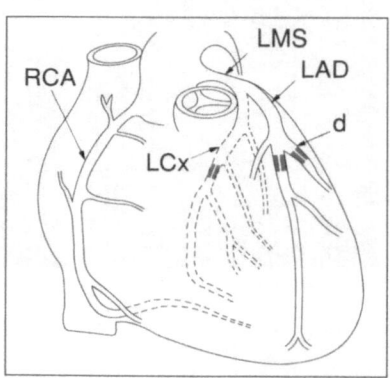

Coronary Angiography

There were stenoses in the proximal left anterior descending artery after the first septal branch and in the proximal left circumflex artery. Left ventricular wall motion was normal.

Conclusion

Extensive ischaemia in the territories of two coronary arteries with reper-fusion, indicating viable myocardium. Because of the extent of ischaemia, this is a high risk scan.

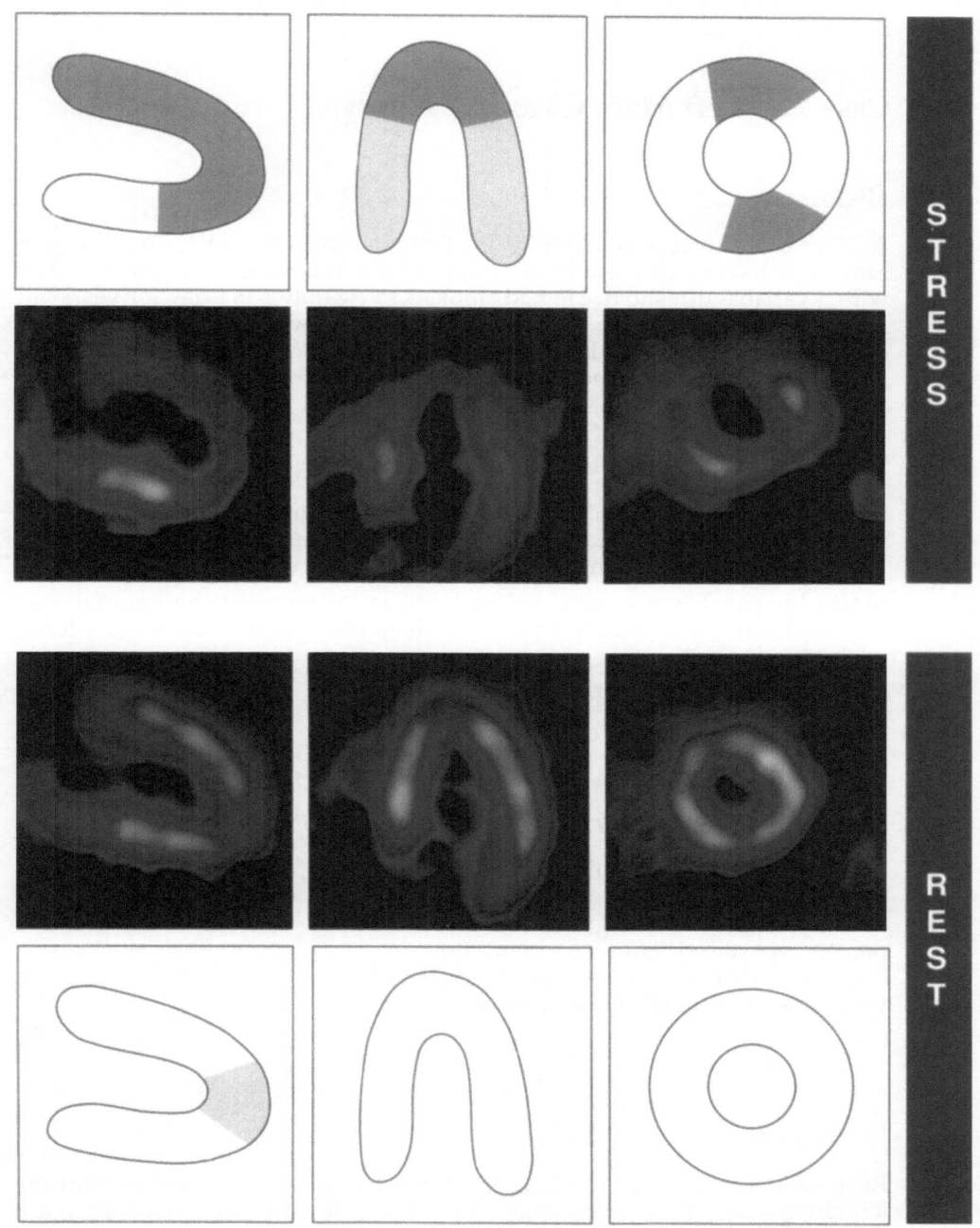

STRESS

REST

In a patient with left ventricular hypertrophy, the significance of exercise-induced ST segment changes can be clarified by thallium imaging.

Case 22 – Left Main Coronary Artery

History

A 51-year-old man was admitted for thallium imaging and coronary angiography following an episode of angina at rest followed by angina of effort with a variable threshold. He had smoked 15 cigarettes per day for years but had no other risk factors. His resting ECG showed inferior Q-waves of doubtful significance and his exercise treadmill test was limited at 5 min because of 2 mm ST segment depression in lead V5 without angina.

Thallium Myocardial Perfusion Tomography

Stress Technique Dipyridamole was infused causing chest pain which did not require intervention. The peak blood pressure and heart rate were 115/80 mmHg and 82/min.

Stress Images There is very reduced uptake of tracer in the anterior wall and apex, and also reduced uptake in the lateral wall and the basal inferior wall.

Rest Images There is improvement in all areas.

Coronary Angiography

The left main stem had two stenoses of 80% and 95%. The left circumflex and left anterior descending arteries were poorly visualised due to poor flow but were thought to be normal. Left ventricular wall motion was normal.

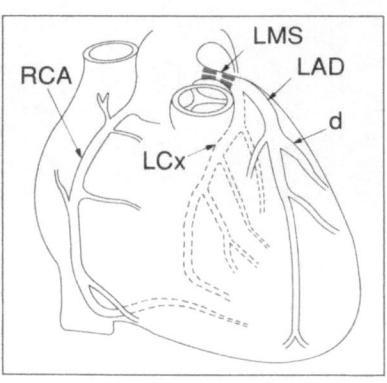

Conclusion

Reversible ischaemia in the territory of the left anterior descending and the left circumflex arteries. The scan confirms that the inferior Q-waves are not the result of infarction. The patient is at high risk of future cardiac events and he underwent urgent coronary artery bypass grafting.

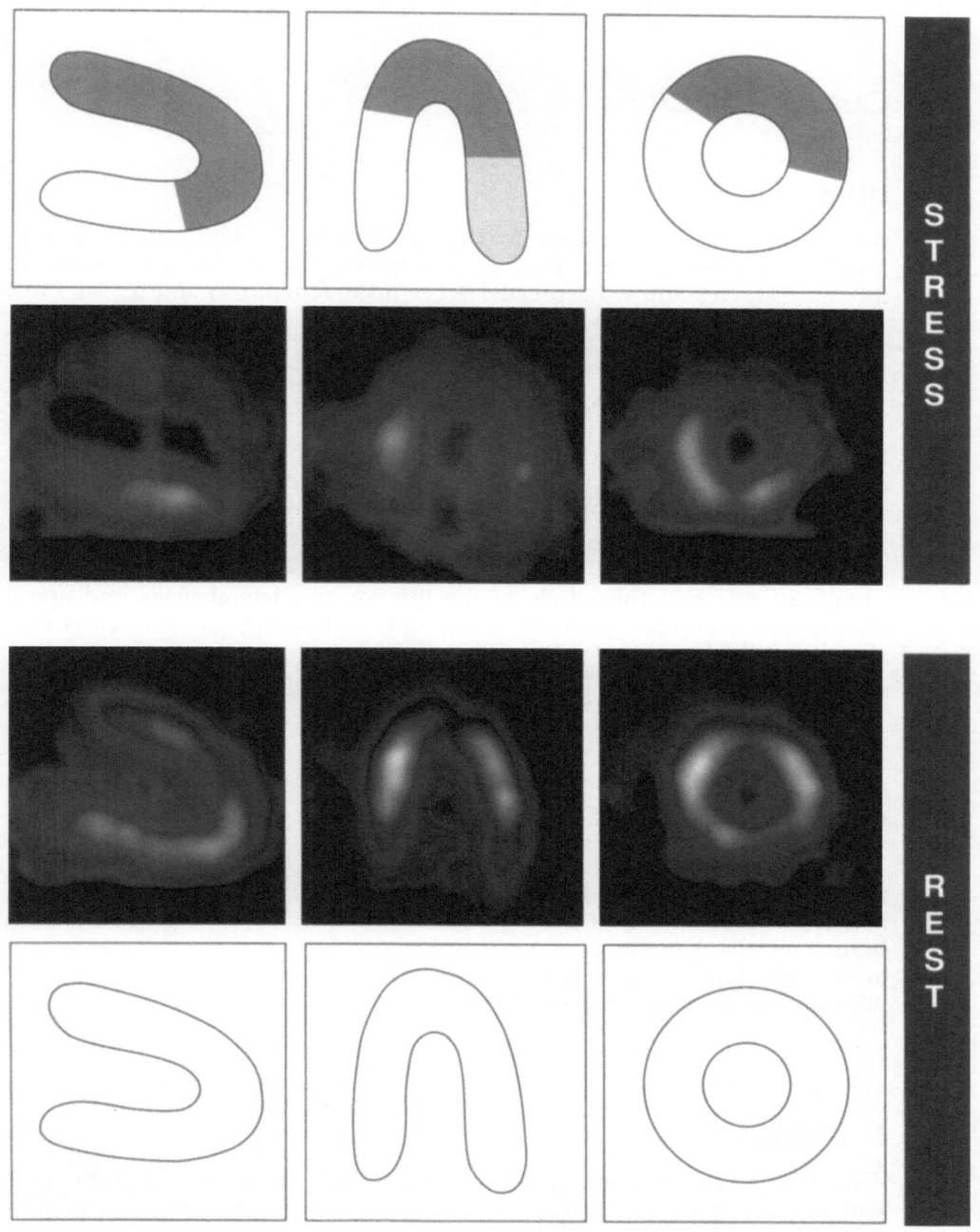

There is no specific pattern of perfusion defect in stenosis of the left main coronary artery. Sparing of septal perfusion in this case implies that it is partly supplied by the right coronary artery.

TWO VESSEL MYOCARDIAL INFARCTION

Case 23 – RCA/LCx

History

A 69-year-old man was referred for thallium imaging 4 weeks after an inferior myocardial infarction. He was asymptomatic. The resting ECG showed inferior Q-waves and widespread T-wave inversion and so an exercise ECG was not performed. He was asthmatic.

Thallium Myocardial Perfusion Tomography

Stress Technique Dipyridamole was not infused because of the history of asthma. Bicycle ergometry was limited at 50 W by dyspnoea without chest pain. The peak blood pressure and heart rate were 130/60 mmHg and 135/min.

Stress Images There was high lung thallium uptake. There is almost absent uptake of tracer in the whole of the inferior and lateral walls and apex. Uptake in the septum is also reduced. The septum appears shortened and thinned at the base.

Rest Images There is improvement in the septum with no change elsewhere.

Coronary Angiography

There were proximal occlusions of the left circumflex and right coronary arteries with a stenosis of the first septal branch of the left anterior descending artery. The left ventricle showed generalised hypokinesis and inferior akinesis.

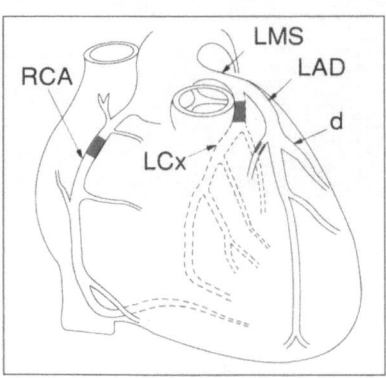

Conclusion

This pattern of infarction in the territories of the left circumflex and the right coronary arteries is unusual given the history of a single infarct. The patient may have had a previous infarction silently, or simultaneous occlusion of two arteries. Reversible ischaemia in the septum is the consequence of left anterior descending disease. The patient underwent coronary artery bypass grafting.

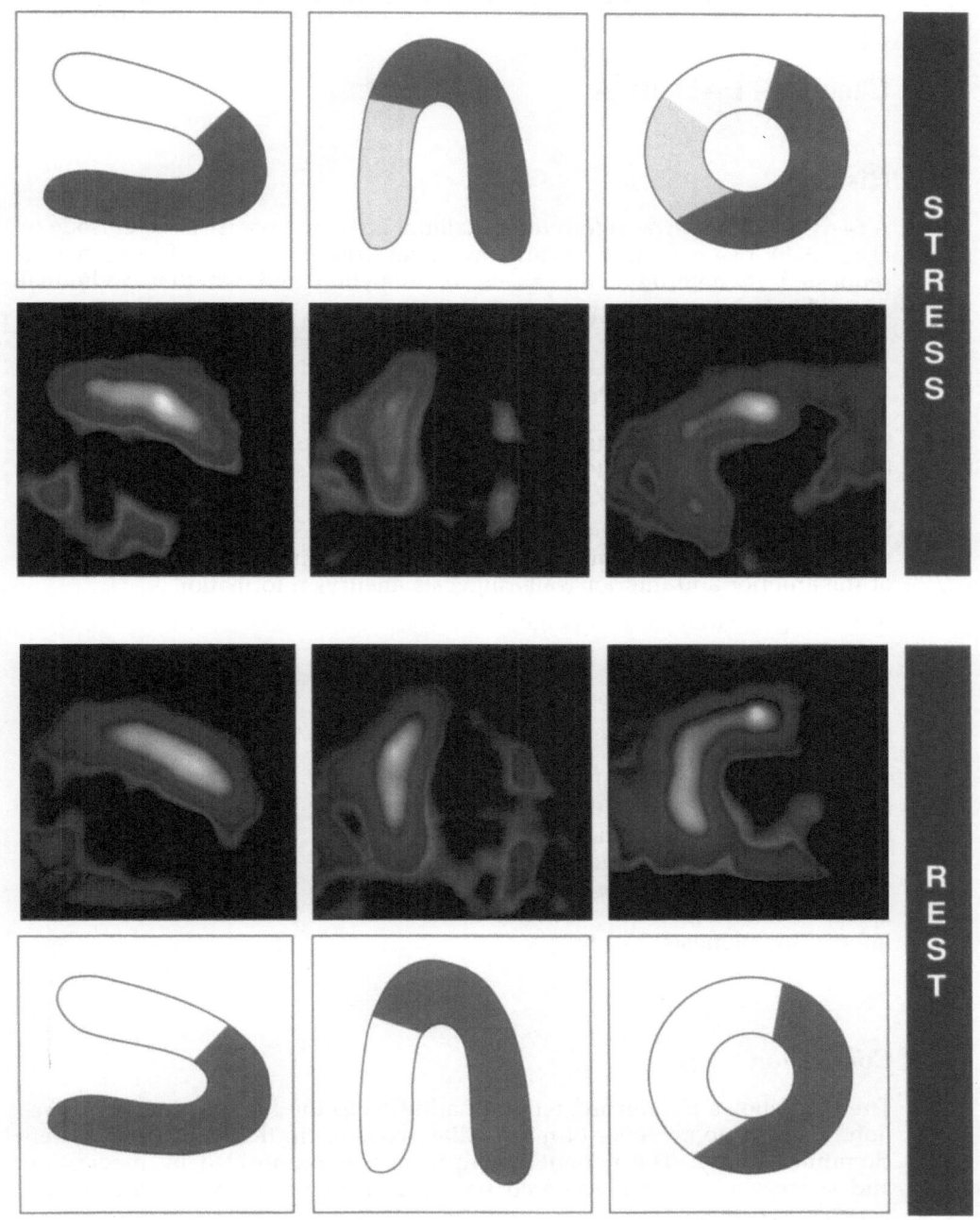

STRESS

REST

A high risk scan with uptake of tracer in the lung, extensive infarction and silent ischaemia.

TWO VESSEL MYOCARDIAL INFARCTION

Case 24 – LAD/RCA

History

A 64-year-old man was referred for thallium imaging because of an episode of chest pain 15 years after an anterior myocardial infarction. The scan was requested to determine the extent of infarction and whether additional reversible ischaemia was present.

Thallium Myocardial Perfusion Tomography

Stress Technique Dipyridamole was infused prior to bicycle exercise to 25 W, limited by fatigue without chest pain. At peak stress the blood pressure and the heart rate were 120/72 mmHg and 104/min.

Stress Images There is almost absent uptake of tracer in the apex with very reduced uptake in the anterior wall, septum, and inferior wall. Divergence of the anterior and inferior walls suggests aneurysm formation.

Rest Images There is no change.

Coronary Angiography

There was a stenosis of the proximal right coronary artery with occlusion of the proximal left anterior descending artery. There were minor stenoses of the left circumflex artery. There was apical dyskinesis with anterior and inferior hypokinesis.

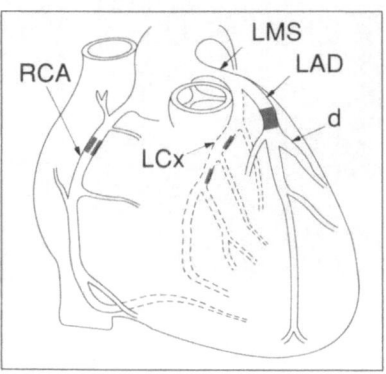

Conclusion

The scan shows inferior infarction in addition to the known anterior infarction. There is no evidence of myocardial ischaemia in the territory of the left circumflex artery. The patient's symptoms were controlled by medication and surgery was not considered beneficial because of the absence of reversible ischaemia.

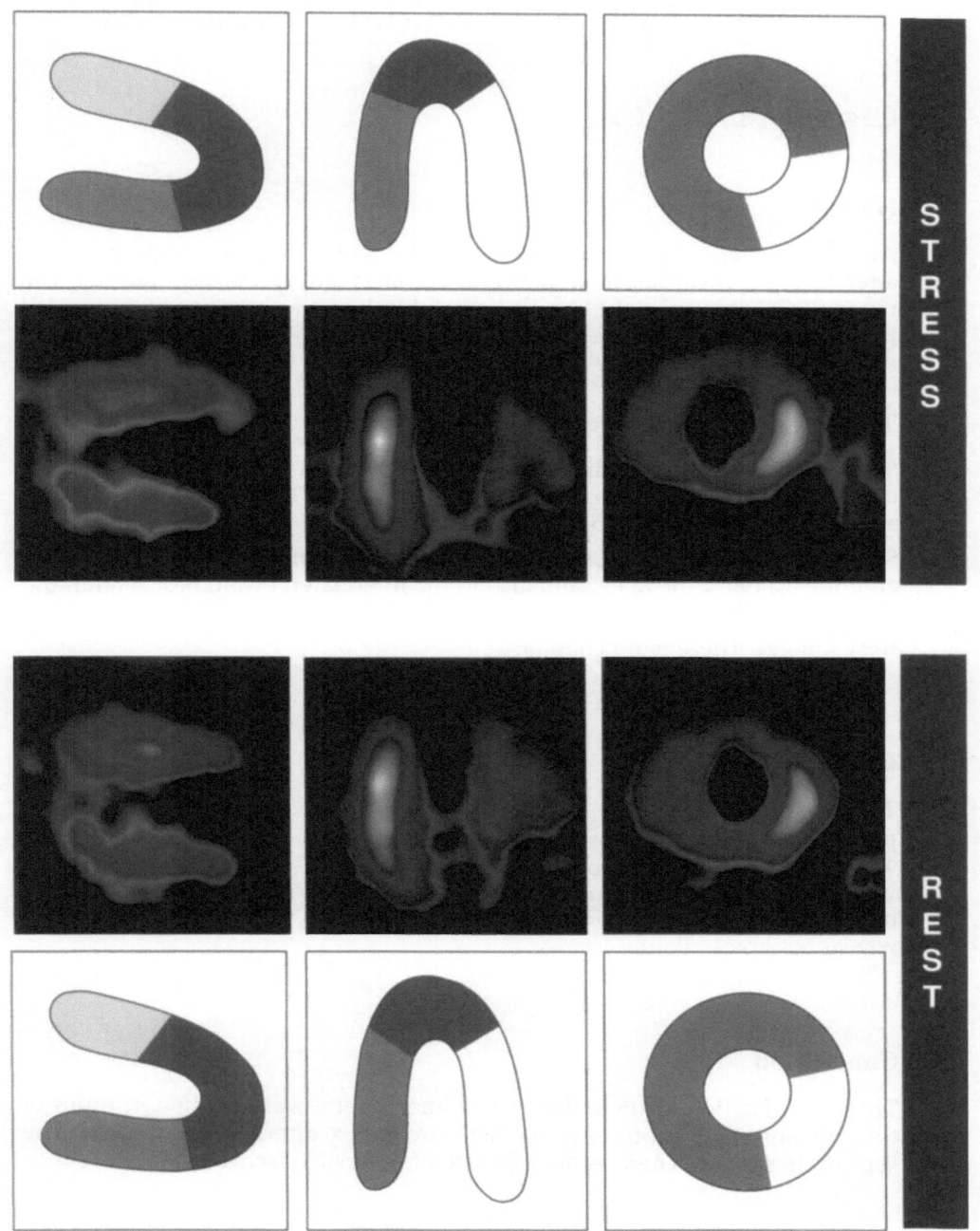

An area of infarction may be subtended by a patent vessel because of recanalisation after the acute event.

TWO VESSEL MYOCARDIAL INFARCTION

Case 25 – LAD/LCx

History

An asymptomatic 61-year-old man was referred for thallium imaging 8 years after apical myocardial infarction and coronary artery bypass grafting. The resting ECG showed right bundle branch block and an exercise ECG was not performed.

Thallium Myocardial Perfusion Tomography

Stress Technique Dipyridamole 40 mg was infused during bicycle exercise to 100 W, limited by fatigue without chest pain. The peak blood pressure and heart rate were 145/85 mmHg and 123/min respectively.

Stress Images There is absent uptake of tracer in the apical portion of the anterior wall and the apex, and also in the inferolateral wall, best seen in the short axis tomogram. Septal uptake is normal.

Rest Images There is no change.

Coronary Angiography

The left circumflex artery was occluded proximally, and the other coronary arteries showed severe disease. There was an occluded left circumflex graft, but the other grafts were patent. There was anteroapical akinesis.

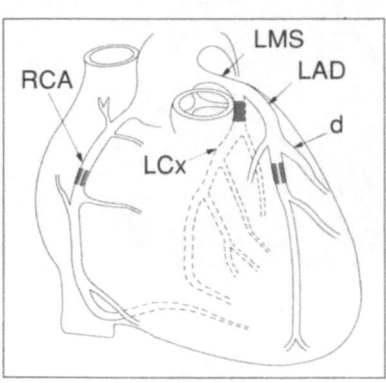

Conclusion

There is infarction of the anterior and inferolateral walls in the territories of the left anterior descending and left circumflex arteries respectively. The septum is spared. There is no evidence of reversible ischaemia.

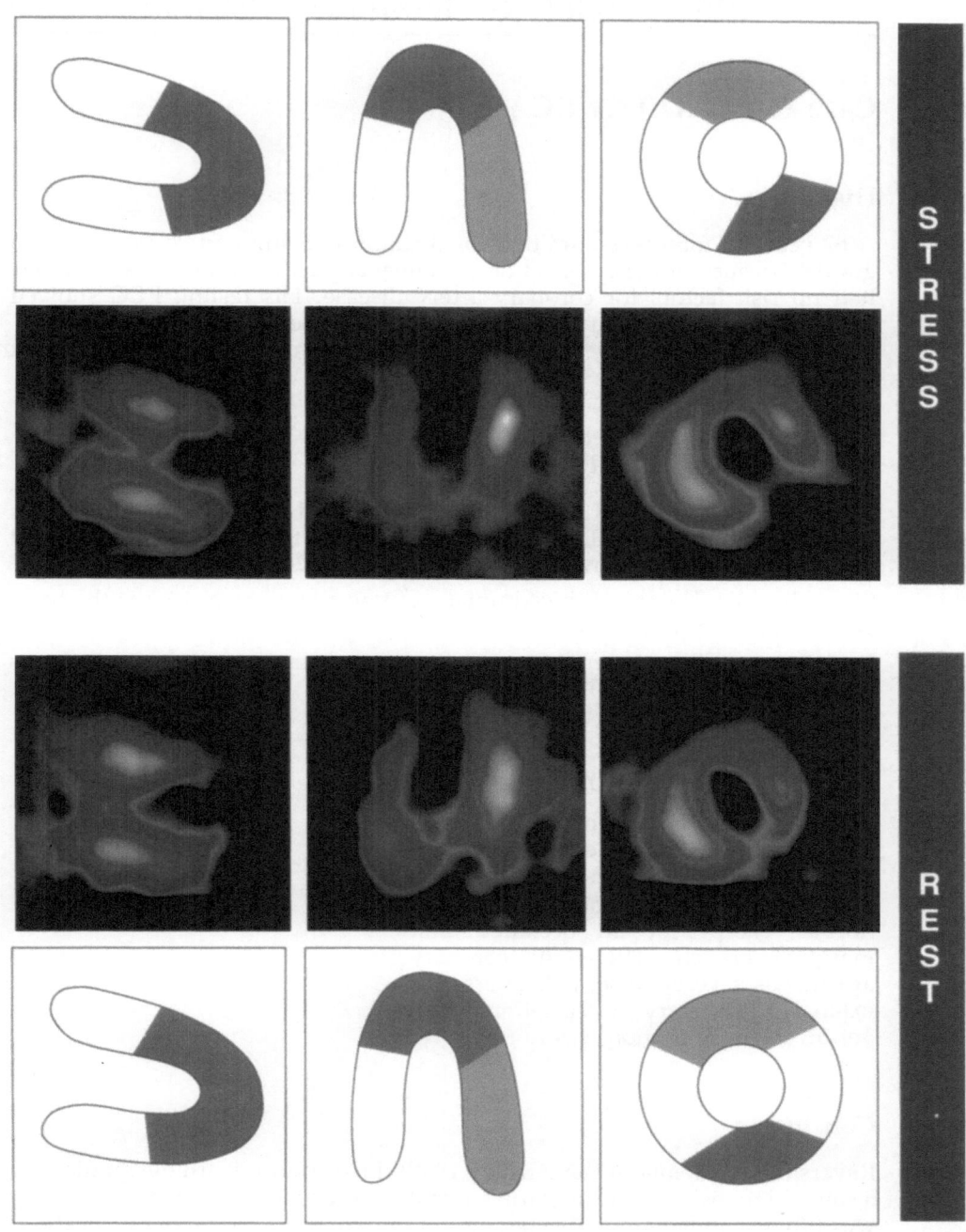

STRESS

REST

Thallium imaging can be used in the follow-up of patients after coronary artery bypass grafting.

Case 26 – LAD/LCx/RCA

History

A 62-year-old man was admitted for thallium imaging and coronary angiography because of recent onset of exertional angina with nocturnal pain. He had no risk factors for coronary artery disease. His resting ECG showed inferolateral ST segment depression. The exercise ECG showed 2 mm ST segment depression in lead V5 at 6 min and exercise was limited by chest pain.

Thallium Myocardial Perfusion Tomography

Stress Technique Dipyridamole infusion caused chest pain which was abolished by aminophylline after injection of the thallium. The peak blood pressure and heart rate were 140/84 mmHg and 124/min.

Stress Images There is reduced uptake of tracer in all areas except the basal portion of the anterior wall.

Rest Images There is improvement in the abnormal areas although this is least marked in the basal inferior wall.

Coronary Angiography

There was a severe stenosis of the proximal left anterior descending artery with occlusion distal to a normal diagonal branch. The left circumflex artery was normal except for an occluded first marginal branch. The right coronary artery was severely diseased. There was extensive coronary calcification. Left ventricular wall motion was normal.

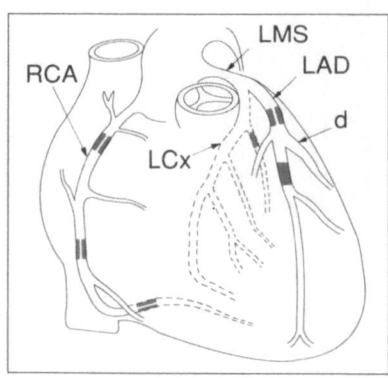

Conclusion

Reversible ischaemia in the territory of all three coronary arteries, indicating a very high risk of future cardiac events. Coronary artery bypass surgery was thought to be impossible because of the extensive coronary calcification.

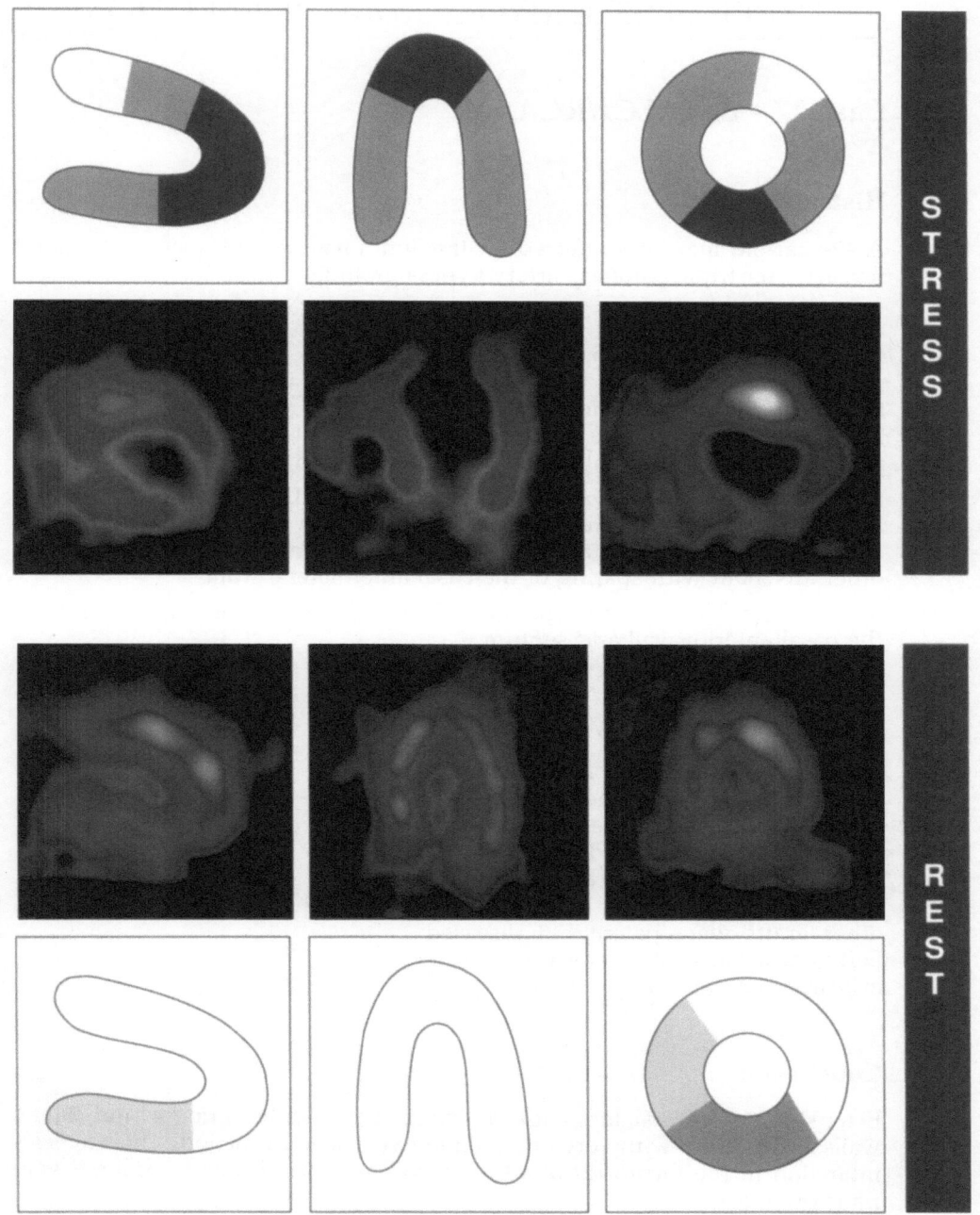

STRESS

REST

Aminophylline is a specific antagonist of dipyridamole and should be used for intolerable side effects. Oral nitrates may also be used to relieve myocardial ischaemia.

THREE VESSEL MYOCARDIAL INFARCTION

Case 27 – LAD/LCx/RCA

History

A 49-year-old man was referred for thallium imaging with recurrent angina 5 years after triple coronary artery bypass grafting.

Thallium Myocardial Perfusion Tomography

Stress Technique Dipyridamole was infused during bicycle exercise to 75 W, limited by fatigue without chest pain. At peak stress the blood pressure and the heart rate were 130/70 mmHg and 130/min.

Stress Images The left ventricle is very large and uptake of tracer in the lungs was seen to be increased in the planar images. There is absent uptake of tracer in the apex and apical anterior wall. There is reduced uptake in all other areas but with sparing of the basal anterolateral wall.

Rest Images There is little change although there is some improvement of the basal anterior wall and septum.

Coronary Angiography

There was occlusion of the left circumflex artery and the left anterior descending artery after a diagonal branch, with severe disease of the right coronary artery. The left anterior descending graft was occluded. The other grafts were patent but diseased. Left ventricular wall motion was globally impaired with apical dyskinesis.

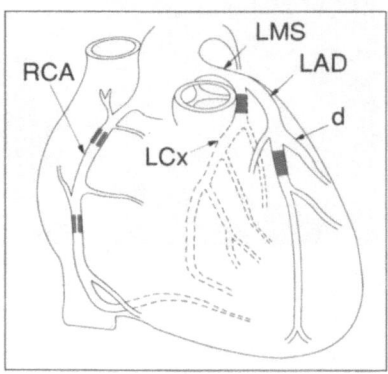

Conclusion

Extensive myocardial infarction affecting the anterior, inferior and lateral walls and septum with very impaired left ventricular function. This suggests infarction in the territories of all three coronary arteries and implies a very poor prognosis.

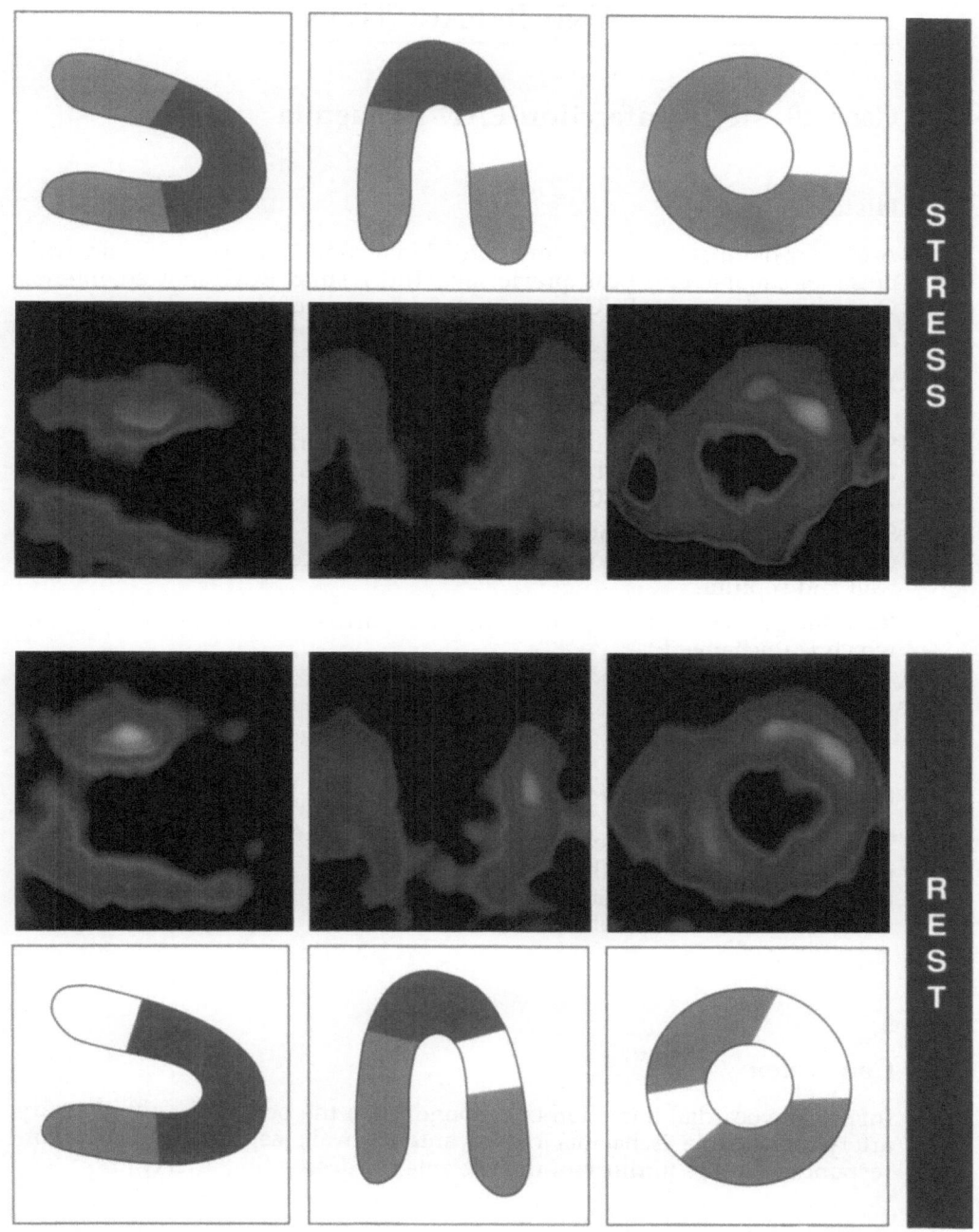

Ventricular dilatation and increased uptake of thallium in the lungs are signs of impaired left ventricular function.

MIXED REVERSIBLE ISCHAEMIA
AND INFARCTION

Case 28 – RCA Infarction/LAD Ischaemia

History

A 65-year-old man suffered a myocardial infarction 12 years previously with onset of angina one year previously. The resting ECG showed inferior Q-waves and exercise ECG was unhelpful because of claudication.

Thallium Myocardial Perfusion Tomography

Stress Technique Dipyridamole was infused during bicycle exercise to 75 W. Stress was limited by fatigue with chest pain. The peak blood pressure and heart rate were 200/96 mmHg and 100/min.

Stress Images There is no uptake of tracer in the apex and anterior wall except in its most basal portion. There is also reduced uptake in the inferior wall and septum.

Rest Images There is improvement in all areas except the inferior wall which is unchanged.

Coronary Angiography

There was an occlusion of the proximal right coronary artery with a stenosis of the proximal left anterior descending artery after the first septal branch.

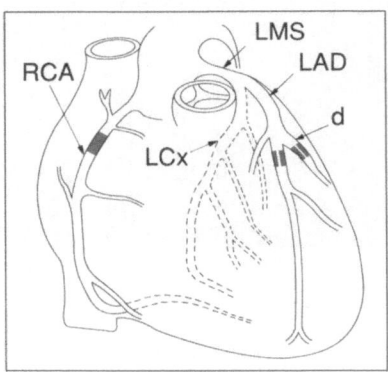

Conclusion

Inferior myocardial infarction corresponding to the occluded right coronary artery. Reversible ischaemia of the anterior wall, septum and apex corresponding to the territory of the left anterior descending artery.

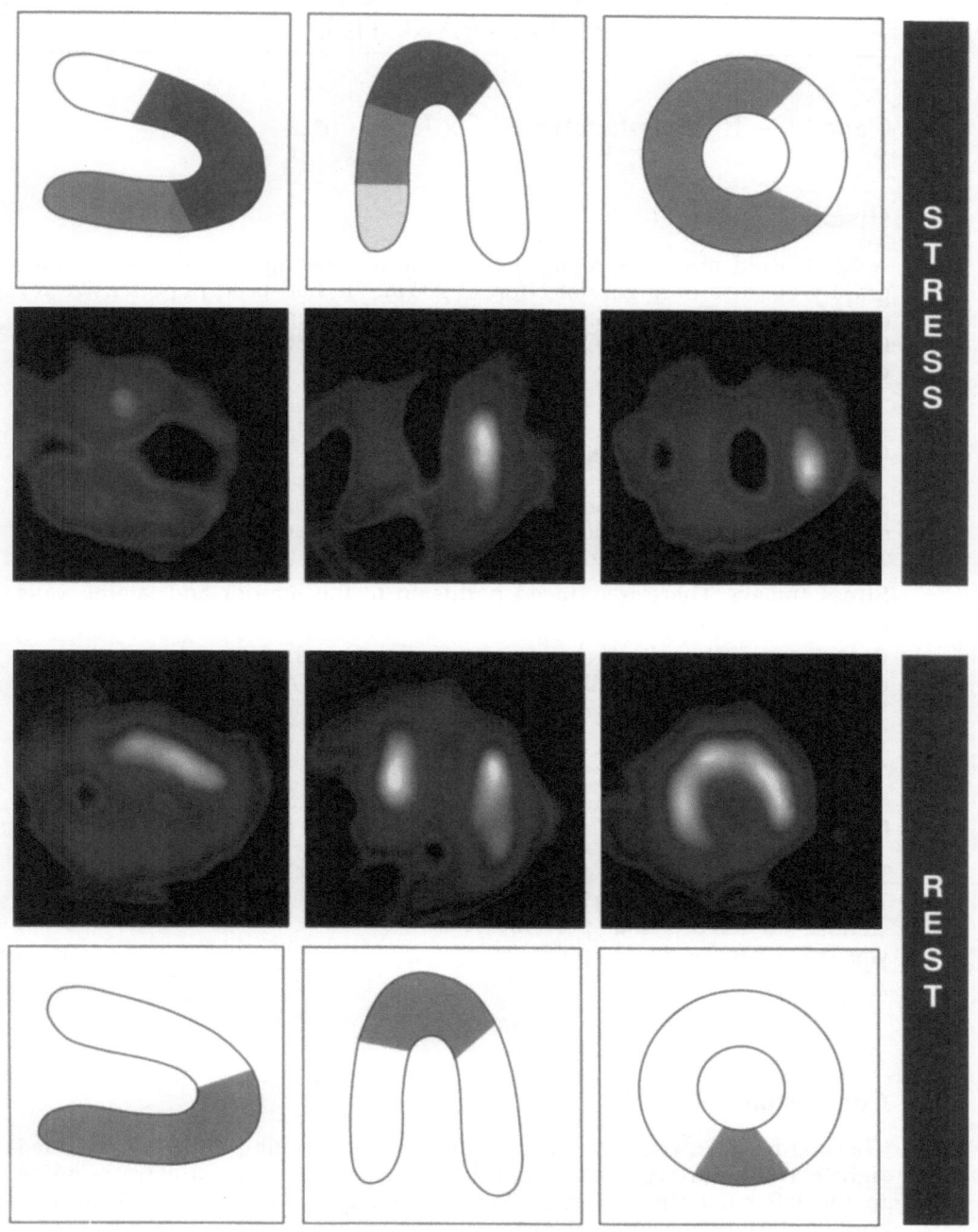

STRESS

REST

Dipyridamole may allow a diagnostic scan to be obtained despite the presence of claudication.

MIXED REVERSIBLE ISCHAEMIA
AND INFARCTION

Case 29 – RCA Infarction/LCx Ischaemia

History

A 58-year-old man was referred for thallium imaging and coronary angio-graphy because of angina of effort at 200 m. He had been hypertensive for 8 years but had no other risk factors. His resting ECG showed inferior Q-waves and his exercise ECG was stopped at 7 min by fatigue with 1 mm of ST segment depression in lead V5.

Thallium Myocardial Perfusion Tomography

Stress Technique Dipyridamole was infused causing chest pain which settled without intervention. The peak blood pressure and heart rate were 120/75 mmHg and 108/min.

Stress Images There is reduced perfusion to the inferior and lateral walls extending into the apex.

Rest Images There is improvement in the lateral wall and apex but no change in the inferior wall.

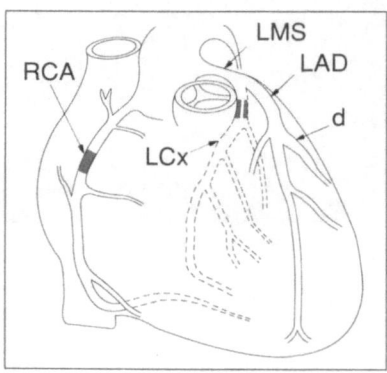

Coronary Angiography

The right coronary artery was occluded. The left circumflex artery had a tight stenosis in its proximal portion. There was basal inferior wall hypokinesis.

Conclusion

There is basal inferior myocardial infarction in keeping with the occluded right coronary artery, and reversible inferolateral ischaemia corresponding to the left circumflex stenosis. Symptoms improved with β-blockade and coronary artery surgery was not offered.

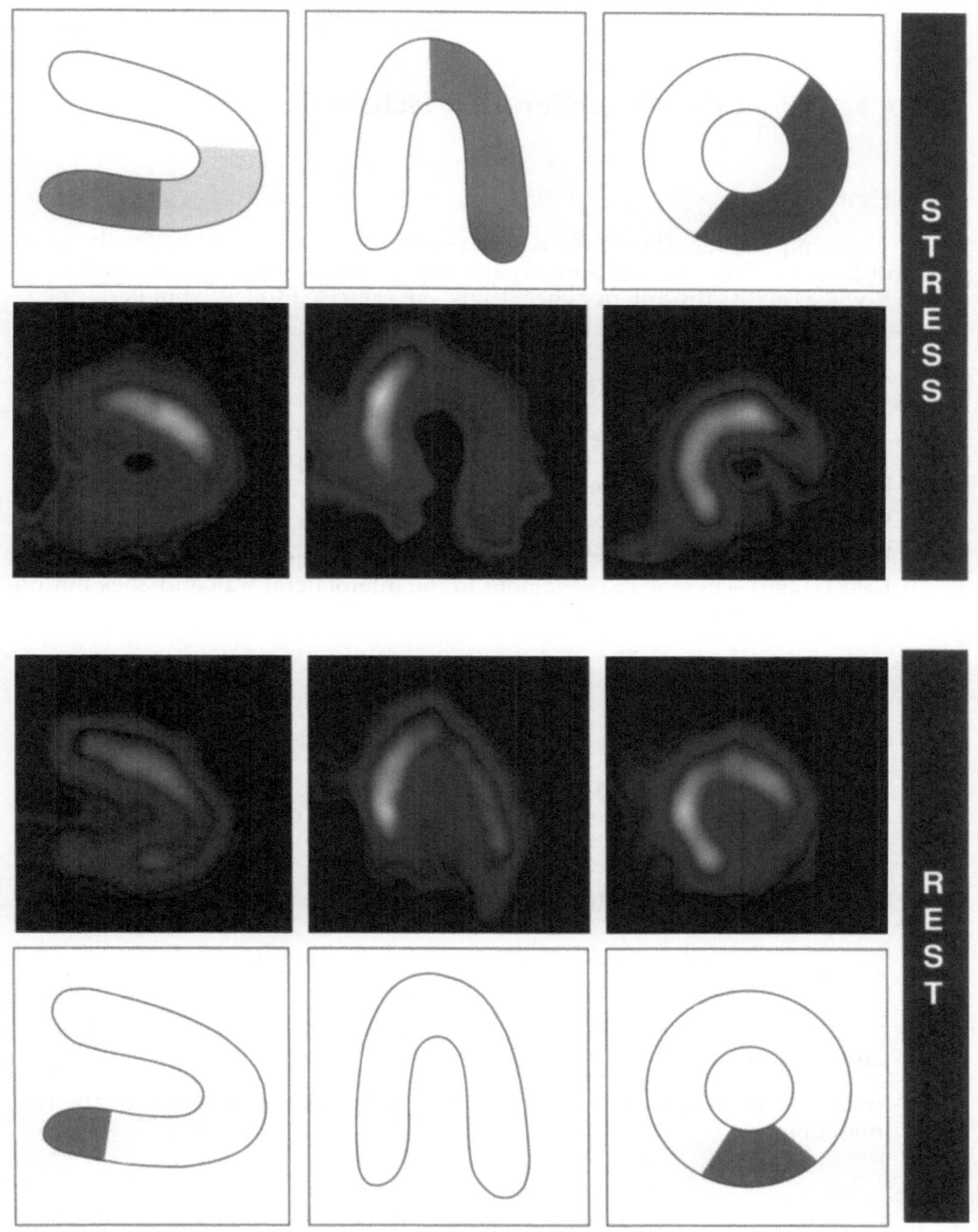

MIXED REVERSIBLE ISCHAEMIA
AND INFARCTION

Case 30 – LAD Infarction/LCx Ischaemia

History

An asymptomatic 60-year-old man was referred for thallium imaging because of longstanding diabetes and hypertension. The resting ECG showed loss of R-waves across the anterior chest leads. An exercise ECG was not performed.

Thallium Myocardial Perfusion Tomography

Stress Technique Dipyridamole was infused during bicycle exercise to 100 W, limited by fatigue without chest pain. The peak blood pressure and heart rate were 200/96 mmHg and 113/min.

Stress Images There is reduced uptake of tracer in the anterior and inferolateral walls extending into the apex.

Rest Images There is improvement in the inferolateral wall and apex but no change in the anterior wall.

Coronary Angiography

There were stenoses in the diagonal artery and an occlusion of the left anterior descending artery after the first septal branch. There was also a stenosis of the proximal left circumflex artery which was dominant.

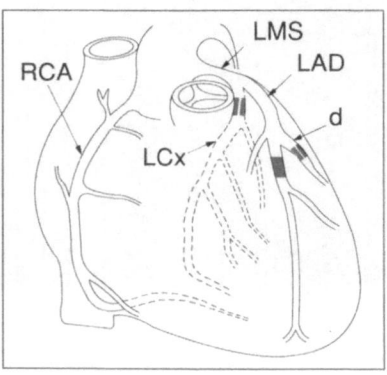

Conclusion

Reversible ischaemia in the territory of the left circumflex artery with anterior infarction.

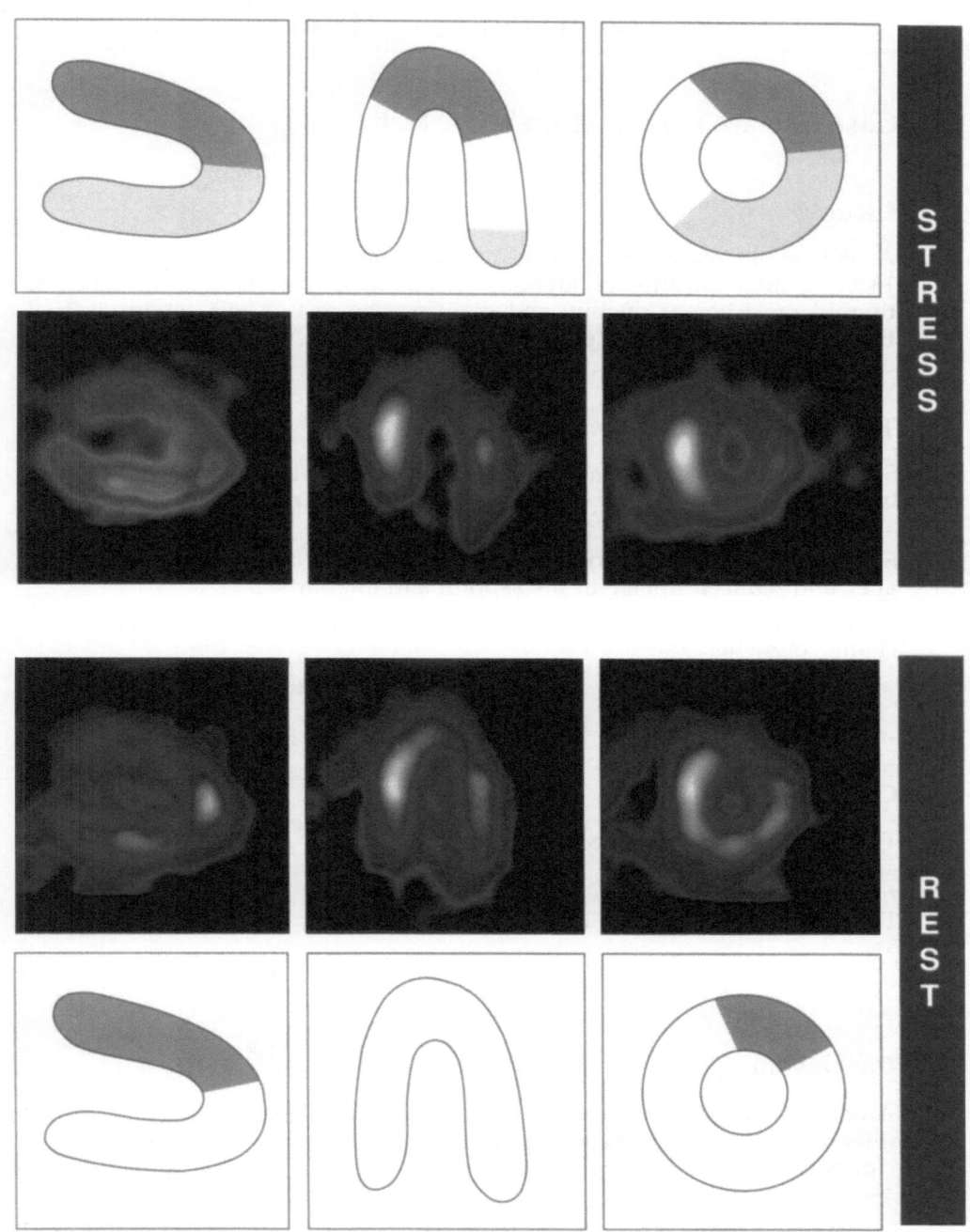

Diabetic patients may suffer significant reversible ischaemia without symptoms.

MIXED REVERSIBLE ISCHAEMIA
AND INFARCTION

Case 31 – LAD Infarction/RCA Ischaemia

History

A 58-year-old man was referred for thallium imaging because of angina 16 years after an anterior myocardial infarction. He was diabetic and on thyroid replacement therapy and digoxin. The resting ECG showed atrial fibrillation and digoxin effect.

Thallium Myocardial Perfusion Tomography

Stress Technique Dobutamine was infused to 20 µg/kg/min and was limited by chest pain. The peak blood pressure and heart rate were 168/74 mmHg and 112/min.

Stress Images There is no uptake of tracer in the distal anterior wall and apex and reduced uptake in the septum and inferior wall.

Rest Images There is improvement in the inferior wall and septum but little change elsewhere.

Coronary Angiography

The proximal left anterior descending artery was occluded and the proximal right coronary artery was stenosed. There was anteroapical akinesis.

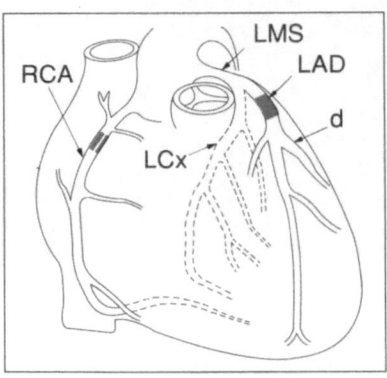

Conclusion

Anterior and apical myocardial infarction with reversible ischaemia of the inferior wall. The reperfusion in the septum is due to supply from the right coronary artery.

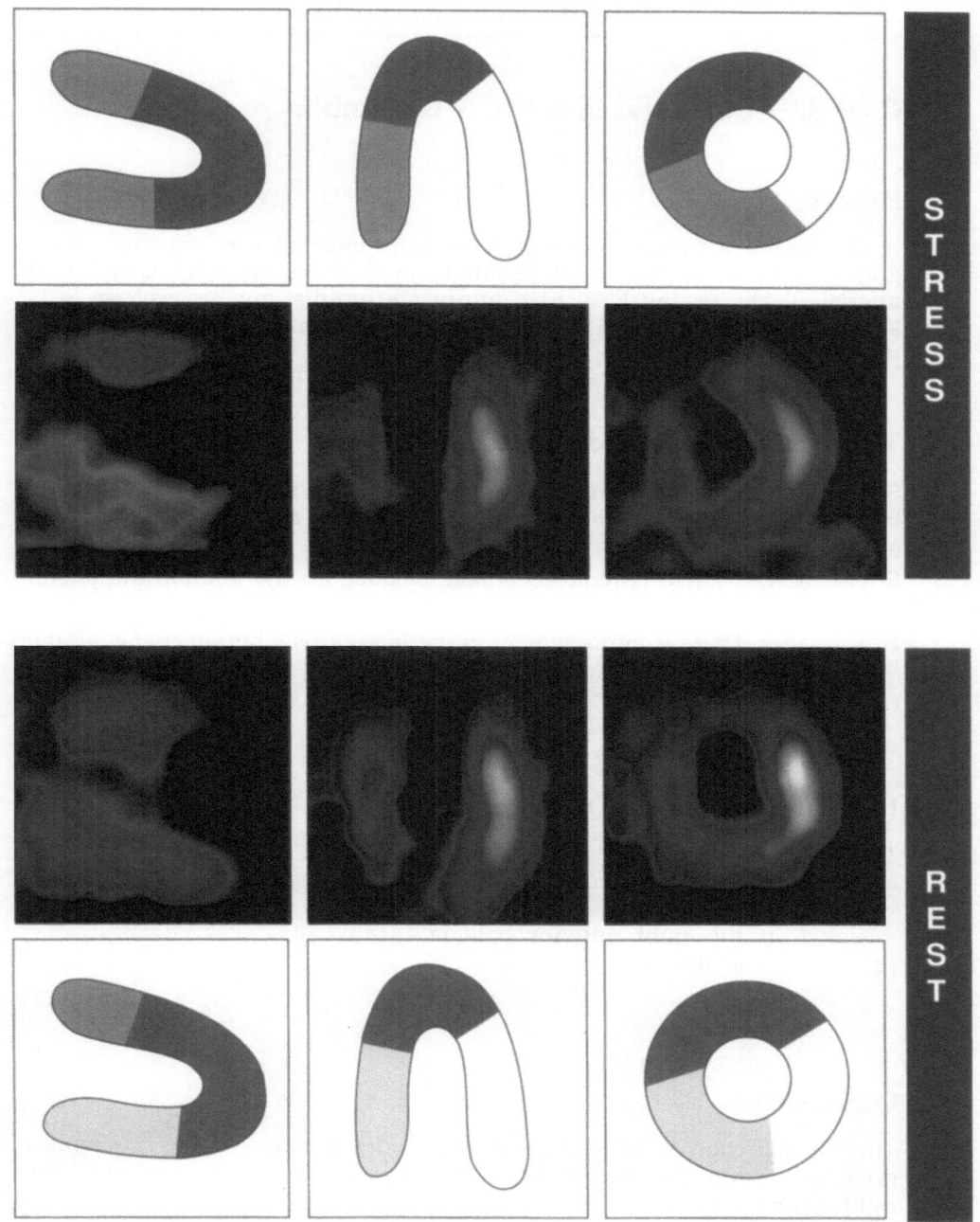

Thallium imaging is a valuable method of assessing ischaemia when the exercise ECG cannot be interpreted because of resting ST segment abnormalities.

MIXED REVERSIBLE ISCHAEMIA
AND INFARCTION

Case 32 – LCx Infarction/RCA Ischaemia

History

A 62-year-old man was referred for thallium imaging and coronary angiography because of the development of angina 7 years after lateral wall infarction. His resting ECG had returned to normal but his exercise ECG showed 3 mm anterior ST depression after 5 min, associated with chest pain.

Thallium Myocardial Perfusion Tomography

Stress Technique Dobutamine was infused to 15 µg/kg/min and was limited by chest pain. The peak blood pressure and heart rate were 158/83 mmHg and 130/min.

Stress Images There is reduced uptake of tracer in the inferior and lateral walls.

Rest Images There is improvement in the inferior wall but no change in the lateral wall.

Coronary Angiography

The left circumflex artery was occluded and the proximal right coronary artery was stenosed. Regional wall motion, assessed in the right anterior oblique projection, was normal.

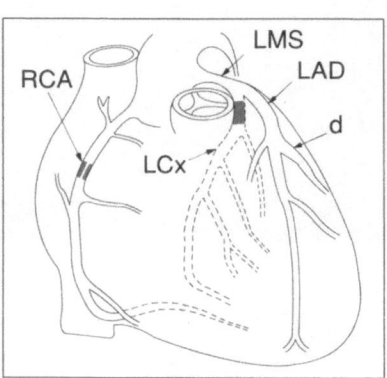

Conclusion

There is infarction of the lateral wall which corresponds to the left circumflex occlusion. Reversible inferior ischaemia is in keeping with disease of the right coronary artery.

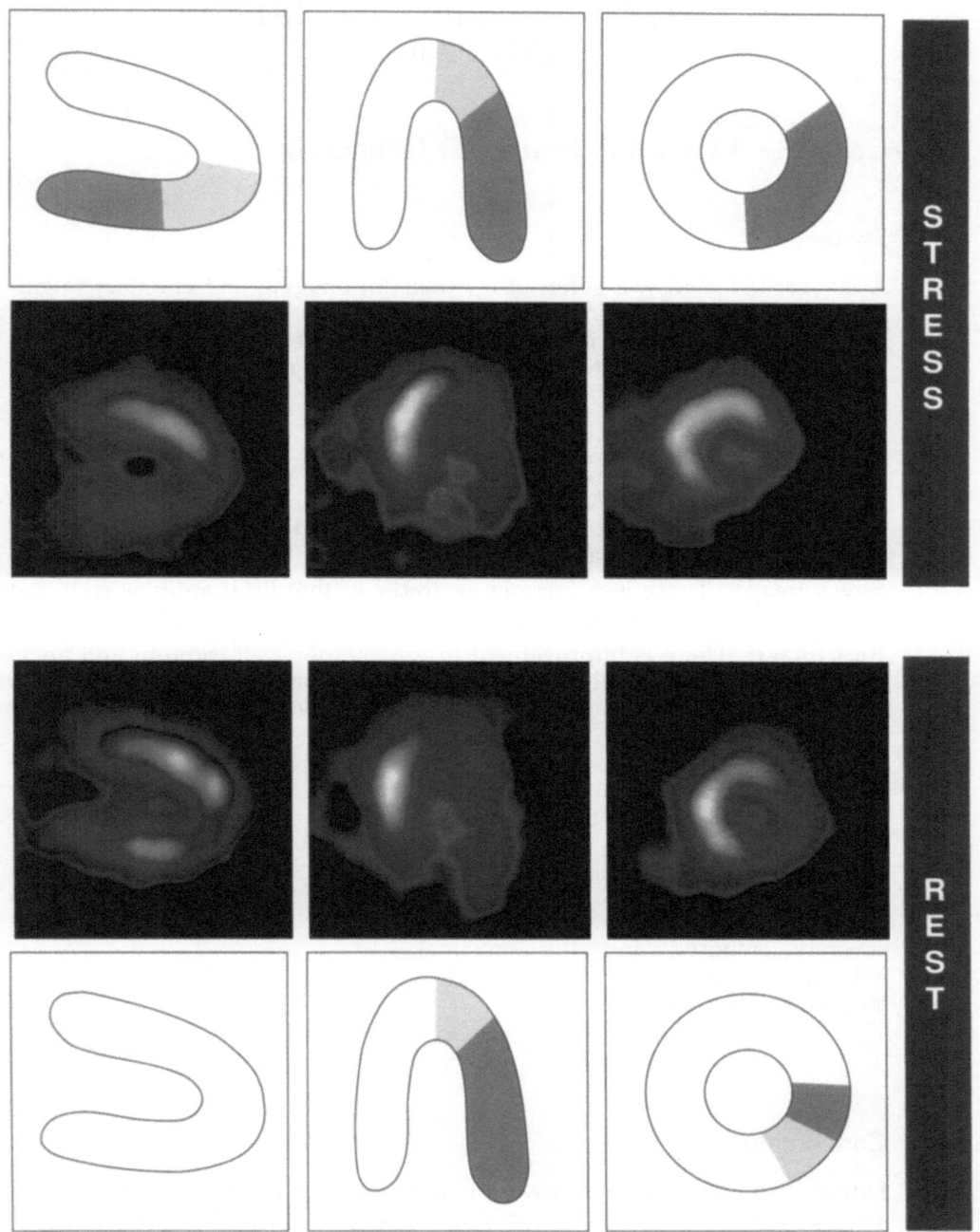

STRESS

REST

The territory of the right coronary and left circumflex arteries overlap. Despite ischaemia in a single myocardial territory, disease of two coronary arteries may be present.

MIXED REVERSIBLE ISCHAEMIA
AND INFARCTION

Case 33 – LCx Infarction/LAD Ischaemia

History

A 60-year-old man was referred for thallium imaging and coronary angio-graphy because of angina after lateral wall infarction. His resting ECG showed T-wave changes in leads 1 and aVl. His exercise ECG showed 3 mm inferior ST depression after 5 min, associated with chest pain.

Thallium Myocardial Perfusion Tomography

Stress Technique Dipyridamole was infused during bicycle exercise to 75 W. Stress was limited by chest pain. The peak blood pressure and heart rate were 150/95 mmHg and 129/min.

Stress Images There is no uptake of tracer in the distal anterior wall and apex, and reduced uptake in the distal septum and lateral wall.

Rest Images There is improvement in the anterior wall, septum and apex, but no improvement in the lateral wall. The appearance of the lateral wall is unusual and review of the planar projections showed patient motion during data acquisition.

Coronary Angiography

The proximal left circumflex artery was severely stenosed and the proximal left anterior descending artery had a long and tight stenosis.

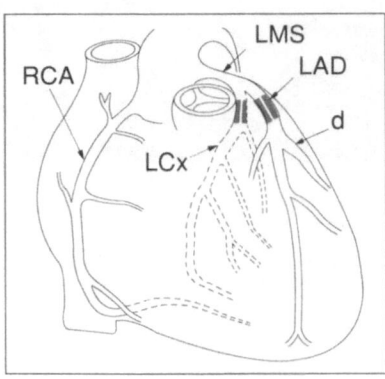

Conclusion

Lateral wall infarction with reversible ischaemia of the anterior wall, septum and apex. The unusual appearance of the lateral wall and the thickening of the inferior wall are the result of patient motion during data acquisition at rest.

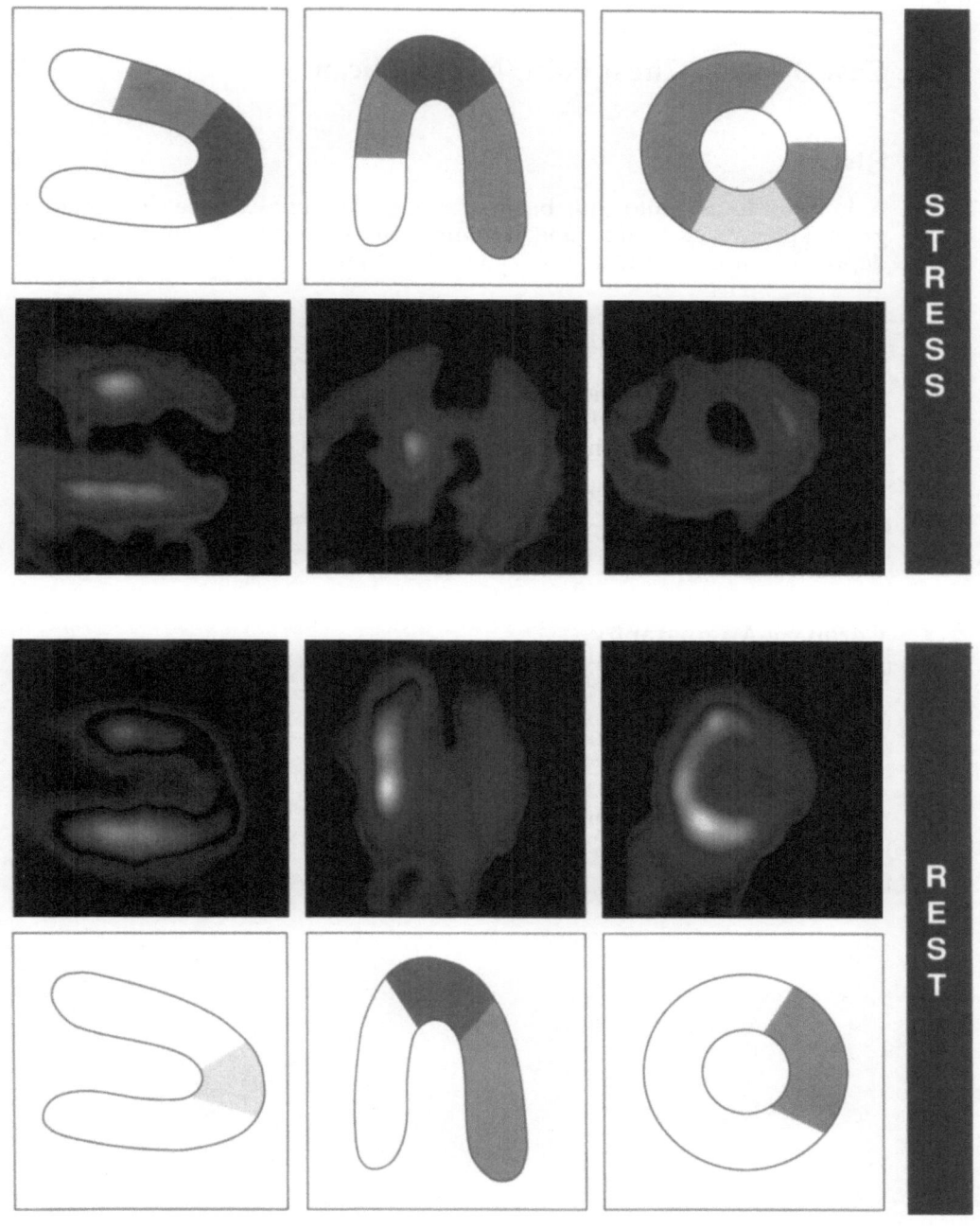

Motion artefact may be recognised from the planar images, but does not always interfere with interpretation of the study.

Case 34 – No Chest Pain, Normal Scan

History

A 44-year-old asymptomatic businessman underwent exercise electrocardiography as part of an insurance examination. There was 3 mm ST segment depression at 12 min with a maximum heart rate of 170/min.

Thallium Myocardial Perfusion Tomography

Stress Technique Dipyridamole was infused during bicycle exercise to 150 W which was limited by leg fatigue without chest pain. At peak stress the blood pressure and the heart rate were 210/100 mmHg and 168/min.

Stress Images The uptake of tracer is normal.

Rest Images Because of the normal stress images, rest imaging was not performed.

Coronary Angiography

This was not performed.

Conclusion

There was no evidence of myocardial ischaemia.

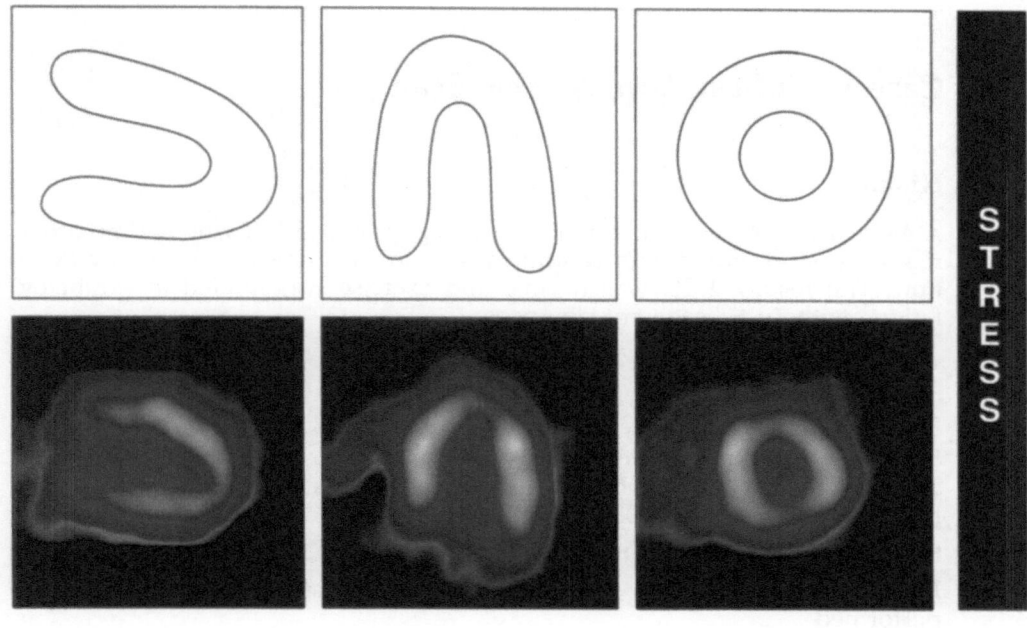

STRESS

Routine exercise ECG in the absence of symptoms is unwarranted but, if an abnormality is encountered, invasive investigation can be avoided with a normal stress thallium scan.

Case 35 – Chest Pain, Normal Scan

History

A 48-year-old obese woman who was a heavy smoker but who had no other risk factors presented with central chest pain sometimes provoked by exertion. The resting ECG was normal and exercise was limited at 4 min by fatigue without ST segment changes.

Thallium Myocardial Perfusion Tomography

Stress Technique Dipyridamole was infused during bicycle exercise to 50 W. Stress was limited by fatigue. At peak stress the blood pressure and the heart rate were 160/100 mmHg and 126/min.

Stress Images Uptake of tracer is normal.

Rest Images Because the stress images were normal, rest imaging was not performed.

Coronary Angiography

This was not performed.

Conclusion

There was no evidence of myocardial ischaemia.

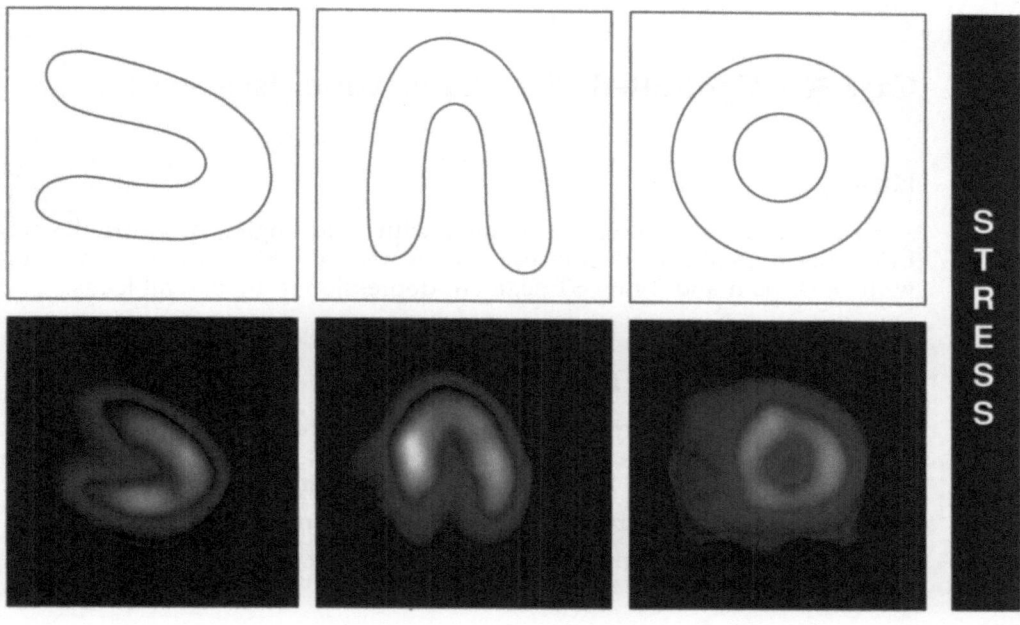

Normal myocardial perfusion during stress is associated with a risk of future cardiac events that is indistinguishable from the normal population.

Case 36 – Controlled Chest Pain, Minor Ischaemia

History

A 55-year-old male smoker presented with mild angina of effort. Resting ECG was normal and during exercise he reached 10 min before stopping with chest pain and 2 mm ST segment depression in the lateral leads.

Thallium Myocardial Perfusion Tomography

Stress Technique Dipyridamole was infused during bicycle exercise to 125 W. Stress was limited by chest pain. At peak stress the blood pressure and the heart rate were 170/95 mmHg and 145/min.

Stress Images There is reduced uptake of tracer in the inferior wall.

Rest Images There is improvement in the inferior wall.

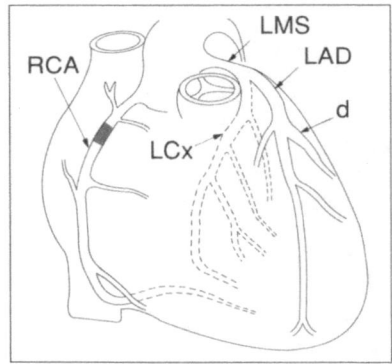

Coronary Angiography

The right coronary artery was occluded. The other vessels were normal.

Conclusion

There is a limited area of reversible ischaemia affecting the inferior wall. Symptoms were abolished on beta-blockers. The patient is being followed.

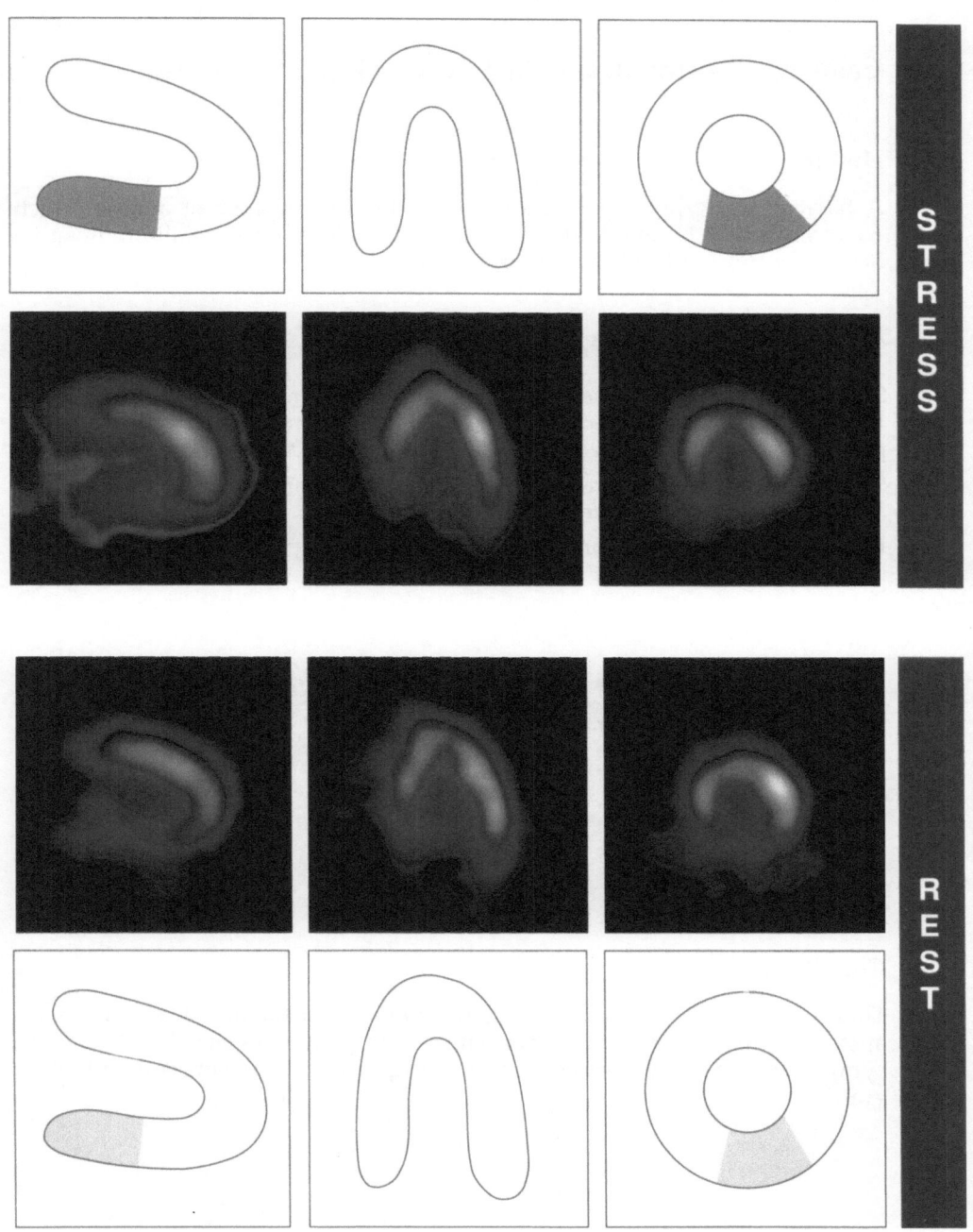

The limited extent of reversible ischaemia implies a good prognosis.

Case 37 – Controlled Chest Pain, Major Ischaemia

History

A 50-year-old hypertensive man with a five-year history of angina which was controlled by medical treatment was referred for thallium imaging because a routine ECG showed inferior Q-waves.

Thallium Myocardial Perfusion Tomography

Stress Technique Dipyridamole was infused during bicycle exercise to 100 W. Stress was limited by fatigue without chest pain. The peak blood pressure and heart rate were 140/105 mmHg and 100/min.

Stress Images There is reduced uptake of tracer in the anterior wall and apex, and also in the inferior wall.

Rest Images There is improvement in all areas except the basal inferior wall.

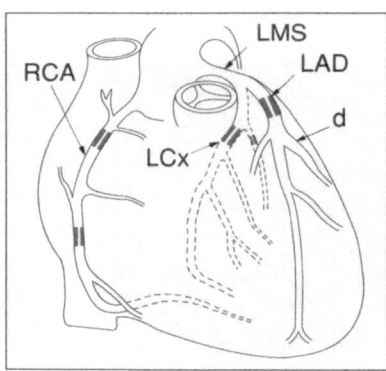

Coronary Angiography

There was significant disease of all three coronary arteries.

Conclusion

There is basal inferior infarction and reversible ischaemia of anterior wall, apex, and inferior wall. The ischaemia is extensive despite the absence of symptoms and he underwent coronary angiography and subsequent bypass grafting.

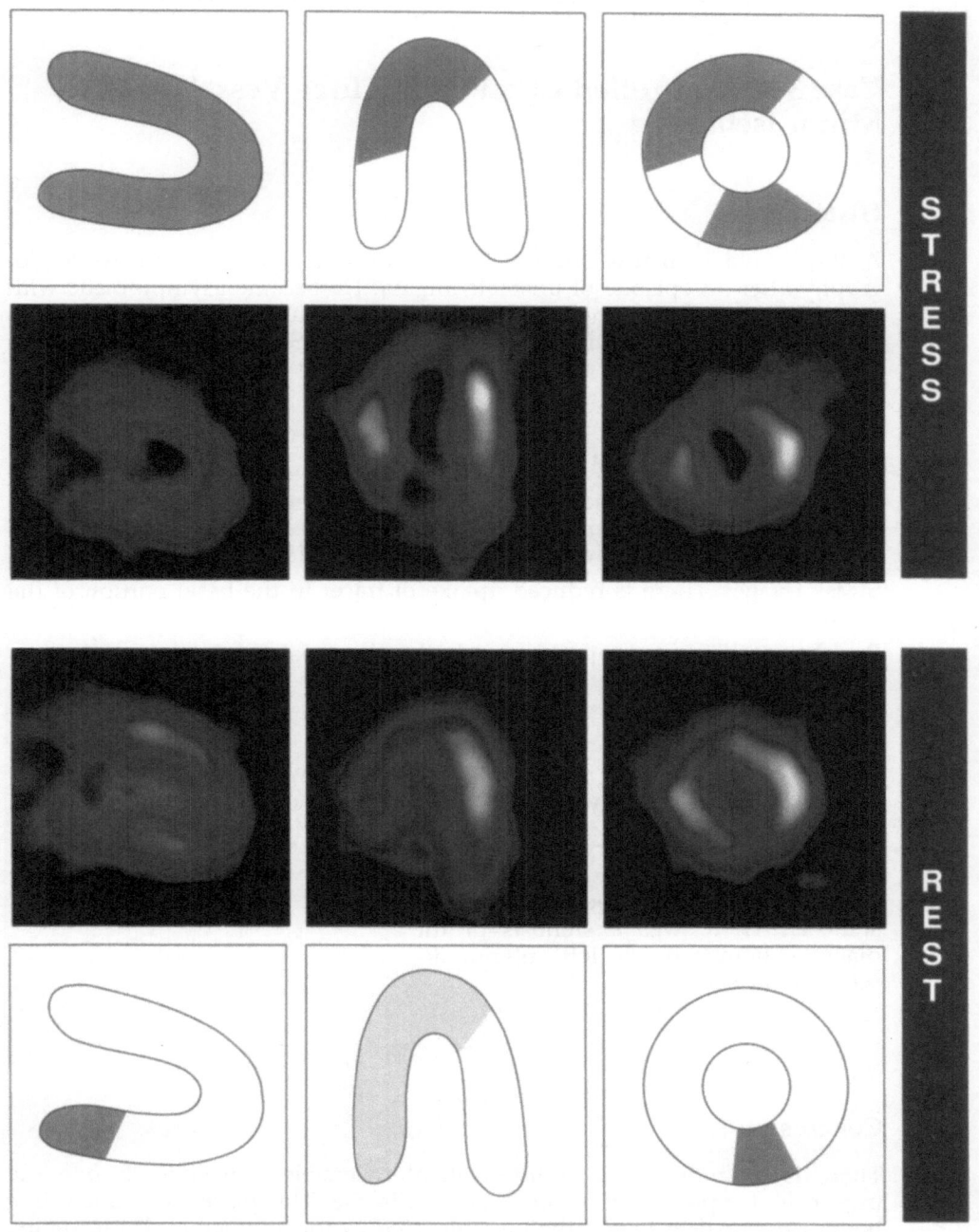

STRESS

REST

In patients with controlled angina, thallium imaging allows the detection of patients at high risk and who warrant invasive investigation.

Case 38 – Controlled Chest Pain, Three Vessel Disease, Minor Ischaemia

History

A 48-year-old man was referred for thallium imaging and coronary angiography after an episode of unstable angina. He became asymptomatic with beta-blockade. The resting ECG was normal and during exercise he reached 8 min before stopping with chest pain and 1 mm ST segment depression in the lateral leads.

Thallium Myocardial Perfusion Tomography

Stress Technique Dipyridamole 40 mg was infused during bicycle exercise to 100 W. Stress was limited by fatigue with chest pain. The peak blood pressure and heart rate were 180/100 mmHg and 154/min respectively.

Stress Images There is reduced uptake of tracer in the basal portion of the inferolateral wall.

Rest Images There is improvement in the abnormal area.

Coronary Angiography

The left circumflex artery was occluded and filled from the right coronary artery which had a moderate proximal stenosis. There was a stenosis of the diagonal branch of the left anterior descending artery.

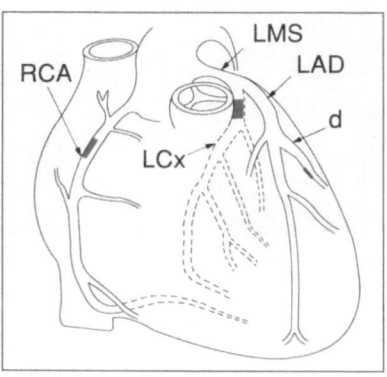

Conclusion

There is a limited area of inferolateral reversible ischaemia despite the presence of triple vessel coronary artery disease. This places the patient in a better prognostic category than is suggested by the angiogram. If the angina can be controlled by medication, surgical intervention may be deferred.

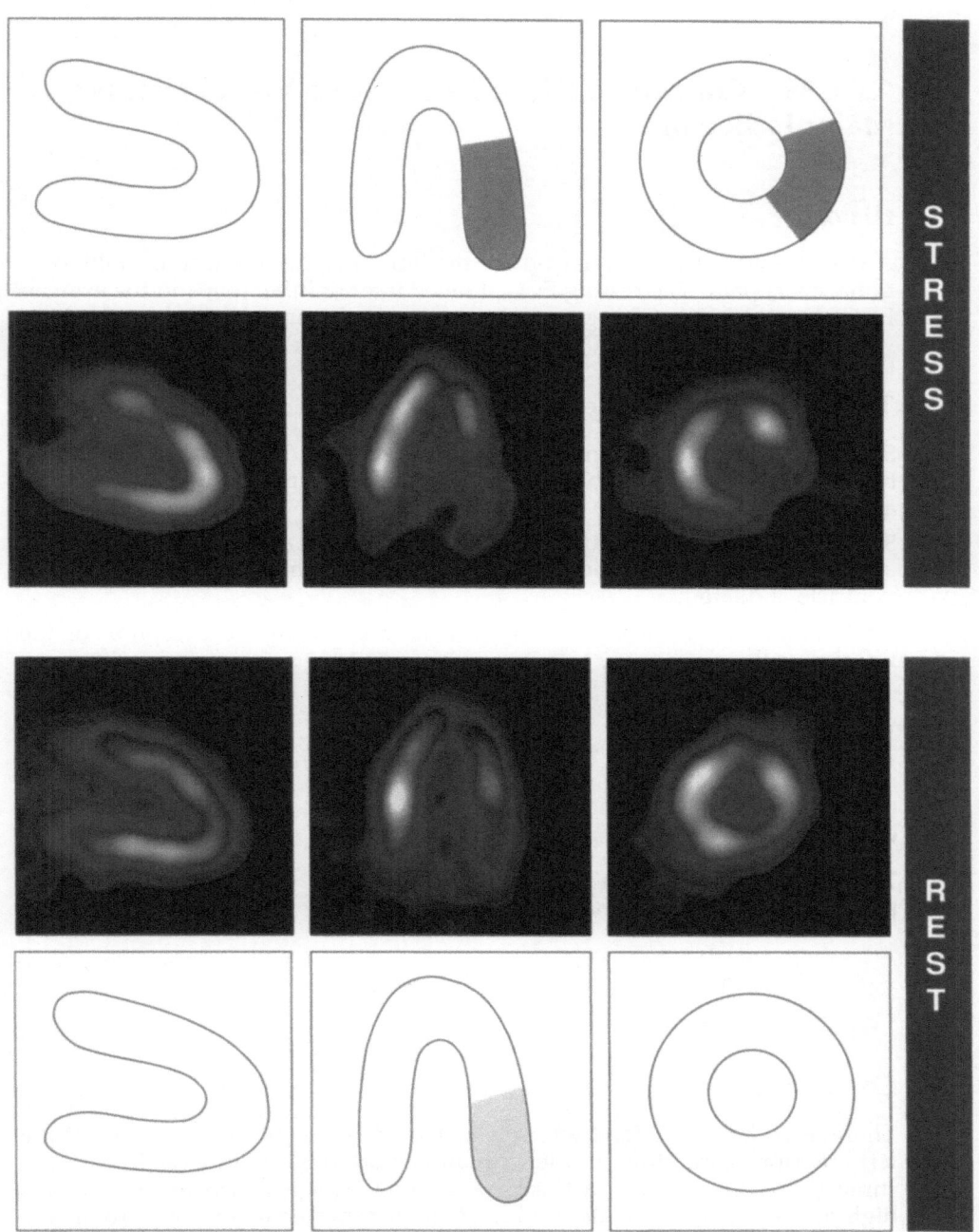

Patients with disease of three vessels may not have ischaemia in all three territories. Prognosis is more closely related to the extent of ischaemia than the number of vessels affected. Contrast with case 39.

Case 39 – Controlled Chest Pain, Three Vessel Disease, Major Ischaemia

History

A 60-year-old man was referred for thallium imaging because of mild exertional chest pain. The resting ECG showed inferior infarction and the exercise ECG showed 3 mm ST segment depression in the anterior leads at 8 min.

Thallium Myocardial Perfusion Tomography

Stress Technique Dobutamine was infused to 20 μg/kg/min and was limited by chest pain. The peak blood pressure and heart rate were 138/64 mmHg and 93/min.

Stress Images There is no uptake of tracer in the apex and inferior walls and reduced uptake in the anterior wall, septum and lateral wall. The left ventricle is dilated.

Rest Images There is improvement in all areas with the exception of the inferior wall.

Coronary Angiography

There were stenoses in the proximal portions of all three coronary arteries.

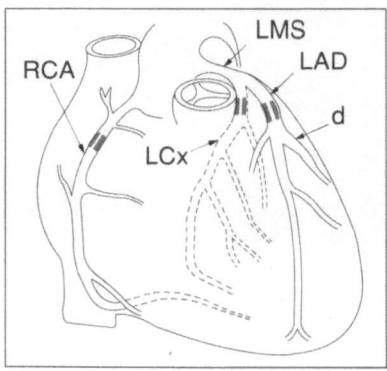

Conclusion

There is an inferior infarct with reversible ischaemia in the territories of the left anterior descending and left circumflex arteries. As in case 38, there is three vessel disease but in this case there is extensive ischaemia. This is a high risk scan and revascularisation would be expected to improve prognosis.

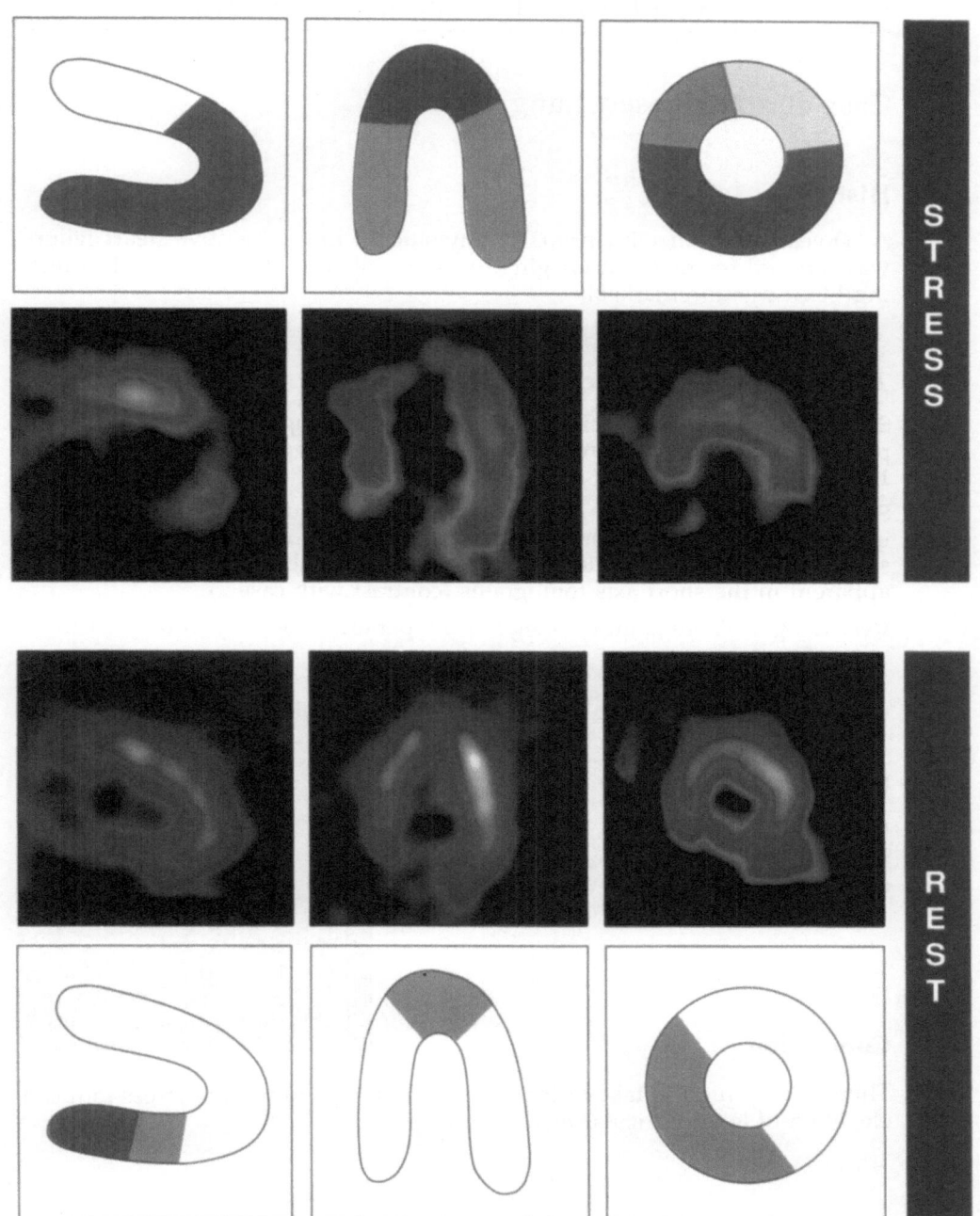

STRESS

REST

Patients with three vessel coronary artery disease do not have a uniformly poor prognosis. The extent of reversible ischaemia is best determined by thallium imaging. Contrast with case 38.

Case 40 – Increased Lung Uptake

History

A 60-year-old man with primary amyloidosis and congestive heart failure was referred for thallium imaging to assess myocardial perfusion. The resting ECG was unremarkable.

Thallium Myocardial Perfusion Tomography

Stress Technique Adenosine was infused to 140 µg/kg/min without chest pain. The peak blood pressure and heart rate were 120/60 mmHg and 100/min.

Stress Images There are minor abnormalities of uptake of tracer in the inferior wall but the pattern is otherwise normal. An anterior planar image showed high uptake of tracer in the lungs (see below) and this is also apparent in the short axis tomograms (contrast with case 2).

Rest Images There is little change in the pattern of activity in the heart.

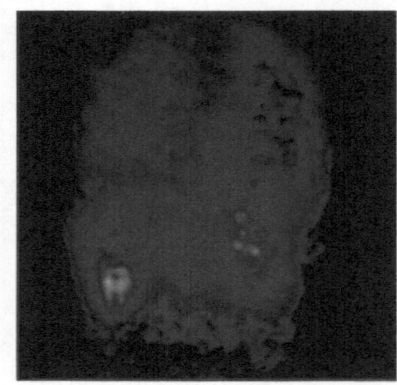

Coronary Angiography

Left ventricular biopsy confirmed amyloid infiltration of the heart without coronary artery disease.

Conclusion

There is very high uptake of thallium in the lungs, indicating stress-induced elevation of left ventricular end-diastolic pressure.

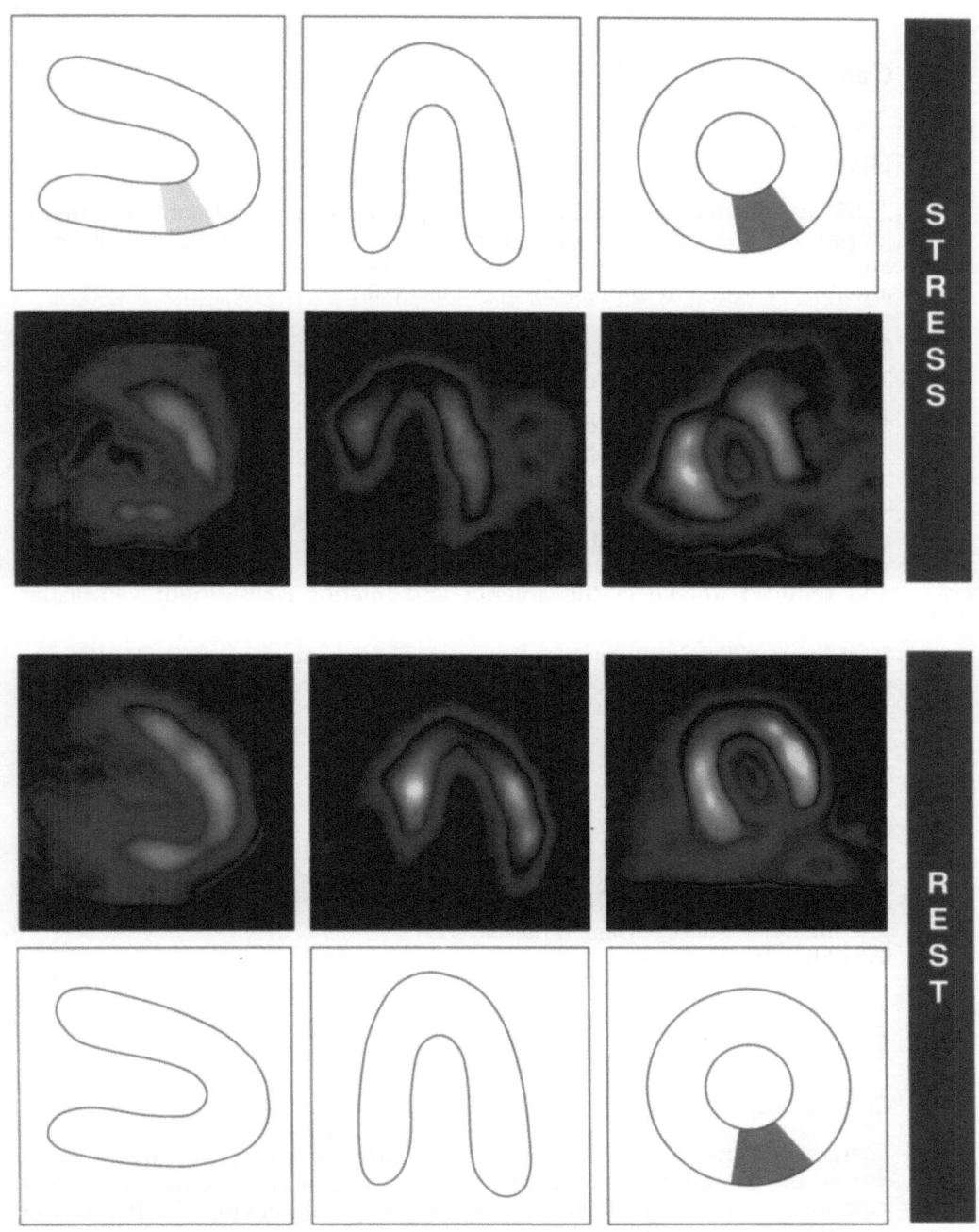

STRESS

REST

In the absence of lung pathology, high uptake of thallium in the lungs is associated with a poor prognosis.

Case 41 – Dilated Left Ventricle on Exercise

History

A 55-year-old man was referred for thallium imaging and coronary angio-graphy because of a 12-month history of angina. His resting ECG showed anterior Q-waves and his exercise ECG was limited at 5 min with 2 mm of anterior ST segment depression and chest pain.

Thallium Myocardial Perfusion Tomography

Stress Technique Dipyridamole was infused during bicycle exercise to 75 W. Stress was limited by chest pain. The peak blood pressure and heart rate were 160/95 mmHg and 130/min.

Stress Images The left ventricle is dilated (*arrows* show size of left ven-tricular cavity). Increased uptake of tracer in the lungs was seen in the planar projections. There is absent uptake of tracer in the apex and septum and reduced uptake in the anterior and inferior walls. Right ventricular uptake is clearly seen.

Rest Images The left ventricle is smaller. There is improvement of uptake in all of the abnormal areas.

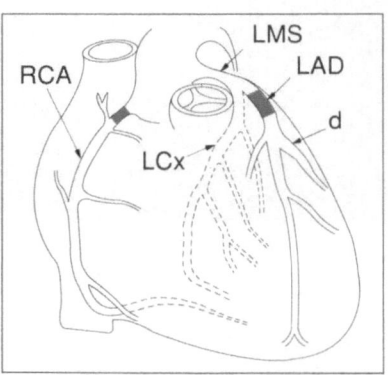

Coronary Angiography

The left anterior descending and right coronary arteries were occluded proximally. There was anteroapical hypokinesis.

Conclusion

There is extensive reversible ischaemia affecting all of the myocardium except the lateral wall. This patient has three indicators of an adverse prognosis: extensive ischaemia, stress-induced dilatation of the left ventricle and increased lung uptake.

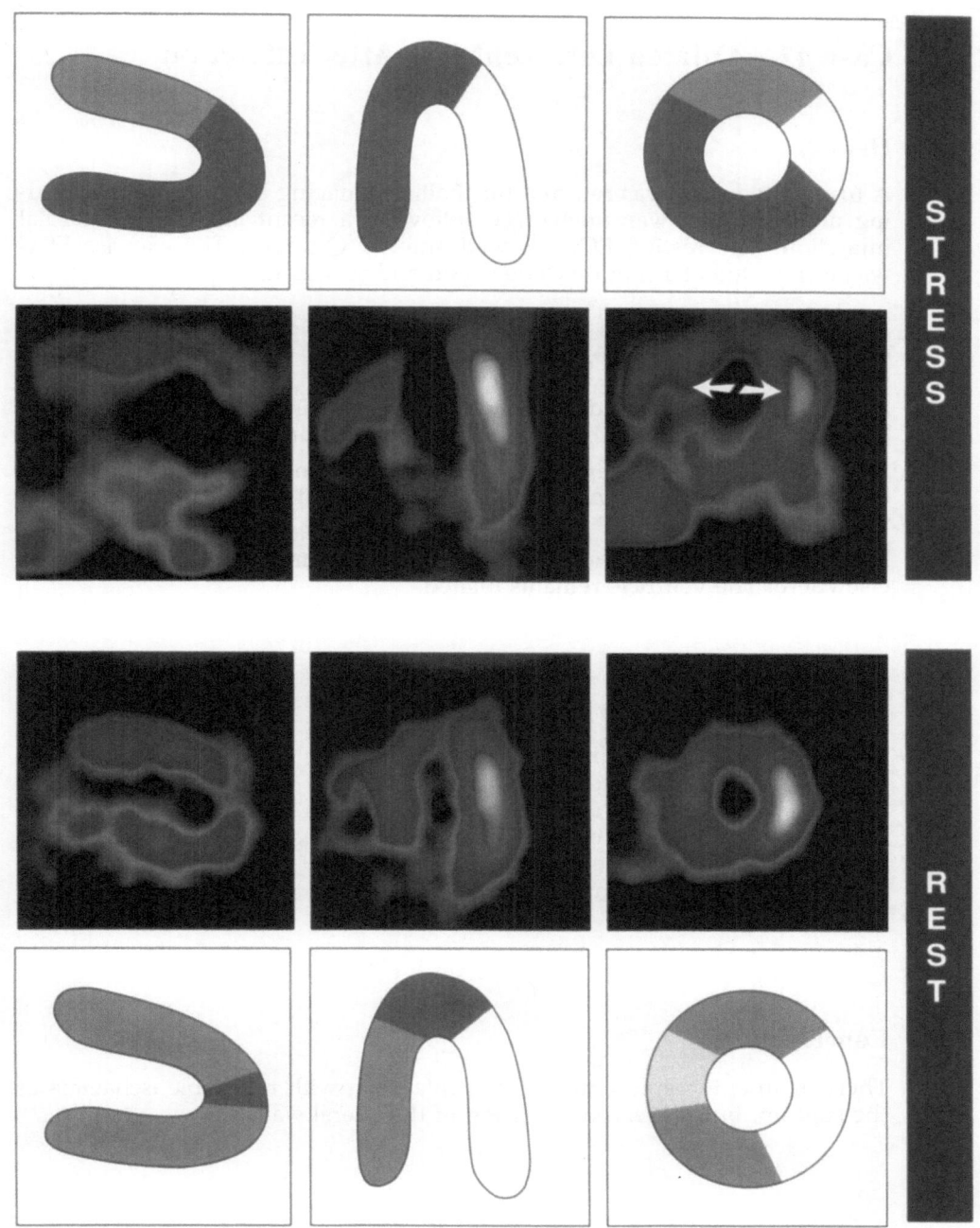

Dilatation of the left ventricle during stress is a poor prognostic sign.

Case 42 – Dilated Left Ventricle After Infarction

History

A 61-year-old man was referred for thallium imaging because of longstanding angina which was unchanged following a recent anterior myocardial infarction. The resting ECG showed anterior Q-waves. The exercise ECG was terminated at 1 min by claudication and so was unhelpful.

Thallium Myocardial Perfusion Tomography

Stress Technique Dipyridamole was infused causing chest pain. The peak blood pressure and heart rate were 140/60 mmHg and 85/min.

Stress Images The left ventricle is dilated. Uptake of tracer in the lungs was increased. There is reduced uptake of tracer in all areas except the lateral wall.

Rest Images There is improvement in the septum, with minor changes elsewhere. The ventricle remains dilated.

Coronary Angiography

The left anterior descending and left circumflex arteries were blocked although a large intermediate (trifurcation) vessel was normal. The right coronary artery was also diseased. The left ventricle was dilated with global hypokinesis and anteroapical akinesis.

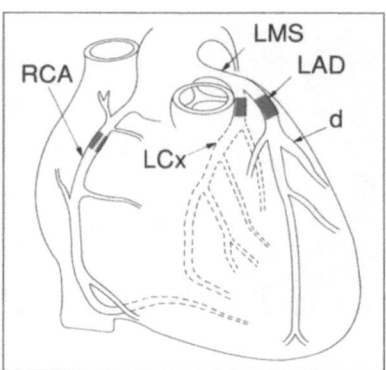

Conclusion

There is an anteroapical and inferior infarction with reversible ischaemia of the septum, but preserved perfusion of the lateral wall.

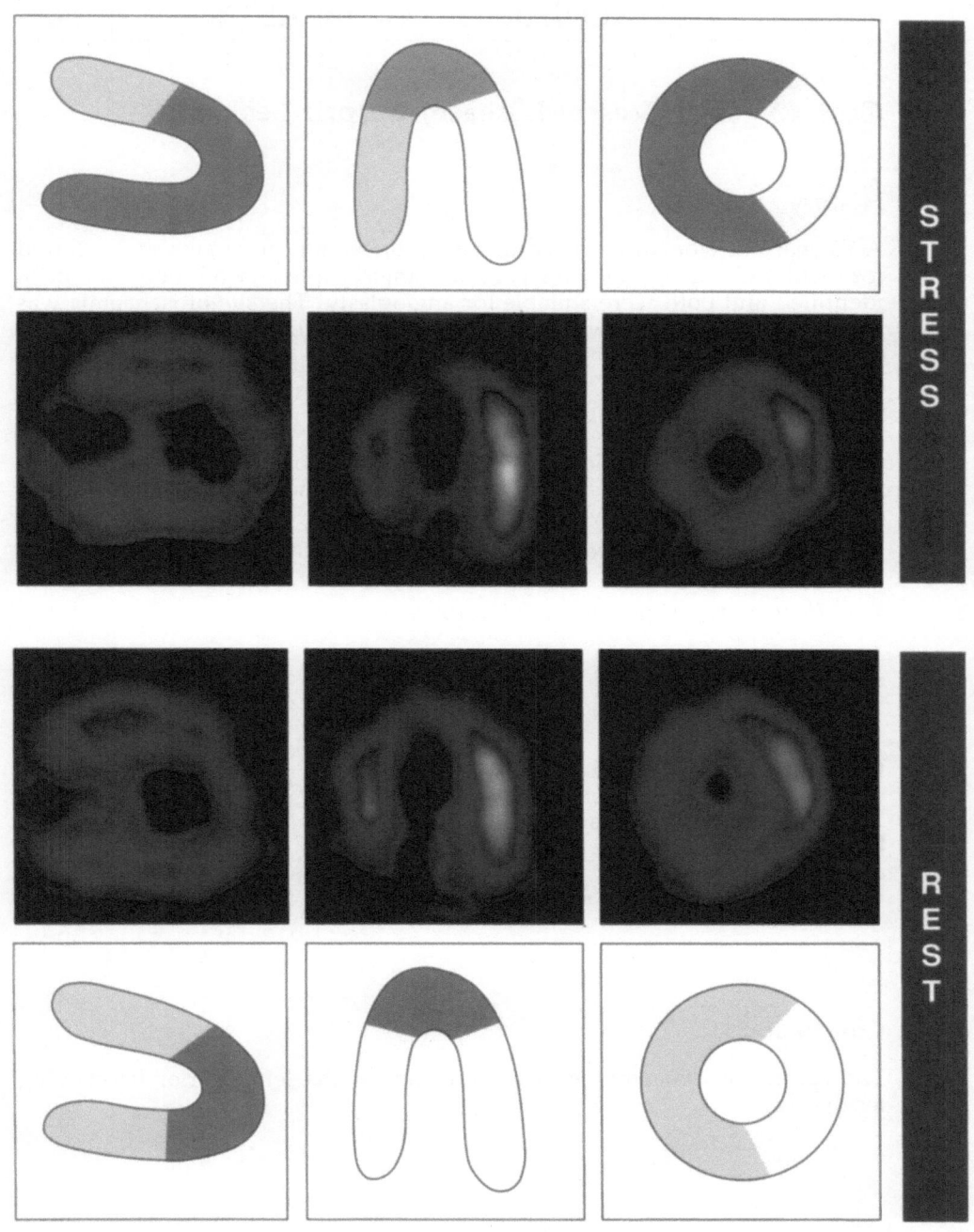

STRESS

REST

Dilatation of the left ventricle at rest is an adverse prognostic sign. Contrast this form of dilatation with the stress-induced dilatation in case 41.

129

CORONARY ANGIOPLASTY

Case 43 – Two Vessel Disease, Culprit Lesion

History

A 73-year-old woman with exertional dyspnoea but no angina was referred for thallium imaging following coronary angiography. Two lesions had been identified and both were suitable for angioplasty. The site of ischaemia was sought in order to plan whether one- or two-vessel dilatation was required.

Thallium Myocardial Perfusion Tomography

Stress Technique Dipyridamole was infused prior to bicycle exercise to 50 W. Exercise was limited by dyspnoea without chest pain. The peak blood pressure and heart rate were 210/100 mmHg and 135/min.

Stress Images There is reduced uptake of tracer in the mid-portion of the anterior wall.

Rest Images The abnormal area improves.

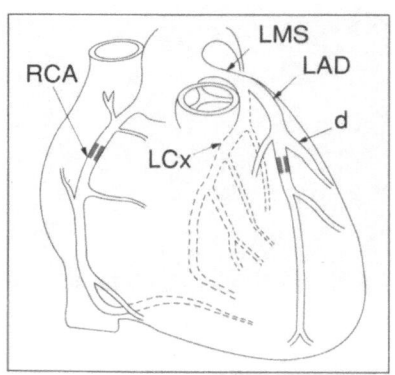

Coronary Angiography

There were 60% stenoses in the left anterior descending and the right coronary artery.

Conclusion

The reversible ischaemia is in the territory of the left anterior descending lesion only.

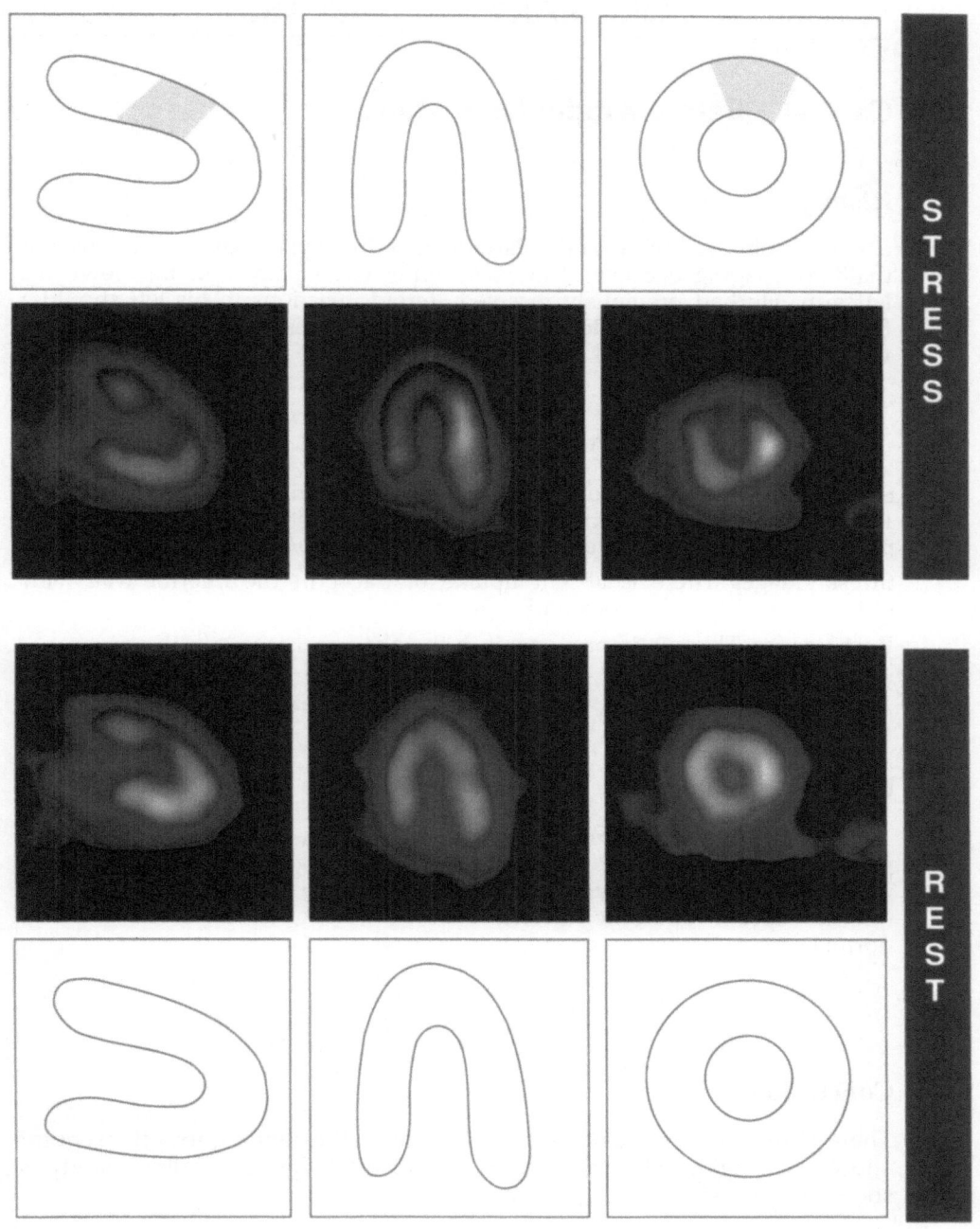

It is difficult to estimate the impairment of coronary flow from the appearance of the arteriogram, particularly if the stenosis is only moderate. Thallium imaging can be used to guide interventional procedures.

Case 44 – Before Angioplasty Study

History

A 48-year-old man with Wolff–Parkinson–White syndrome was referred for thallium imaging because of atypical upper chest pain radiating down his left arm. He had previously received steroid injections to his left shoulder for the same complaint. Because of the abnormal resting ECG, exercise was not performed.

Thallium Myocardial Perfusion Tomography

Stress Technique Dipyridamole was infused during bicycle exercise to 100 W. Stress was limited by dyspnoea with chest pain. The peak blood pressure and heart rate were 140/90 mmHg and 100/min.

Stress Images There is absent uptake of tracer in the inferior wall with reduced uptake in the apex and septum.

Rest Images There is improvement in the abnormal areas.

Coronary Angiography

There was a tight stenosis of the proximal right coronary artery which was a large vessel supplying part of the inferior septum. The other arteries were normal.

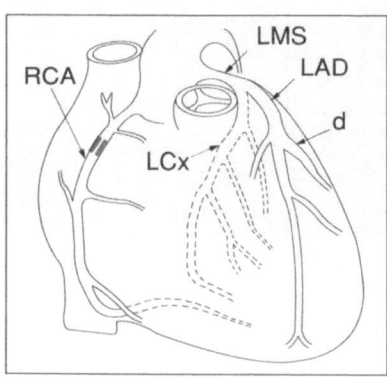

Conclusion

There is reversible ischaemia of the inferior wall extending into the septum and apex. Angioplasty was performed and the follow-up thallium study is shown in case 45.

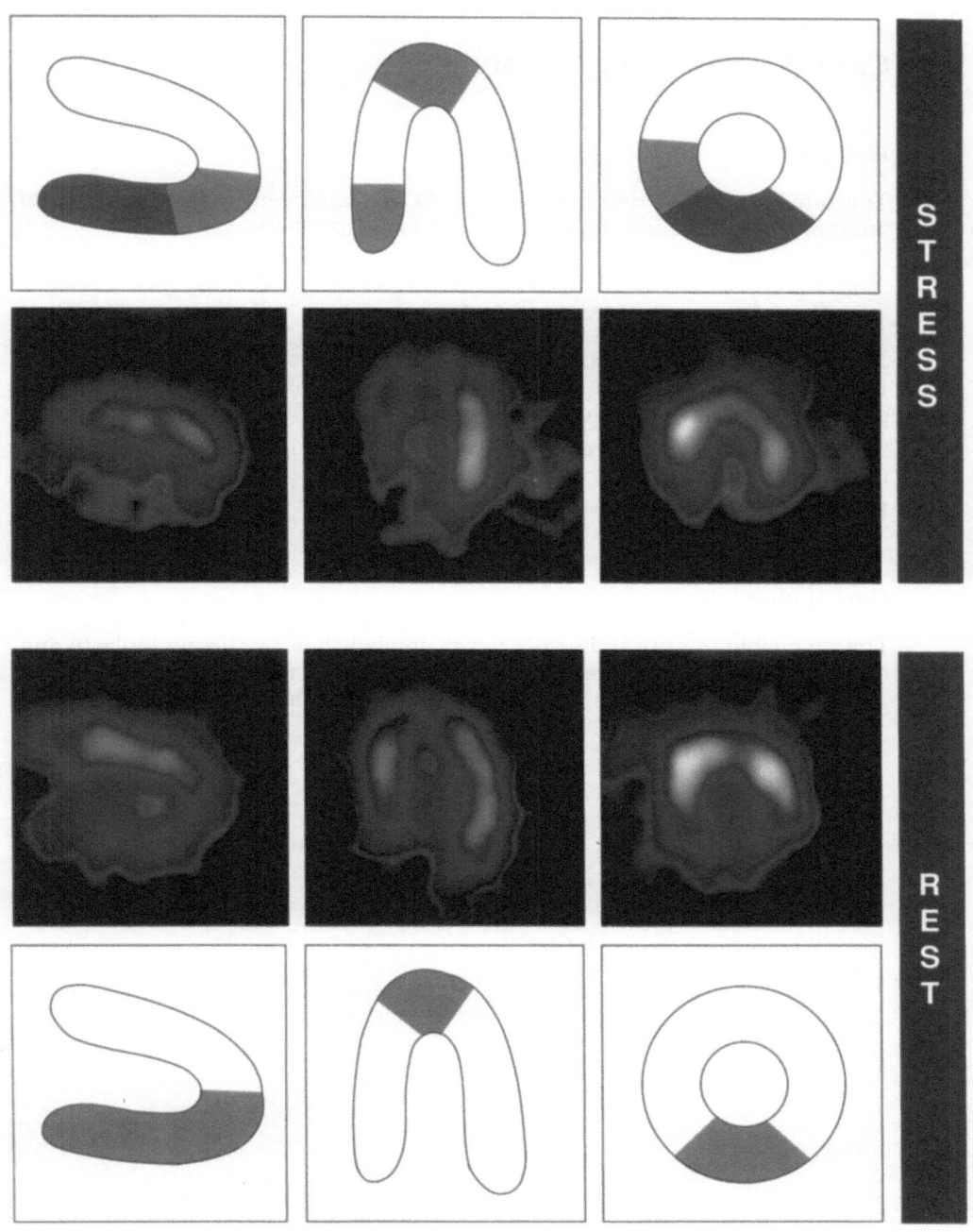

STRESS

REST

Thallium imaging should be performed before intervention as a guide for future management.

Case 45 – After Angioplasty Study

History

The same patient as described in case 44 was followed-up six months after angioplasty by thallium imaging. He was asymptomatic.

Thallium Myocardial Perfusion Tomography

Stress Technique Dipyridamole was infused during bicycle exercise to 125 W. Stress was limited by leg fatigue without chest pain. The peak blood pressure and heart rate were 166/88 mmHg and 143/min.

Stress Images There is reduced uptake of tracer in the apex but normal inferior wall uptake.

Rest Images There is improvement in the apex.

Conclusion

The reversible inferior ischaemia has been abolished by the angioplasty and exercise tolerance has improved (double product increasing from 14.0 to 23.2 $\times$ 10^3 mmHg/min). There is some residual reversible ischaemia of the apex.

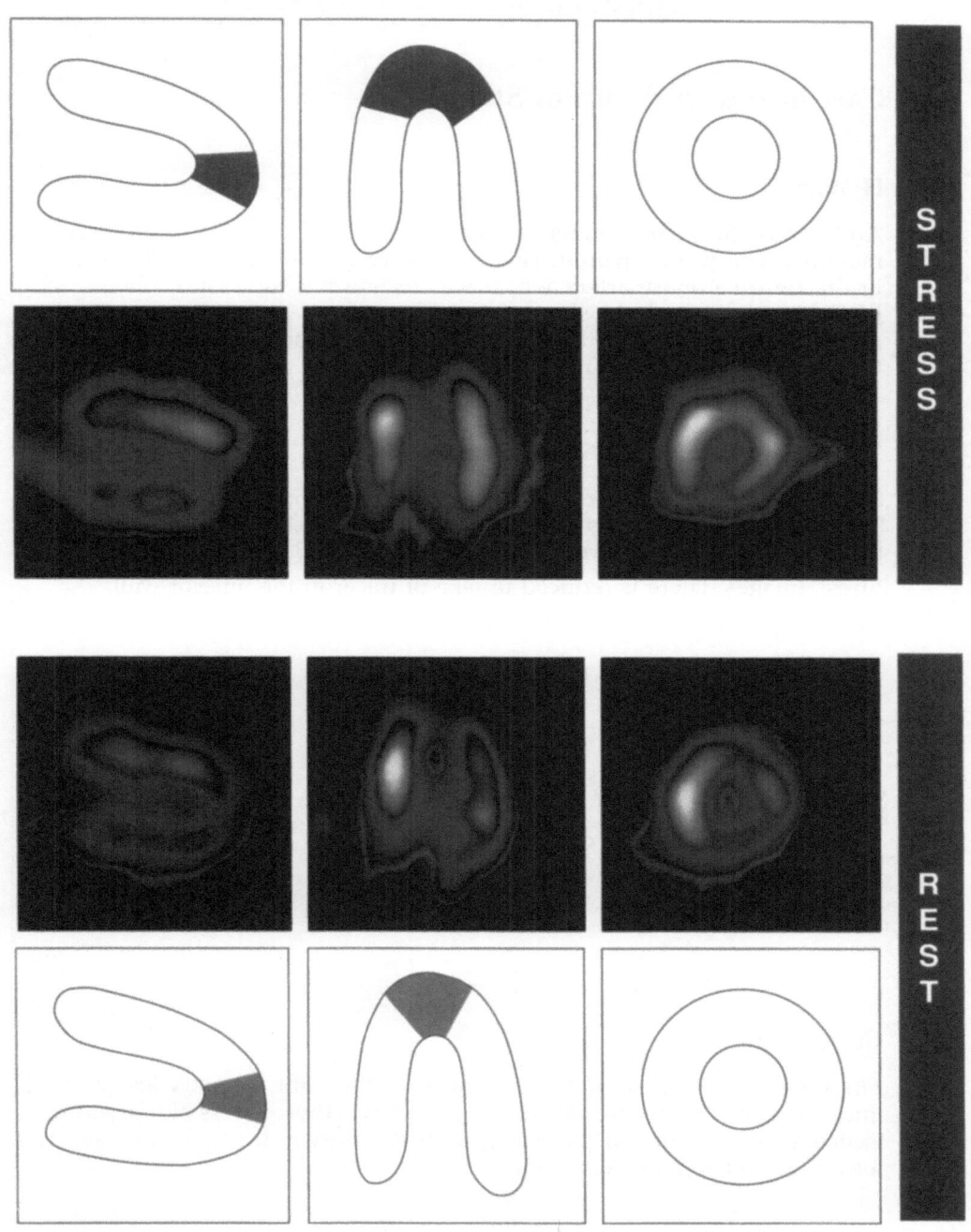

STRESS

REST

Objective evidence of improved perfusion after angioplasty can be obtained by thallium imaging.

Case 46 – Recurrence of Stenosis

History

An 80-year-old woman underwent thallium imaging because of the development of atypical chest pain three months after angioplasty of an 80% stenosis in the right coronary artery which was technically successful. The exercise ECG before angioplasty showed no ST segment changes at 6 min. Two months after angioplasty there were still no ST segment changes and exercise time had reduced to 4 min, limited by fatigue.

Thallium Myocardial Perfusion Tomography

Stress Technique Dipyridamole was infused prior to bicycle exercise to 50 W. Stress was limited by fatigue without chest pain. The peak blood pressure and heart rate were 160/80 mmHg and 111/min.

Stress Images There is reduced uptake of tracer in the inferior wall.

Rest Images The abnormal area improves.

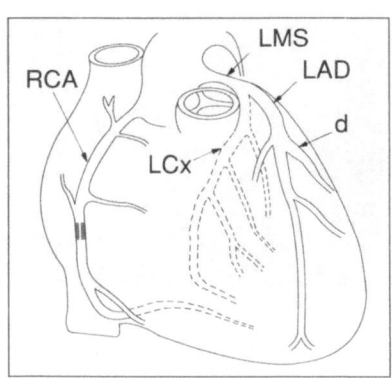

Coronary Angiography

The stenosis of the right coronary artery had recurred.

Conclusion

The inferior ischaemia implies restenosis of the right coronary lesion. Thallium imaging is useful in determining whether reversible myocardial ischaemia is present and if it relates to the territory of the treated vessel. The lesion was dilated a second time.

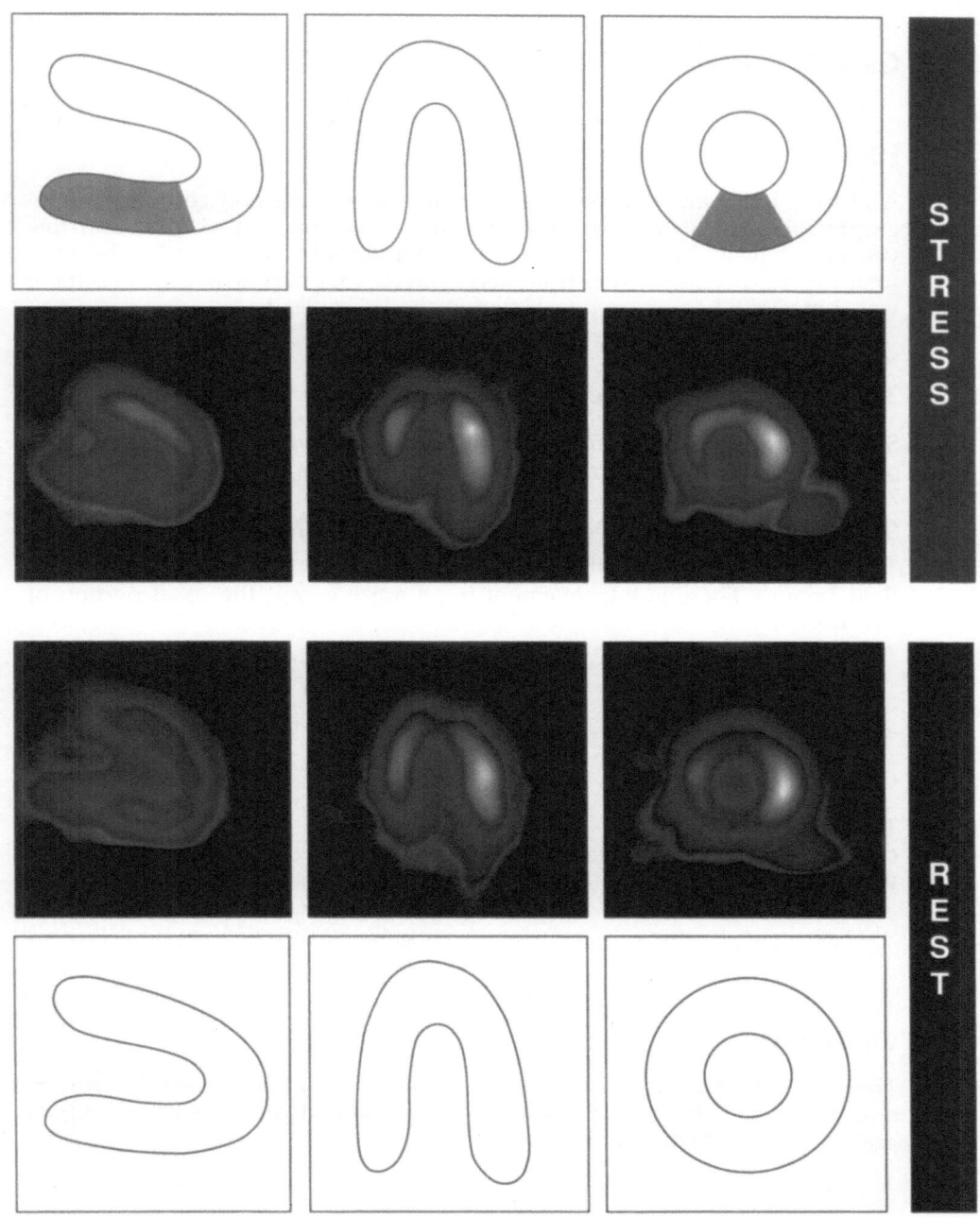

One-third of stenoses recur within six months of angioplasty and may present with atypical pain.

Case 47 – Preoperative Study

History

A 65-year-old man was referred for thallium imaging and coronary angiography because of angina following an inferior myocardial infarction five years previously. The resting ECG showed inferior Q-waves. He had bilateral total hip replacements which limited exercise to 4 min at which time there was 3 mm of ST segment depression in the lateral leads.

Thallium Myocardial Perfusion Tomography

Stress Technique Dobutamine was infused to 20 µg/kg/min and was limited by chest pain. At peak stress the blood pressure and heart rate were 160/78 mmHg and 112/min.

Stress Images There is reduced uptake of tracer in the anterior wall and apex, and in the inferior and lateral walls.

Rest Images There is improvement in all areas except the basal portion of the inferior wall.

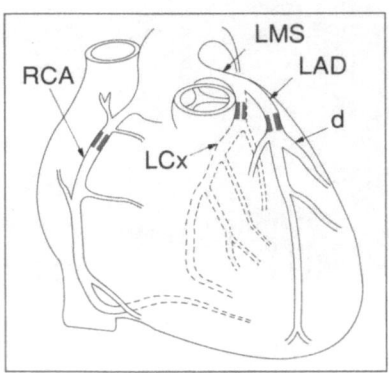

Coronary Angiography

The proximal portions of all three coronary arteries were stenosed. There was inferior hypokinesis.

Conclusion

There is extensive reversible ischaemia suggesting three vessel coronary artery disease. This indicates a poor prognosis and coronary artery bypass grafting was undertaken. See case 48.

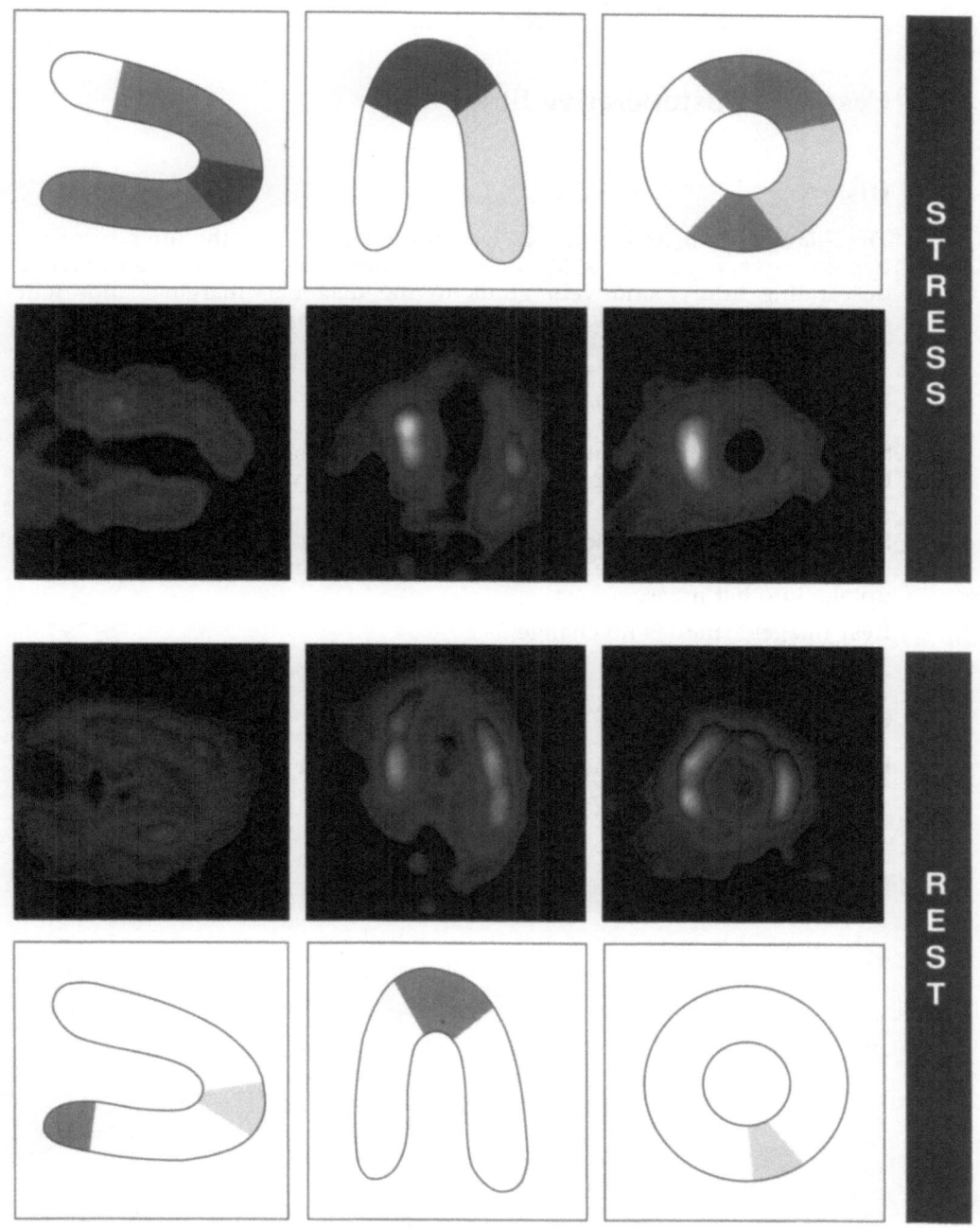

Thallium imaging reveals the extent of ischaemia prior to coronary artery bypass grafting and is useful as a baseline for follow-up.

Case 48 – Postoperative Study

History

The same patient as in case 47 was restudied six months after coronary bypass surgery. He had a left internal mammary graft to the left anterior descending artery, and vein grafts to the diagonal, marginal and right coronary arteries. He was asymptomatic.

Thallium Myocardial Perfusion Tomography

Stress Technique Dobutamine was infused to 20 µg/kg/min without symptoms. The peak blood pressure and heart rate were 165/85 mmHg and 115/min.

Stress Images The ventricle is not as dilated as in the preoperative study. There is reduced uptake of tracer in the basal inferior wall but normal uptake in other areas.

Rest Images There is no change.

Conclusion

Basal inferior infarction but good perfusion in other areas.

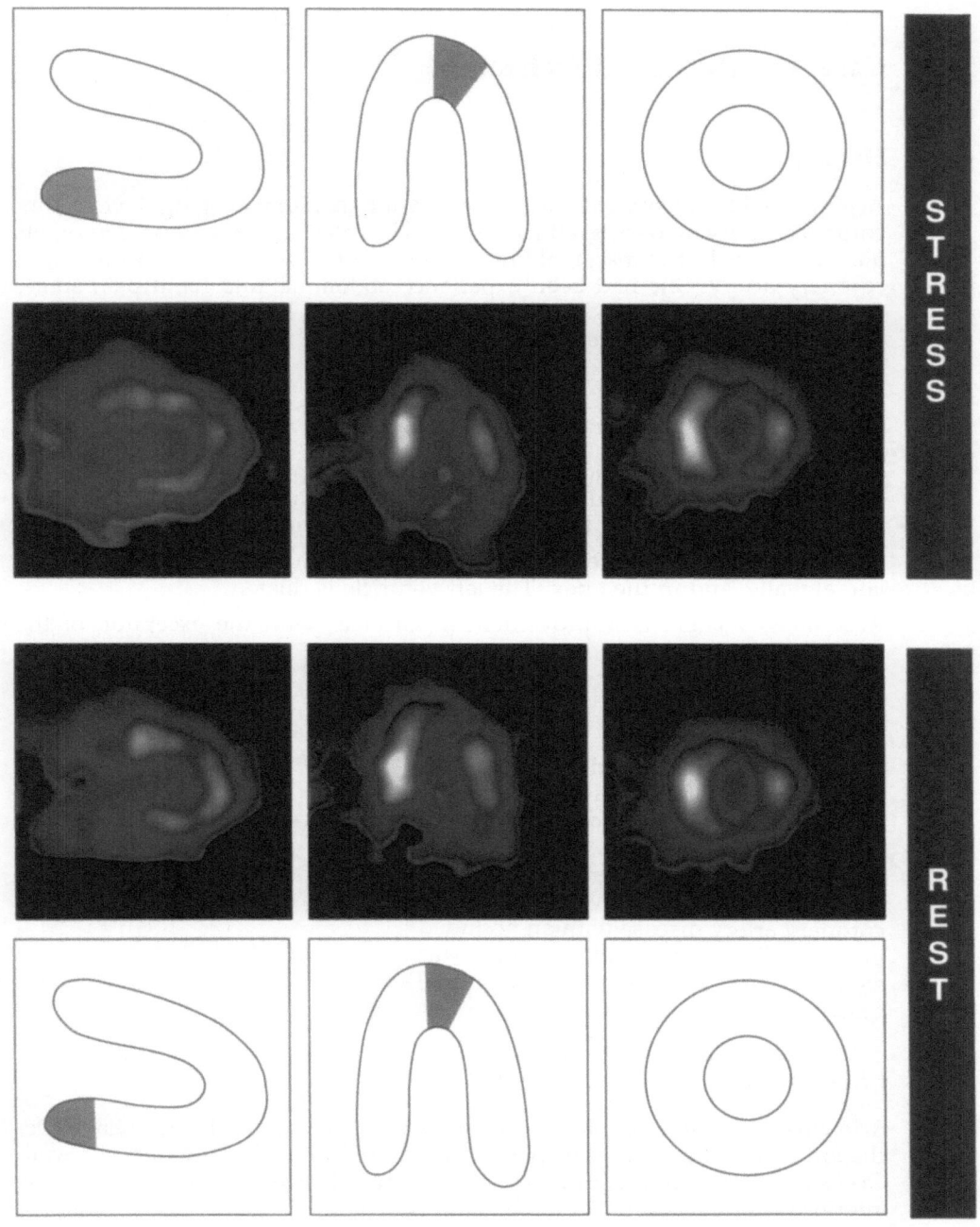

Thallium imaging can be used to confirm the abolition of ischaemia after bypass surgery.

Case 49 – Recurrent Ischaemia

History

A 60-year-old diabetic lady was referred for thallium imaging 1 year after coronary artery bypass grafting to the left anterior descending artery, its diagonal branch, the marginal branch of the circumflex artery, and the right coronary artery. She had been experience abdominal and hand pain sometimes related to exercise. The resting ECG showed left bundle branch block and her exercise tolerance was poor.

Thallium Myocardial Perfusion Tomography

Stress Technique Dipyridamole was infused prior to bicycle exercise to 50 W. Stress was limited by fatigue with abdominal and hand pain. The peak blood pressure and heart rate were 170/90 mmHg and 125/min.

Stress Images There is reduced uptake of tracer in the anterior and inferolateral walls, and in the apex. The left ventricle is dilated.

Rest Images There is improvement in all areas with the exception of the mid-portion of the anterior wall.

Coronary Angiography

The left anterior descending artery was occluded distal to the diagonal branch which was stenosed and to which the vein graft had occluded. The distal left anterior descending artery filled from a patent vein graft. There was native right coronary artery disease with an occluded graft. The left circumflex artery was stenosed but with a patent marginal graft.

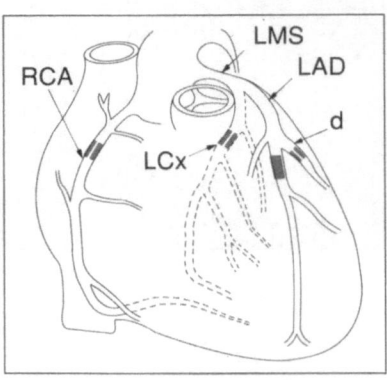

Conclusion

Extensive reversible ischaemia of the anterior and inferolateral walls. Occlusion of the diagonal graft has led to infarction in the mid-anterior wall. Occlusion of the right coronary graft has caused reversible ischaemia of the inferior wall.

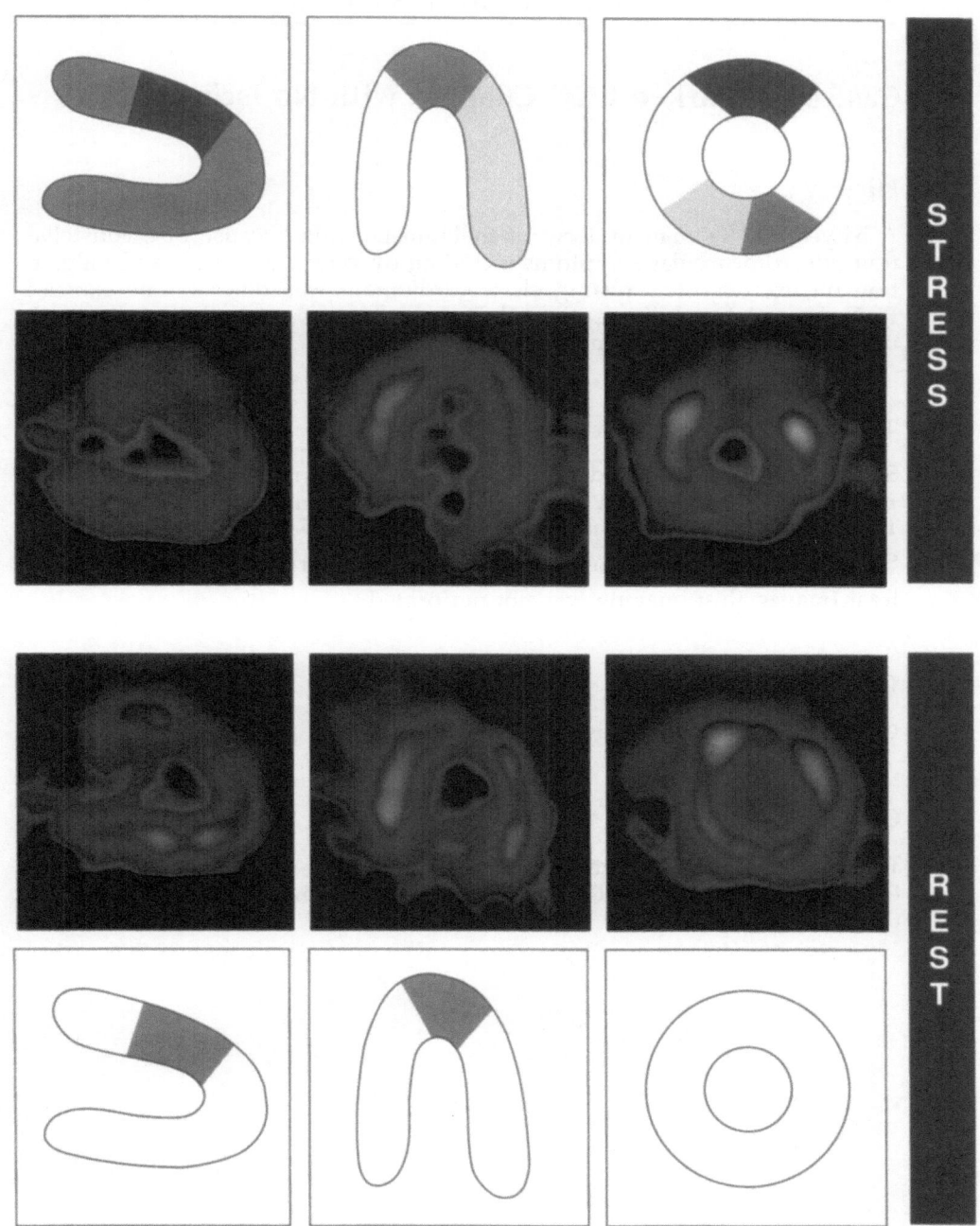

STRESS

REST

Thallium imaging is useful for the follow-up of patients after coronary artery bypass grafting. Diabetic patients may have atypical manifestations of myocardial ischaemia.

Case 50 – Marked ECG Changes with No Ischaemia

History

A 54-year-old woman underwent thallium imaging because of a constellation of cardiovascular symptoms including dyspnoea, faintness and palpitation on exercise. The resting electrocardiogram was normal. The exercise ECG showed 2 mm of inferolateral ST depression after 10 min despite a lack of symptoms other than fatigue.

Thallium Myocardial Perfusion Tomography

Stress Technique Dipyridamole was infused during bicycle exercise to 100 W. Stress was limited by palpitation and giddiness without chest pain. The peak blood pressure and heart rate were 150/95 mmHg and 124/min.

Stress Images The pattern of uptake of tracer is normal.

Rest Images Rest imaging was not performed.

Coronary Angiography

Coronary angiography was normal.

Conclusion

There is no significant myocardial ischaemia despite the symptoms. Despite the abnormal exercise ECG, the probability of coronary artery disease after thallium imaging was low.

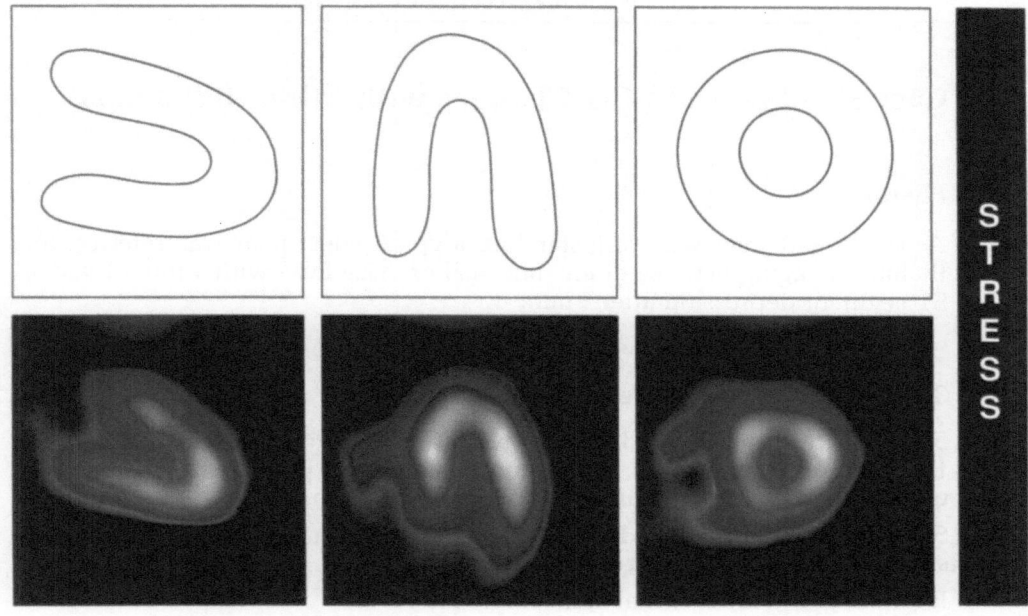

Exercise electrocardiography has a poorer specificity (approximately 70%) than thallium emission tomography (approximately 90%) for the detection of coronary artery disease.

Case 51 – Marked ECG Changes with Minor Ischaemia

History

A 54-year-old man with longstanding atypical chest pain was referred for thallium imaging because of an abnormal exercise ECG with 4 mm of lateral ST segment depression after 9 min.

Thallium Myocardial Perfusion Tomography

Stress Technique Dipyridamole was infused during bicycle exercise to 125 W. Stress was limited by fatigue without chest pain. Peak blood pressure and heart rate were 210/110 mmHg and 135/min.

Stress Images There is reduced uptake of tracer in the basal portions of the septum and of the inferior and lateral walls.

Rest Images The abnormal areas improve.

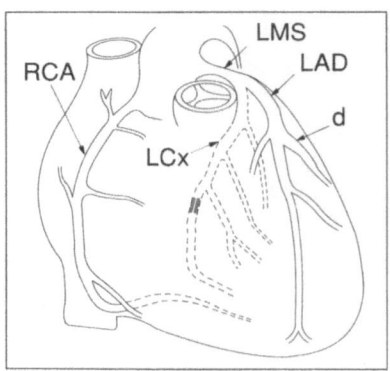

Coronary Angiography

There was a stenosis in the distal left circumflex artery.

Conclusion

There is minor reversible ischaemia of the basal septum and basal inferior and lateral walls.

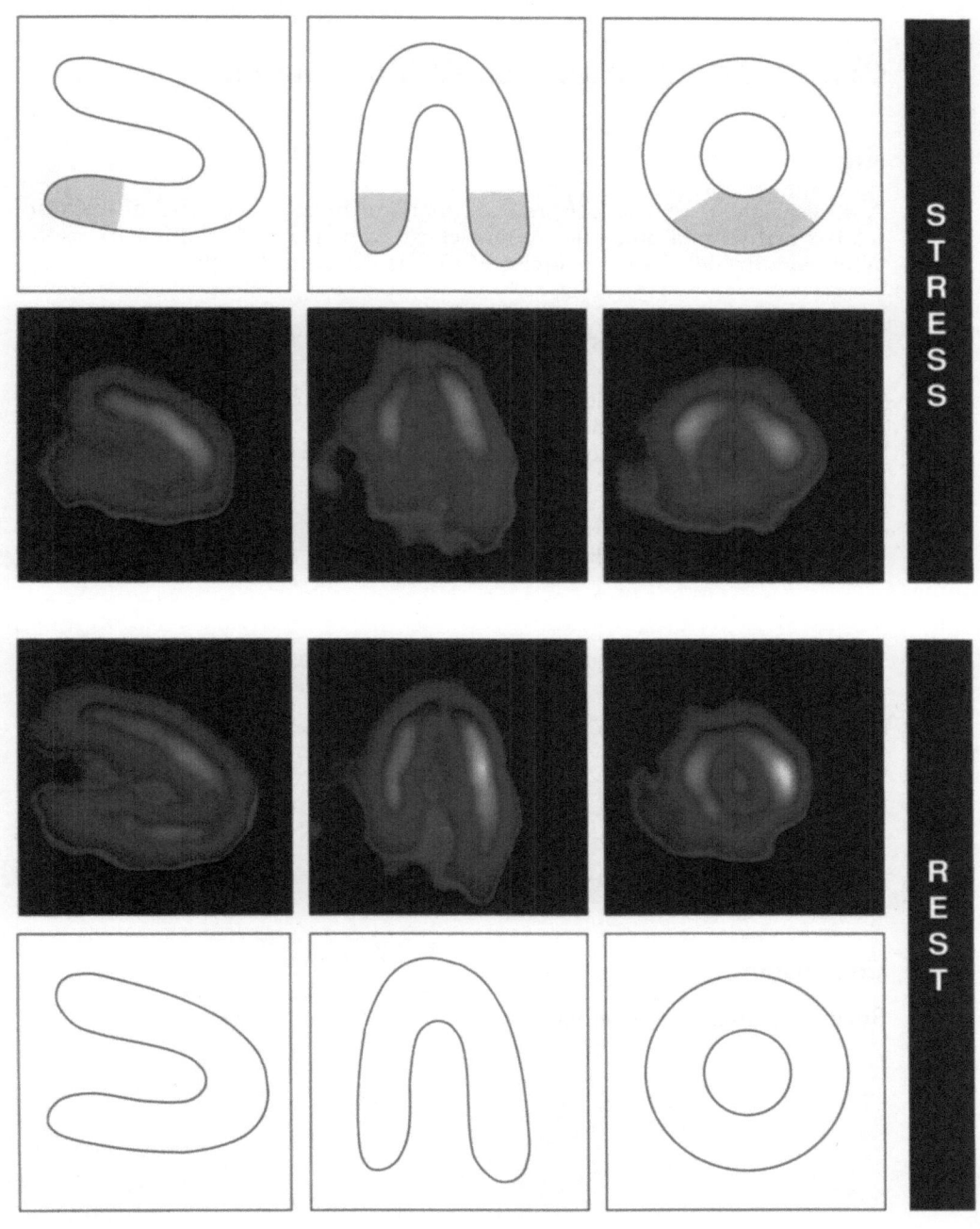

Profound ST segment changes do not always indicate extensive ischaemia.

Case 52 – Wolff–Parkinson–White Syndrome

History

A 49-year-old man was referred for thallium imaging because of exercise-related arrhythmia and intermittent chest pain. He had Wolff–Parkinson–White syndrome and the exercise ECG was therefore unhelpful.

Thallium Myocardial Perfusion Tomography

Stress Technique Dipyridamole was infused during bicycle exercise to 100 W. Stress was limited by fatigue without chest pain. At peak stress the blood pressure and the heart rate were 120/80 mmHg and 135/min.

Stress Images There is reduced uptake of tracer in the inferior wall extending into the apex.

Rest Images The abnormal area improves.

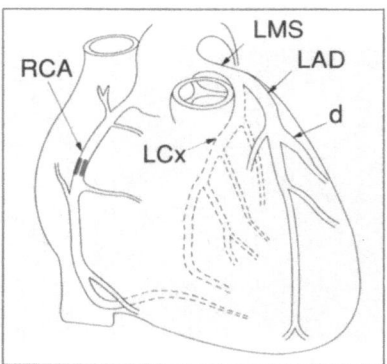

Coronary Angiography

There was a stenosis of the right coronary artery.

Conclusion

Reversible inferior ischaemia.

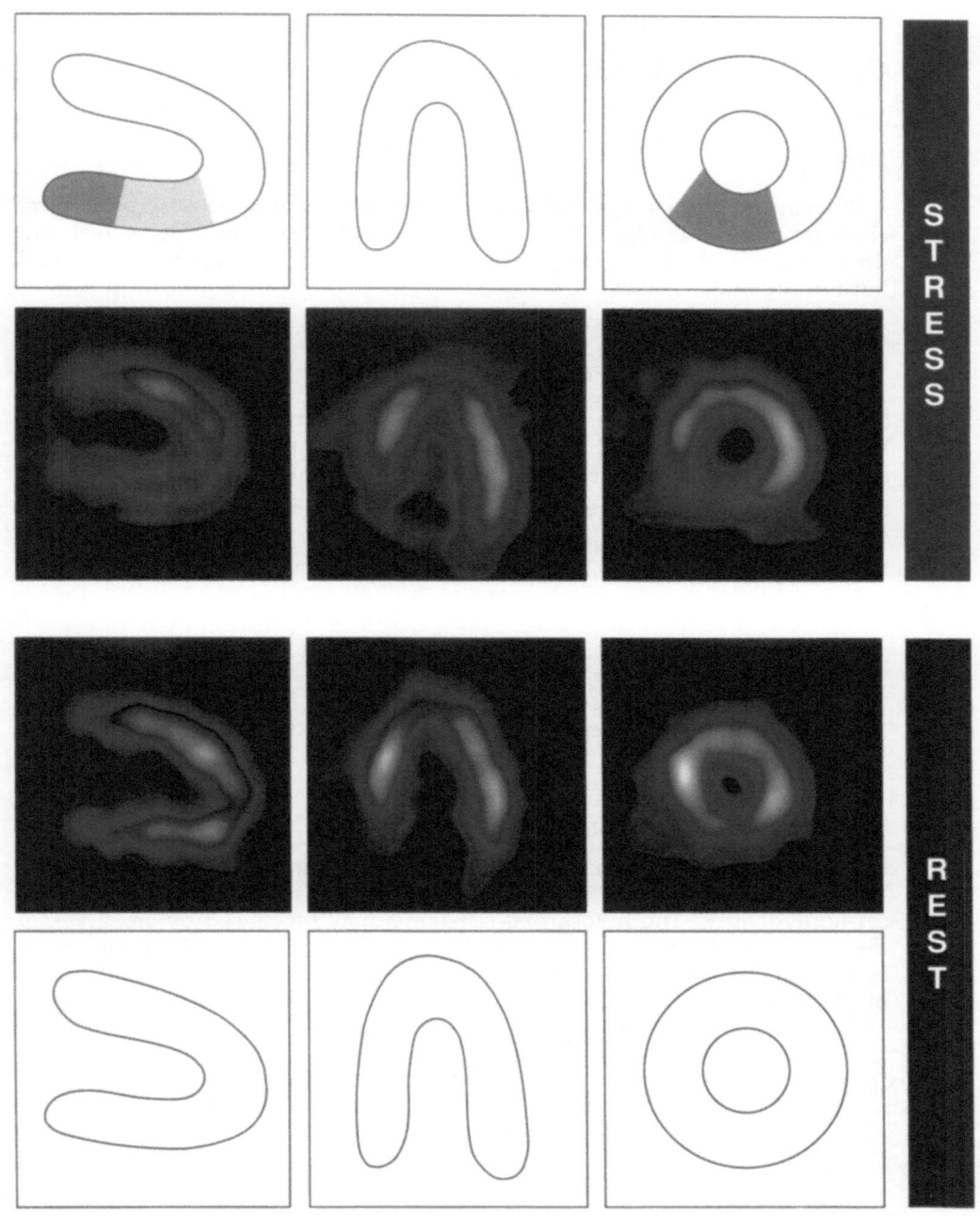

STRESS

REST

Thallium imaging is particularly useful when an abnormality of the resting ECG prevents interpretation of exercise-induced changes.

Case 53 – Left Bundle Branch Block

History

A 49-year-old woman was referred for thallium imaging because of atypical chest pain and a family history of early heart disease. The ECG at rest and during exercise had previously been normal but she had recently developed left bundle branch block.

Thallium Myocardial Perfusion Tomography

Stress Technique Dipyridamole was infused during bicycle exercise to 100 W. Stress was limited by fatigue without chest pain. At peak stress the blood pressure and the heart rate were 170/110 mmHg and 150/min.

Stress Images There is reduced uptake of tracer in the anterior wall and septum.

Rest Images The abnormal areas improve.

Coronary Angiography

The coronary arteries were normal although the left anterior descending artery was small and tapering. Left ventricular function was normal.

Conclusion

Despite the normal coronary arteries, the distribution of tracer is abnormal. The cause of this is unclear. Possible causes are myocardial ischaemia or cardiomyopathy. The myocardial ischaemia may be caused by small vessel disease, by minor coronary artery atheroma leading to distal embolisation, or by reduced diastolic coronary perfusion caused by the delay in relaxation of the septum.

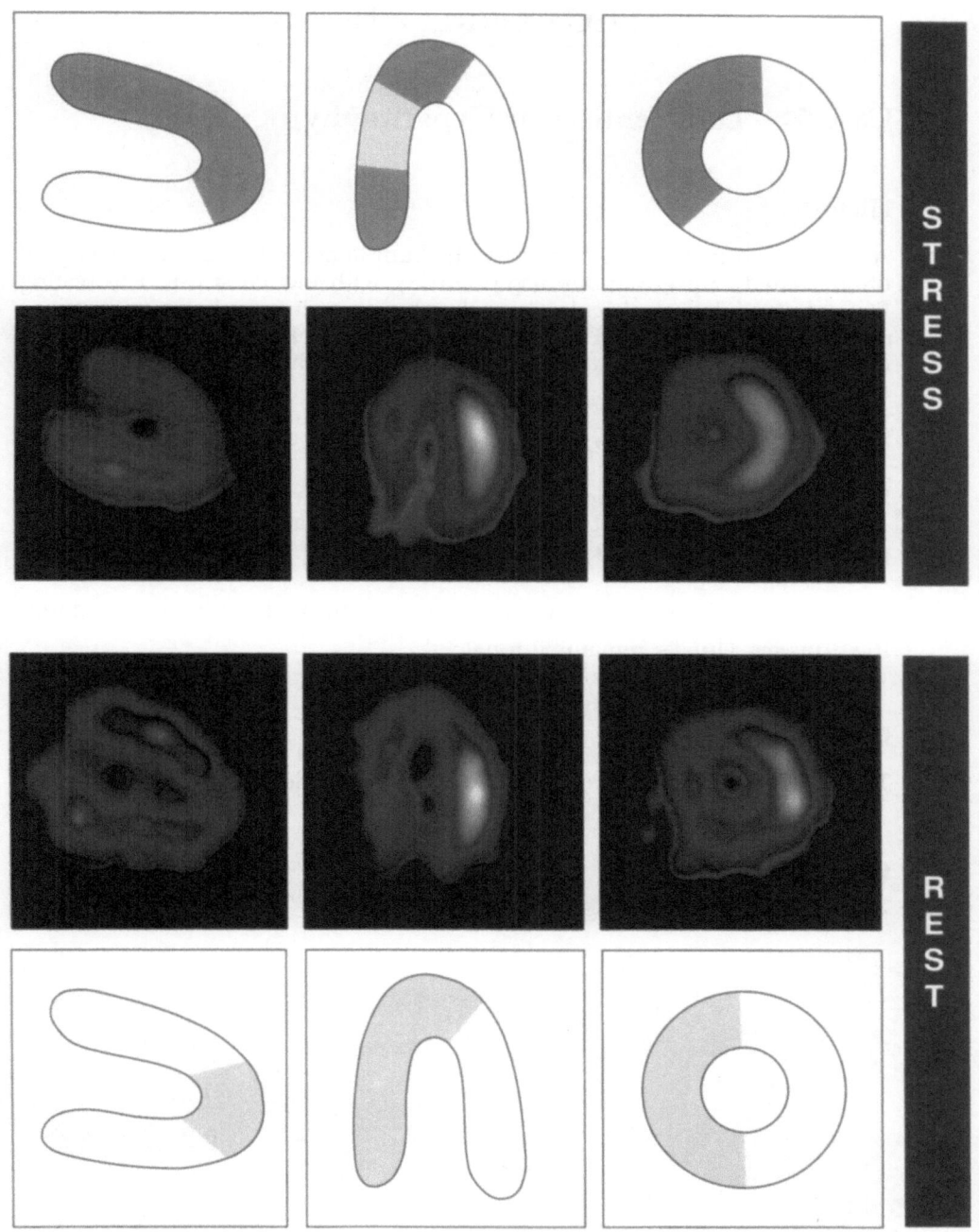

Great care must be exercised in the interpretation of thallium abnormalities in left bundle branch block. A normal thallium scan, however, remains helpful.

Case 54 – Left Ventricular Hypertrophy

History

A 41-year-old man was referred for thallium imaging because of chest pain often related to exercise but also occurring with mental stress. The resting ECG showed left ventricular hypertrophy on voltage criteria with minor repolarisation changes. Exercise was limited at 12 min by fatigue with dyspnoea. The patient practised karate for several hours each day.

Thallium Myocardial Perfusion Tomography

Stress Technique Dipyridamole was infused during bicycle exercise to 150 W. Stress was limited by fatigue and dyspnoea without chest pain. At peak stress the blood pressure and the heart rate were 200/80 mmHg and 138/min.

Stress Images There is normal uptake of tracer throughout the myocardium.

Rest Images Uptake remains normal.

Coronary Angiography

The coronary arteries were normal. The left ventricle was hypertrophied.

Conclusion

Normal myocardial perfusion.

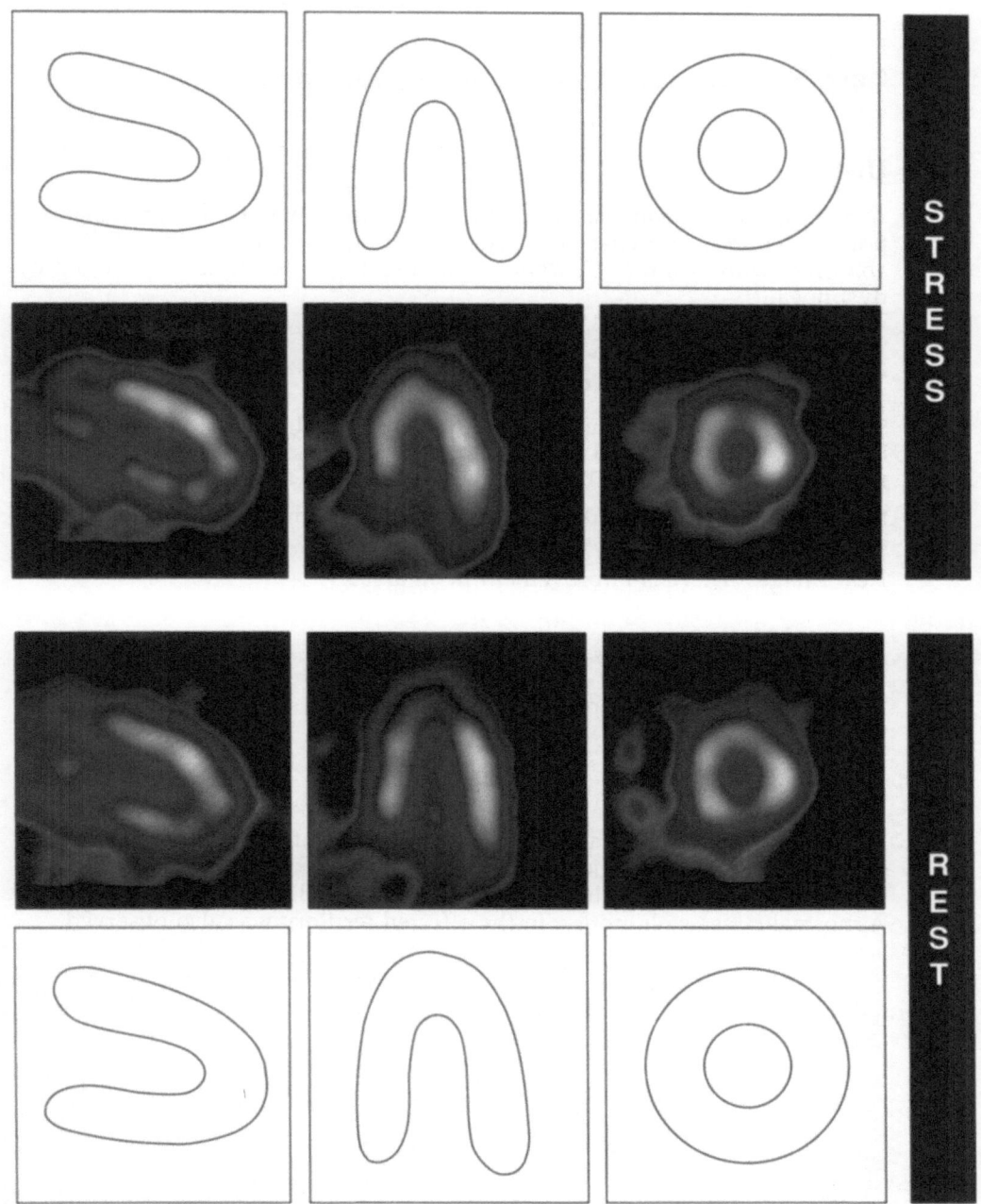

The exercise ECG is unhelpful for the assessment of myocardial ischaemia if there are resting repolarisation abnormalities as in left ventricular hypertrophy.

Case 55 – Normal Angiogram, Syndrome X

History

A 58-year-old woman was referred for thallium imaging because of exertional dyspnoea and chest pain suggesting angina. The exercise ECG was abnormal with 2 mm of ST depression after 1 min. Exercise was limited by dyspnoea.

Thallium Myocardial Perfusion Tomography

Stress Technique Dobutamine was infused up to 10 µg/kg/min. Stress was limited by chest pain and dyspnoea. At peak stress the blood pressure and the heart rate were 152/70 mmHg and 105/min.

Stress Images There is reduced uptake of tracer in the anterior wall, septum, and apex.

Rest Images There is improvement in all areas.

Coronary Angiography

The coronary arteries were normal.

Conclusion

There is reversible myocardial ischaemia in the anteroseptal region despite the normal coronary angiogram. The combination of angina, normal coronary arteries and myocardial ischaemia leads to a diagnosis of syndrome X. Abnormal stress wall motion in the affected territory was also observed.

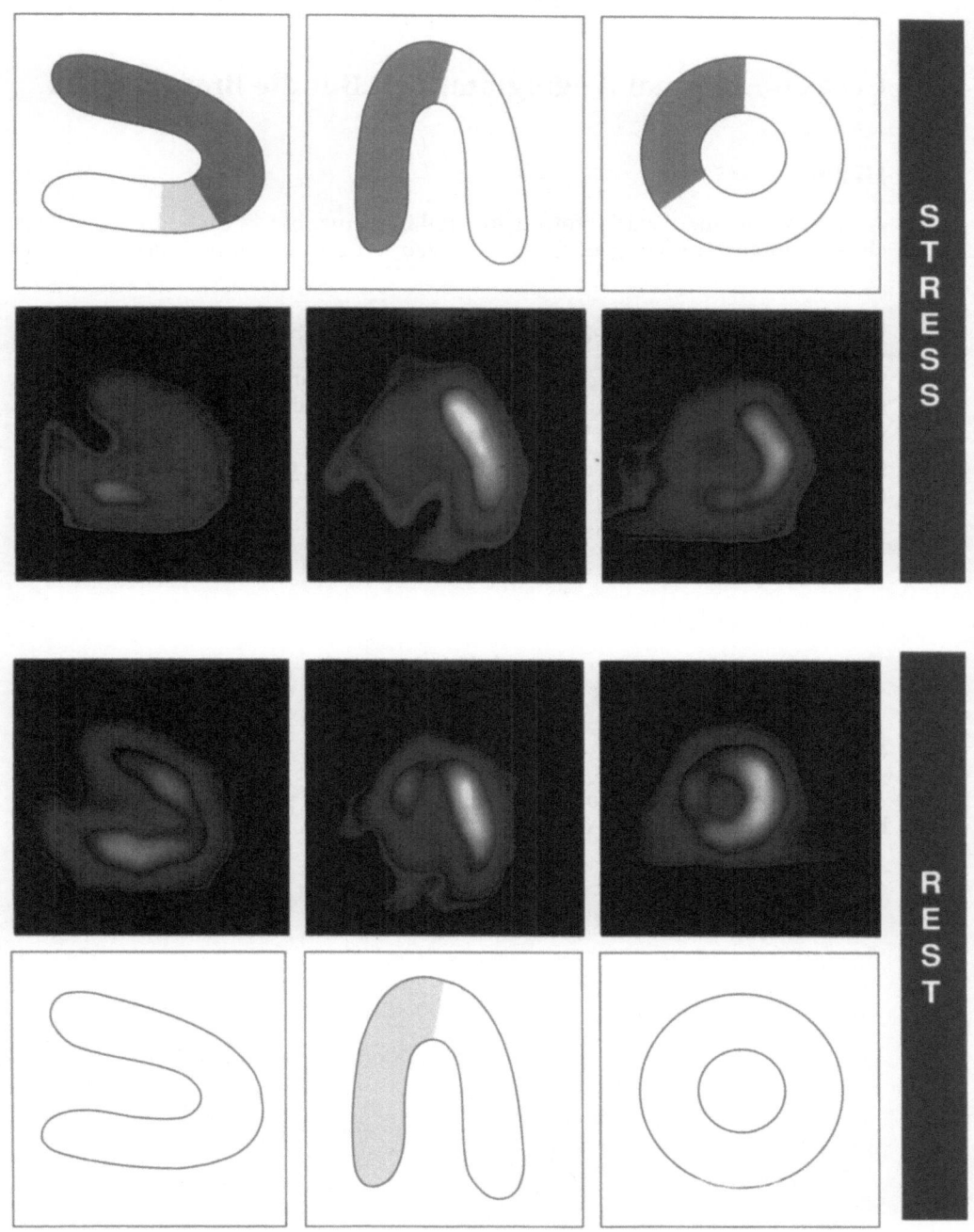

STRESS

REST

Impaired uptake of thallium is not always caused by disease of the epicardial coronary arteries.

Case 56 – Normal Angiogram, Left Bundle Branch Block

History

A 57-year-old man was referred for thallium imaging because of exertional chest pain and a resting ECG that showed left bundle branch block.

Thallium Myocardial Perfusion Tomography

Stress Technique He reached 125 W of bicycle exercise and was limited by fatigue and chest pain. At peak stress the blood pressure and the heart rate were 162/100 mmHg and 130/min.

Stress Images There is reduced uptake of tracer in the septum extending to the inferior wall.

Rest Images The abnormal area improves.

Coronary Angiography

The coronary arteries were normal. Left ventricular contraction was normal.

Conclusion

There is reversible inferoseptal ischaemia in the presence of left bundle branch block and normal coronary arteries.

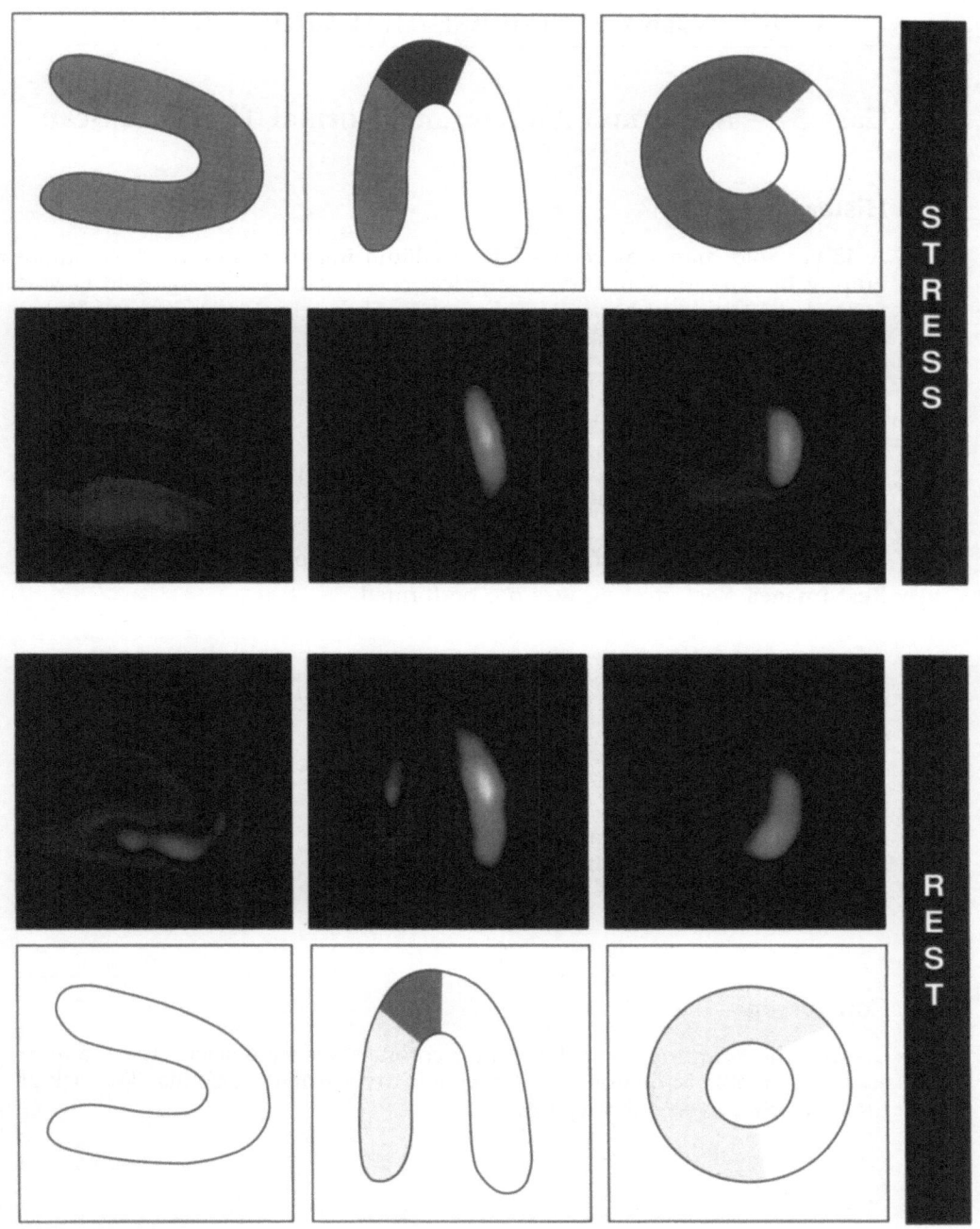

STRESS

REST

Left bundle branch block may be associated with abnormal uptake of thallium despite normal coronary arteries. This may reflect true ischaemia.

CORONARY ANGIOGRAM CORRELATIONS

Case 57 – Abnormal Angiogram, Normal Thallium Scan

History

A 43-year-old man was referred for thallium imaging and coronary angio-graphy because of a history of atypical chest pain. An exercise ECG was normal at 12 min but because of the nature of the chest pain, it was felt that coronary artery disease had not been excluded.

Thallium Myocardial Perfusion Tomography

Stress Technique Dobutamine was infused to 20 μg/kg/min without chest pain. At peak stress the blood pressure and the heart rate were 178/ 64 mmHg and 104/min.

Stress Images There is normal myocardial uptake of tracer.

Rest Images Rest imaging was not performed.

Coronary Angiography

The left circumflex artery was occluded but was non-dominant. There was a mild stenosis in a diagonal branch of the left anterior descending artery.

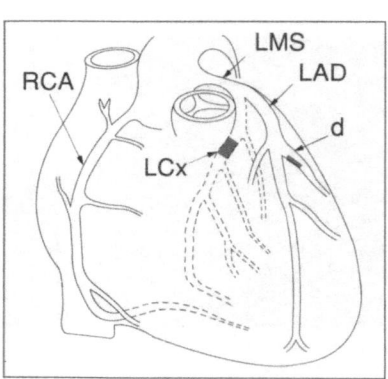

Conclusion

Despite the symptoms and the minor coronary artery disease, the thallium scan was unable to demonstrate reversible myocardial ischaemia. The risk of future cardiac events is very low.

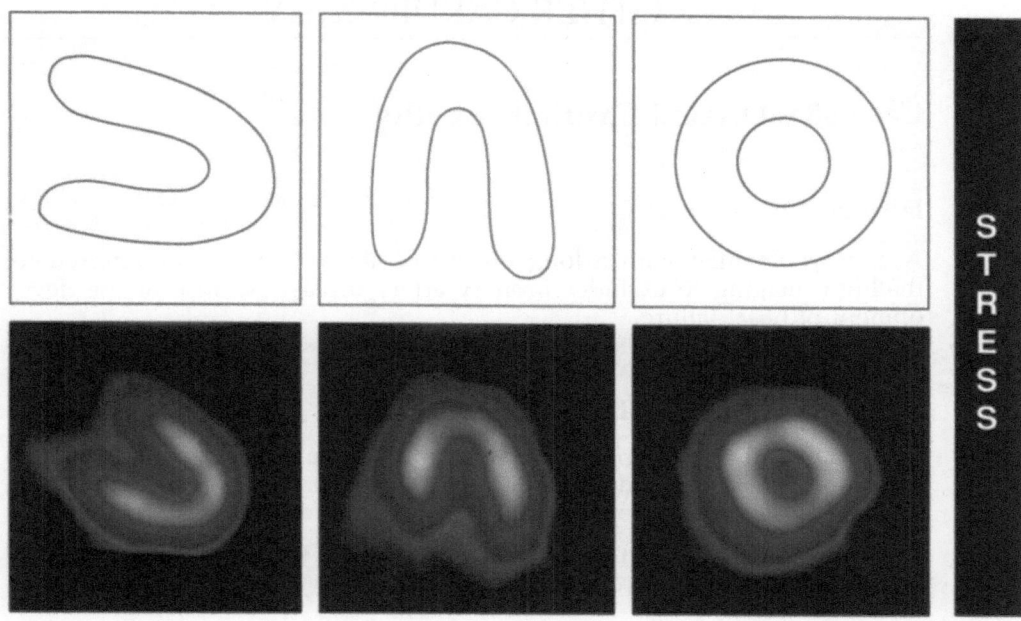

STRESS

Abnormal coronary anatomy may not limit myocardial perfusion.

Case 58 – Dilated Cardiomyopathy

History

A 47-year-old man with a long history of alcohol abuse was referred for thallium imaging to exclude coronary artery disease because of the development of heart failure.

Thallium Myocardial Perfusion Tomography

Stress Technique Dipyridamole was infused during bicycle exercise to 100 W. Stress was limited by fatigue and dyspnoea. At peak stress the blood pressure and the heart rate were 140/90 mmHg and 182/min.

Stress Images The left ventricle is dilated. Uptake of tracer is normal.

Rest Images There is no change.

Coronary Angiography

The coronary arteries were normal. There was global hypokinesis.

Conclusion

Normal myocardial perfusion compatible with alcoholic cardiomyopathy. The resting ejection fraction was 18%.

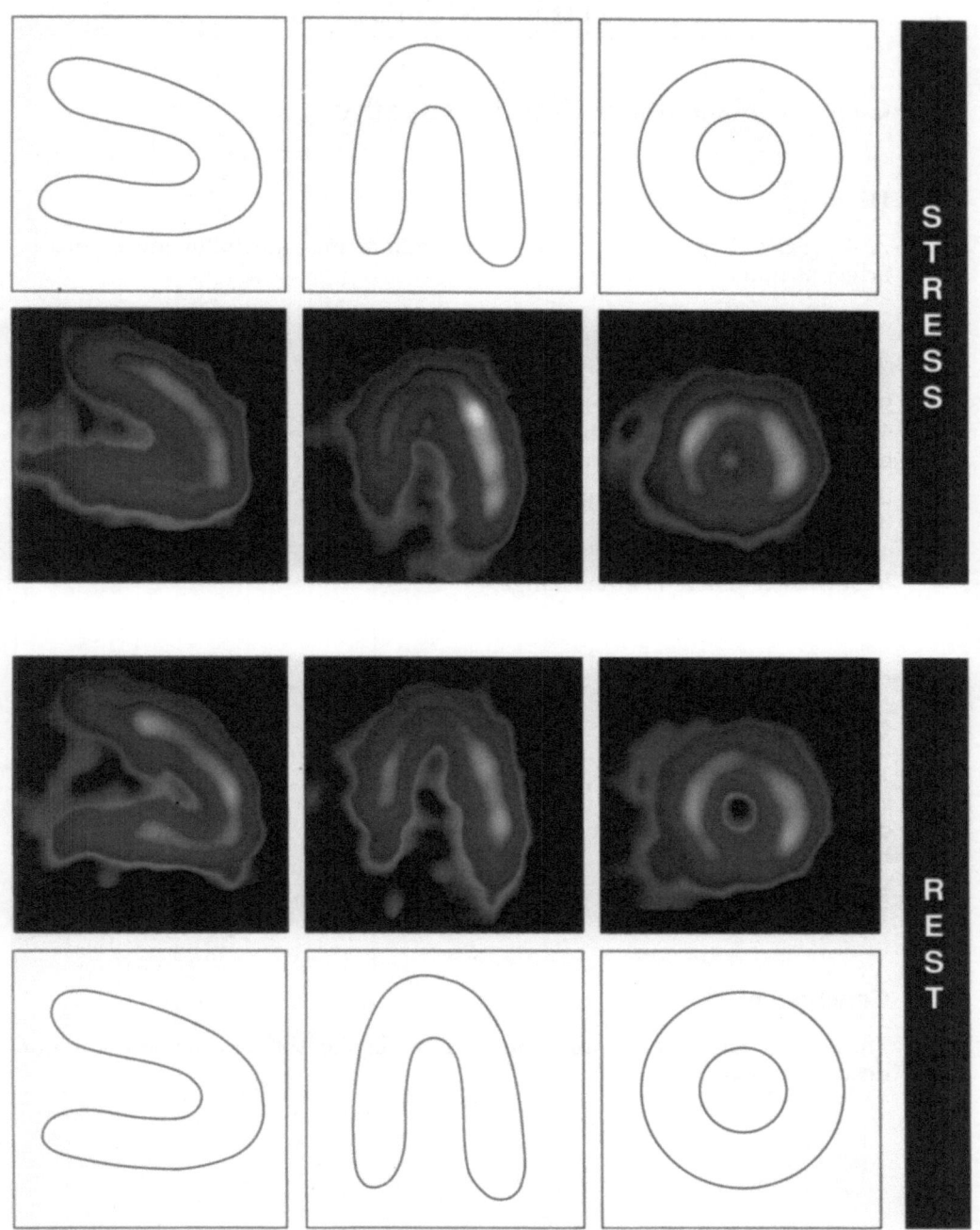

Dilated cardiomyopathy of any cause may have normal or heterogeneous uptake of thallium. Defects simulating reversible ischaemia are rare.

Case 59 – Ischaemic Cardiomyopathy

History

A 45-year-old man was referred for thallium imaging following a cardiac arrest at home.

Thallium Myocardial Perfusion Tomography

Stress Technique Dipyridamole was infused during bicycle exercise to 50 W. Stress was limited by fatigue without chest pain. At peak stress the blood pressure and the heart rate were 152/98 mmHg and 130/min.

Stress Images The left ventricle is dilated. There is very reduced uptake of tracer in the anterior wall and apex sparing the most basal portion of the anterior wall. Uptake in other areas is normal.

Rest Images There is little change.

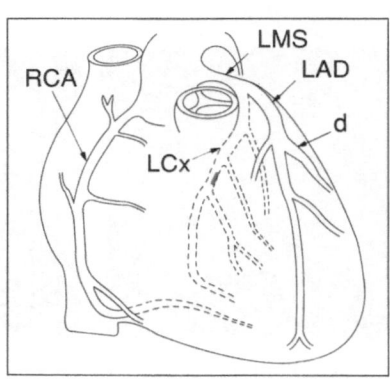

Coronary Angiography

The coronary arteries were normal except for a stenosis in the mid-left circumflex artery. There was global hypokinesis.

Conclusion

There is a large anteroapical infarction despite the normal left anterior descending artery.

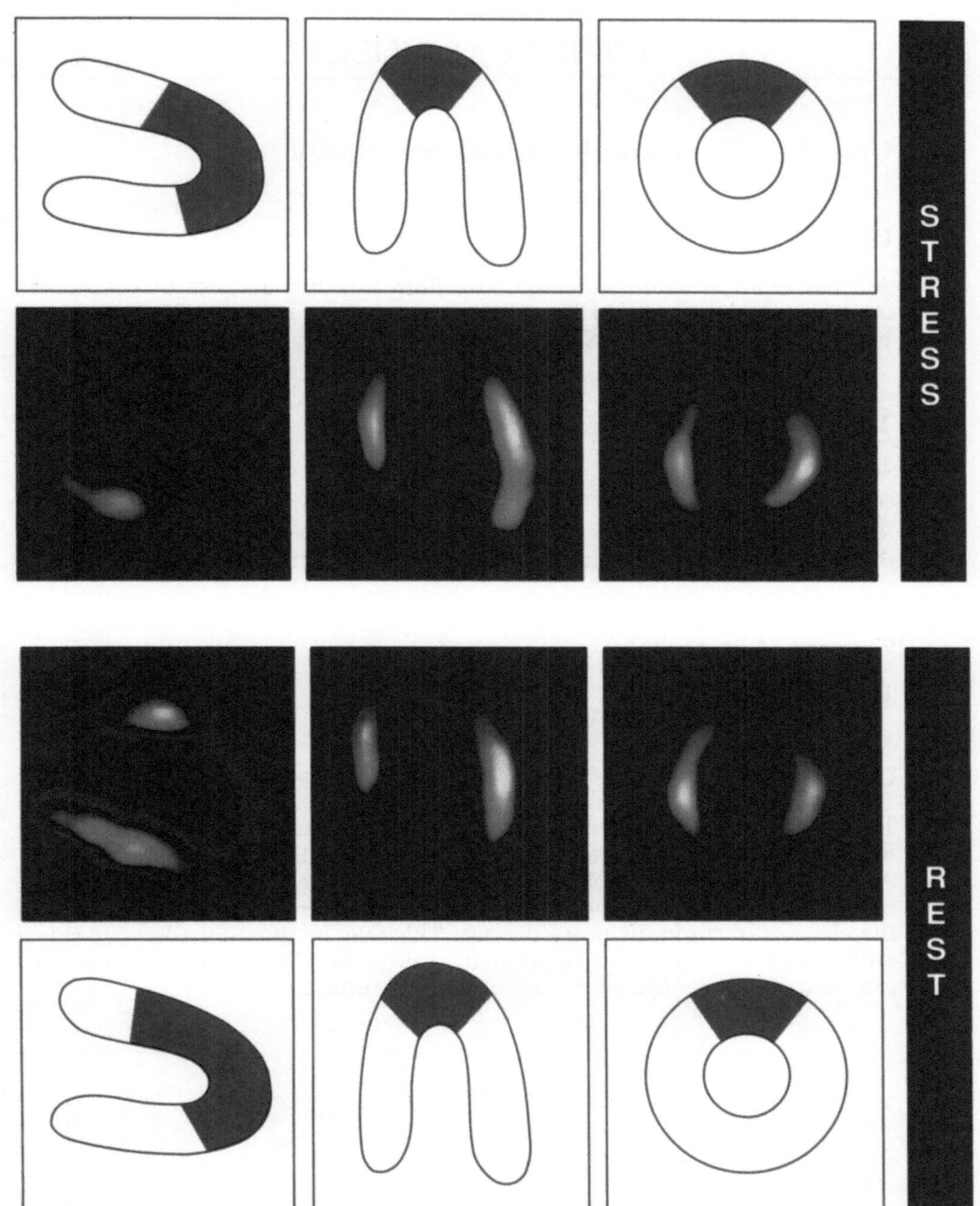

Myocardial infarction may occur despite normal appearance of the coronary arteries. Thrombosis and spontaneous thrombolysis on the surface of an anatomically insignificant lesion may be the explanation, but coronary embolism is an alternative.

Case 60 – Hypertrophic Cardiomyopathy

History

A 75-year-old woman underwent thallium imaging because of exertional chest pain and dyspnoea. Her resting electrocardiogram showed right bundle branch block. Her echocardiogram showed septal hypertrophy.

Thallium Myocardial Perfusion Tomography

Stress Technique In view of the echocardiographic findings, exercise was not performed and thallium was injected at rest.

Rest Images The septum and apex are abnormally thickened (*arrows*) but there are no defects of uptake of tracer.

Coronary Angiography

This was not performed.

Conclusion

Thickened septum and apex compatible with hypertrophic cardiomyopathy. Radionuclide ventriculography showed a high resting ejection fraction of 75%, with poor septal motion and delayed diastolic filling. Thallium imaging in hypertrophic cardiomyopathy can show reversible or fixed defects in the absence of coronary artery disease. This may be due to inadequate subendocardial perfusion caused by high wall stress. The same phenomenon can occur in concentric left ventricular hypertrophy.

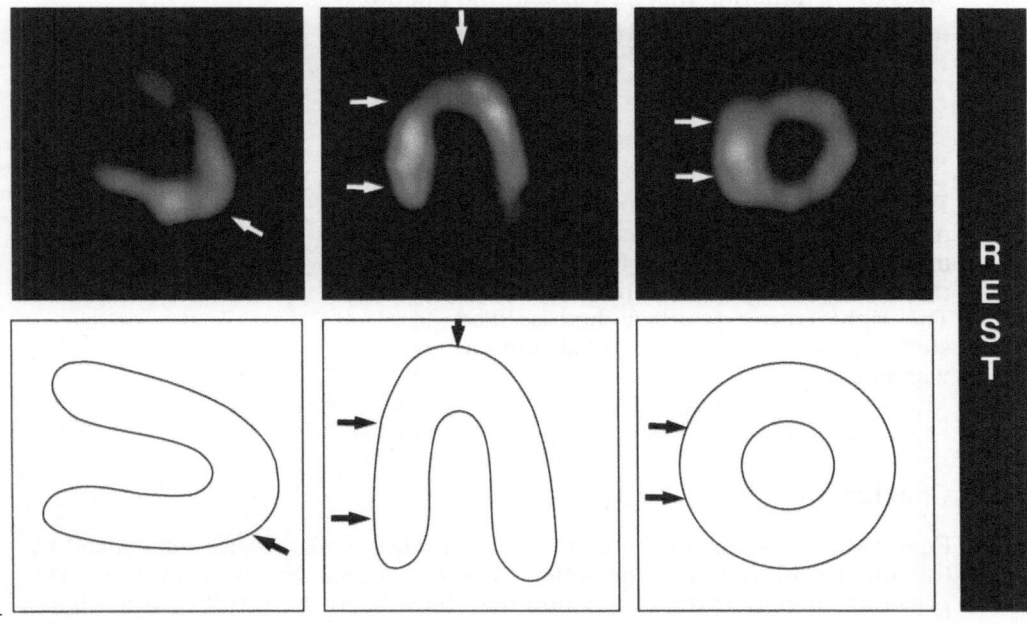

Thallium imaging is not a principal investigation for the diagnosis of hypertrophy, but thickened muscle is sometimes seen. Normal uptake may exclude an ischaemic cause of symptoms.

Case 61 – Coronary Muscle Bridge

History

A 51-year-old man was admitted for thallium imaging and coronary angio-graphy because of mild angina and anxiety following an anterior subendo-cardial infarction. He was a moderately heavy smoker. His resting ECG showed inverted T-waves in the lateral leads. His exercise ECG was stopped at 10 min because of 2 mm ST segment depression in leads V2–4, without chest pain.

Thallium Myocardial Perfusion Tomography

Stress Technique Dobutamine was infused to 20 µg/kg/min. Stress was limited by chest pain. At peak stress the blood pressure and the heart rate were 156/96 mmHg and 120/min.

Stress Images There is reduced uptake of tracer in the mid and basal por-tions of the anterior wall and also in the inferior wall.

Rest Images There is improvement in the abnormal areas.

Coronary Angiography

The left anterior descending artery was normal in diastole but became stenosed in systole in its mid-portion. The ap-pearance was typical of a muscle bridge. The right coronary artery had a fixed stenosis. Left ventricular wall motion was normal.

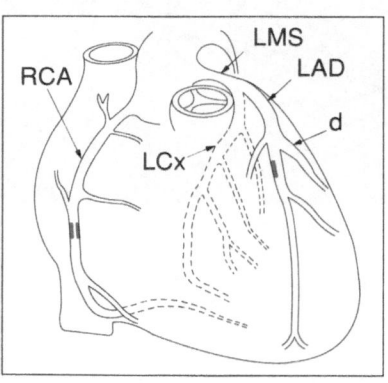

Conclusion

Reversible ischaemia of the anterior and inferior walls, the former caused by the muscle bridge and the latter by conventional coronary disease. The previous subendocardial infarction may have been the result of thrombosis on a minor plaque at the site of the muscle bridge. Because of the mild symptoms, the patient was treated medically.

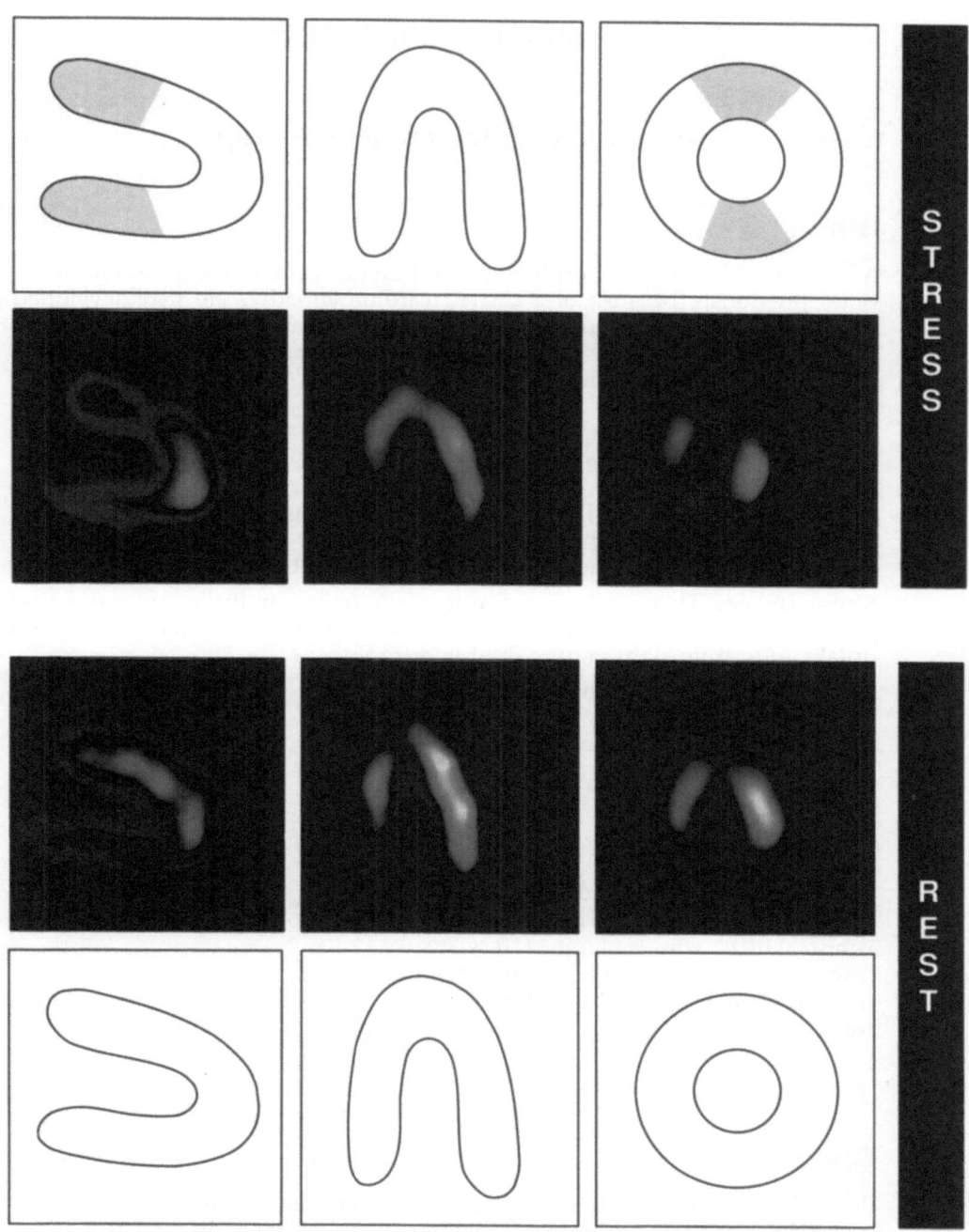

It has been suggested that muscle bridges do not limit coronary flow because they constrict the artery only in systole. This case demonstrates that reversible ischaemia may occur.

Case 62 – Orthotopic Cardiac Transplantation

History

A 50-year-old man had undergone orthotopic cardiac transplantation six years previously because of a dilated cardiomyopathy. He had developed atheroma of the donor coronary arteries which had been treated by angioplasty of the left anterior descending artery. He had no angina but exercise was limited by fatigue and dyspnoea.

Thallium Myocardial Perfusion Tomography

Stress Technique Dipyridamole was infused during bicycle exercise to 75 W. Stress was limited by fatigue without chest pain. At peak stress the blood pressure and the heart rate were 130/90 mmHg and 140/min.

Stress Images There is reduced uptake of tracer in the apex and apical portion of the inferior wall. Right ventricular uptake is similar to left-sided uptake indicating right ventricular hypertrophy.

Rest Images There is improvement of the apical inferior wall and lesser improvement of the apex.

Coronary Angiography

There was a discrete stenosis in the mid-portion of the left anterior descending artery which was a large artery extending around the apex. The other arteries were irregular but without discrete stenoses.

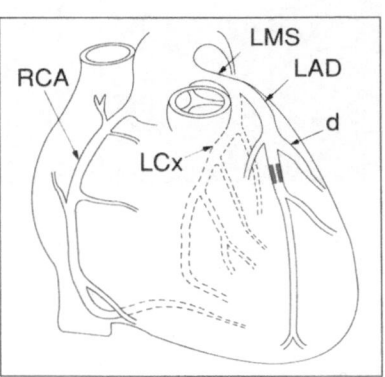

Conclusion

Reversible ischaemia caused by recurrent stenosis of the left anterior descending artery. Experience of thallium imaging following cardiac transplantation is limited and the cause of the increased right ventricular uptake is unknown.

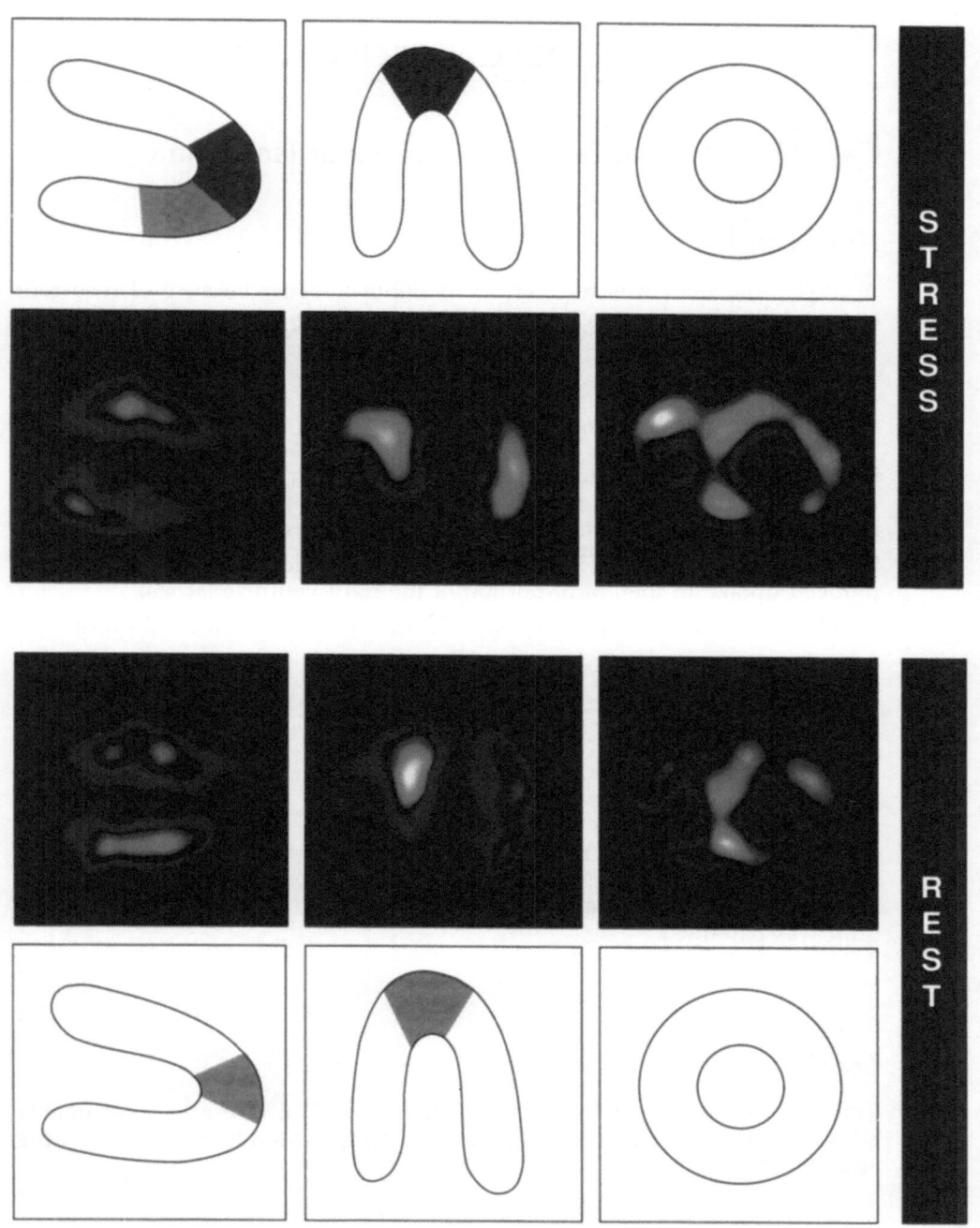

STRESS

REST

Accelerated coronary atheroma may occur after cardiac transplantation. The distinction between perfusion abnormalities caused by atheroma and the effects of chronic rejection is difficult but thallium imaging was helpful in this case.

Case 63 – Reversible Right Ventricular Ischaemia

History

A 60-year-old man was referred for thallium imaging because of recurrent angina following coronary artery bypass grafting and repair of an atrial septal defect.

Thallium Myocardial Perfusion Tomography

Stress Technique Dipyridamole was infused during bicycle exercise to 75 W. Stress was limited by fatigue without chest pain. At peak stress the blood pressure and the heart rate were 140/80 mmHg and 106/min.

Stress Images Uptake of tracer in the left ventricle is normal but there is reduced uptake in the apical portion of the right ventricle (*arrow*).

Rest Images There is improvement in the abnormal area of the right ventricle.

Coronary Angiography

There was disease of the native left anterior descending artery with a patent graft. Disease of the right coronary artery affected the origin of a large right ventricular branch but the right coronary graft was patent.

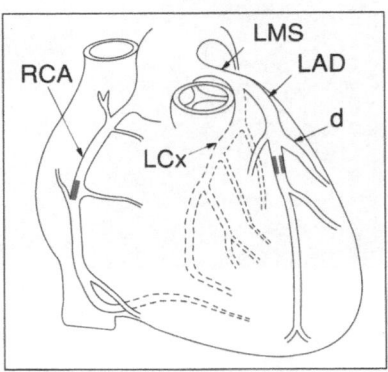

Conclusion

Reversible ischaemia of the right ventricle. This is a rare case, presumably arising because of right ventricular hypertrophy caused by the longstanding atrial septal defect.

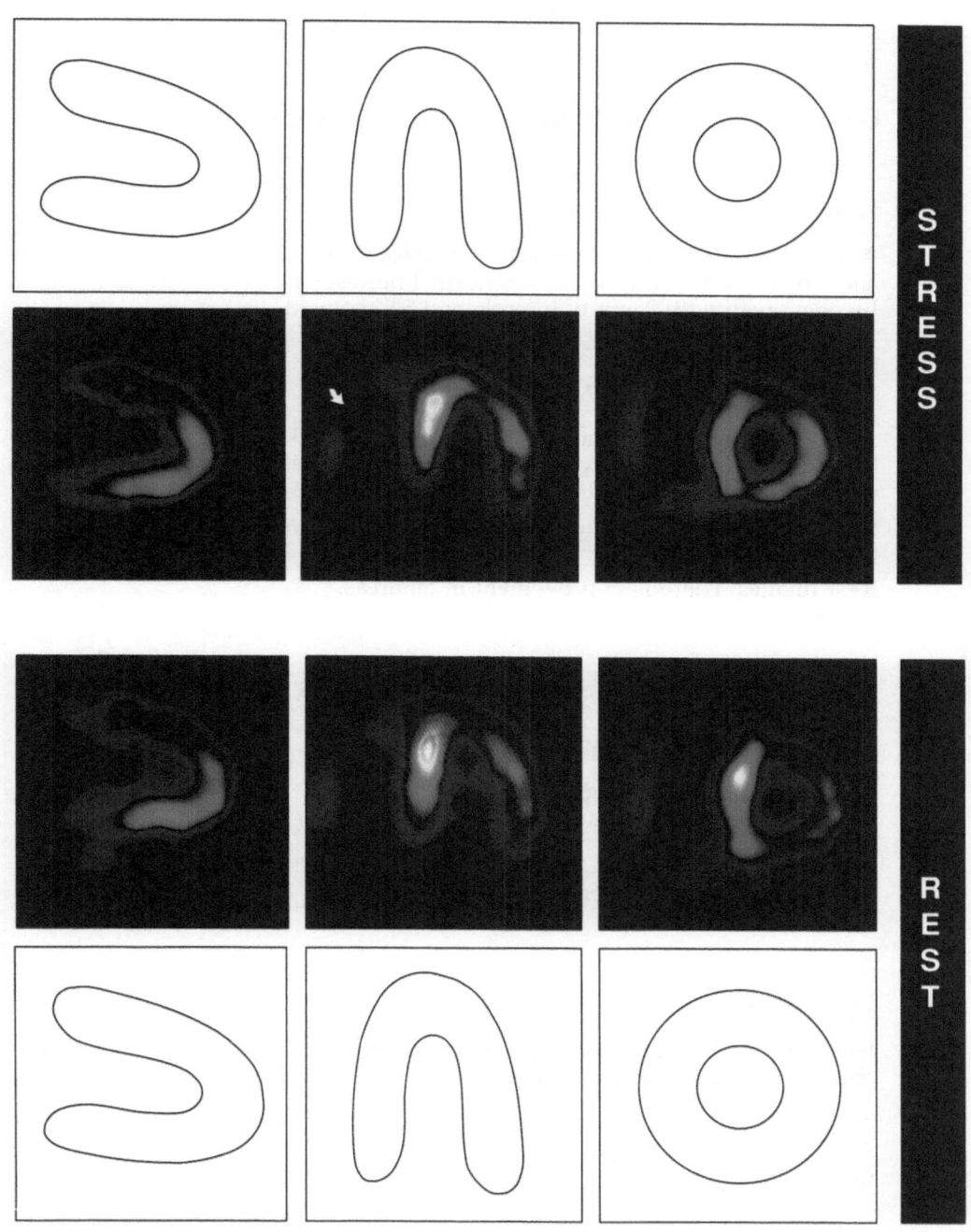

STRESS

REST

Reversible right ventricular ischaemia may be detected by thallium imaging in the presence of right ventricular hypertrophy.

Case 64 – Unusual Coronary Artery Anatomy

History

A 40-year-old man was referred for thallium imaging because of exertional chest pain. The resting ECG was normal but exercise was stopped at 9 min by chest pain with 2 mm of inferolateral ST segment depression.

Thallium Myocardial Perfusion Tomography

Stress Technique Dobutamine was infused to 15 μg/kg/min. Stress was limited by chest pain. At peak stress the blood pressure and the heart rate were 196/92 mmHg and 142/min.

Stress Images There is reduced uptake of tracer in all walls with the exception of the lateral wall.

Rest Images There is improvement in all areas.

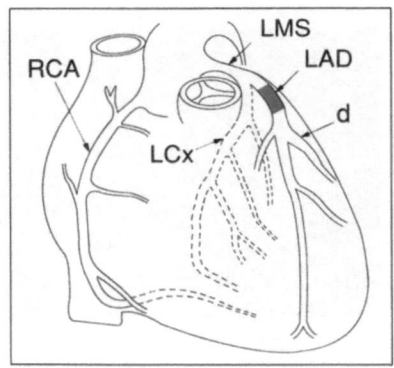

Coronary Angiography

The left anterior descending artery was very large and was occluded. The other arteries were normal.

Conclusion

Extensive reversible ischaemia affecting the inferior wall as well as the characteristic territory of the left anterior descending artery.

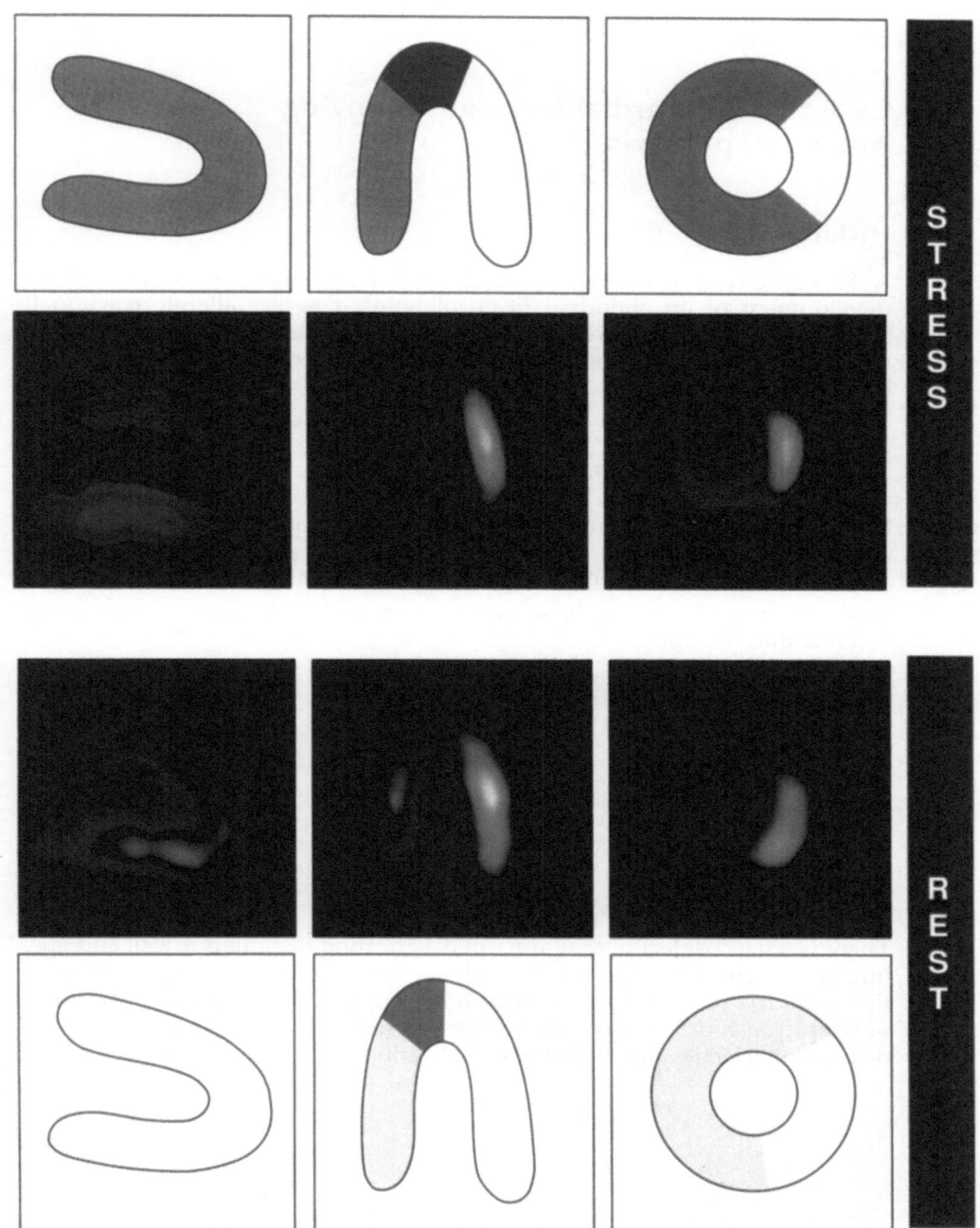

Disease of only the left anterior descending artery may produce very extensive reversible ischaemia which includes the inferior wall.

Case 65 – Myocardial Damage Following Acute Anaphylaxis

History

A 52-year-old woman was referred for thallium imaging because of the development of an abnormal ECG following a severe allergic reaction to amoxycillin associated with severe chest pain. The resting ECG showed widespread anterior T-wave inversion. She was treated with streptokinase but the ECG changes did not resolve.

Thallium Myocardial Perfusion Tomography

Stress Technique Dipyridamole was infused during bicycle exercise to 75 W. Stress was limited by fatigue without chest pain. At peak stress the blood pressure and the heart rate were 170/100 mmHg and 140/min.

Stress Images There is reduced uptake of tracer in the anterior wall which extends into the apex.

Rest Images There is no change.

Coronary Angiography

Coronary angiography was not performed.

Conclusion

There is a fixed defect of thallium uptake affecting the anterior wall and apex implying myocardial damage. The planar projections did not show attenuation from the breasts. It is not known if the myocardial damage is the result of anaphylaxis or coronary artery disease. In the absence of symptoms and of reversible ischaemia, invasive investigation was not performed.

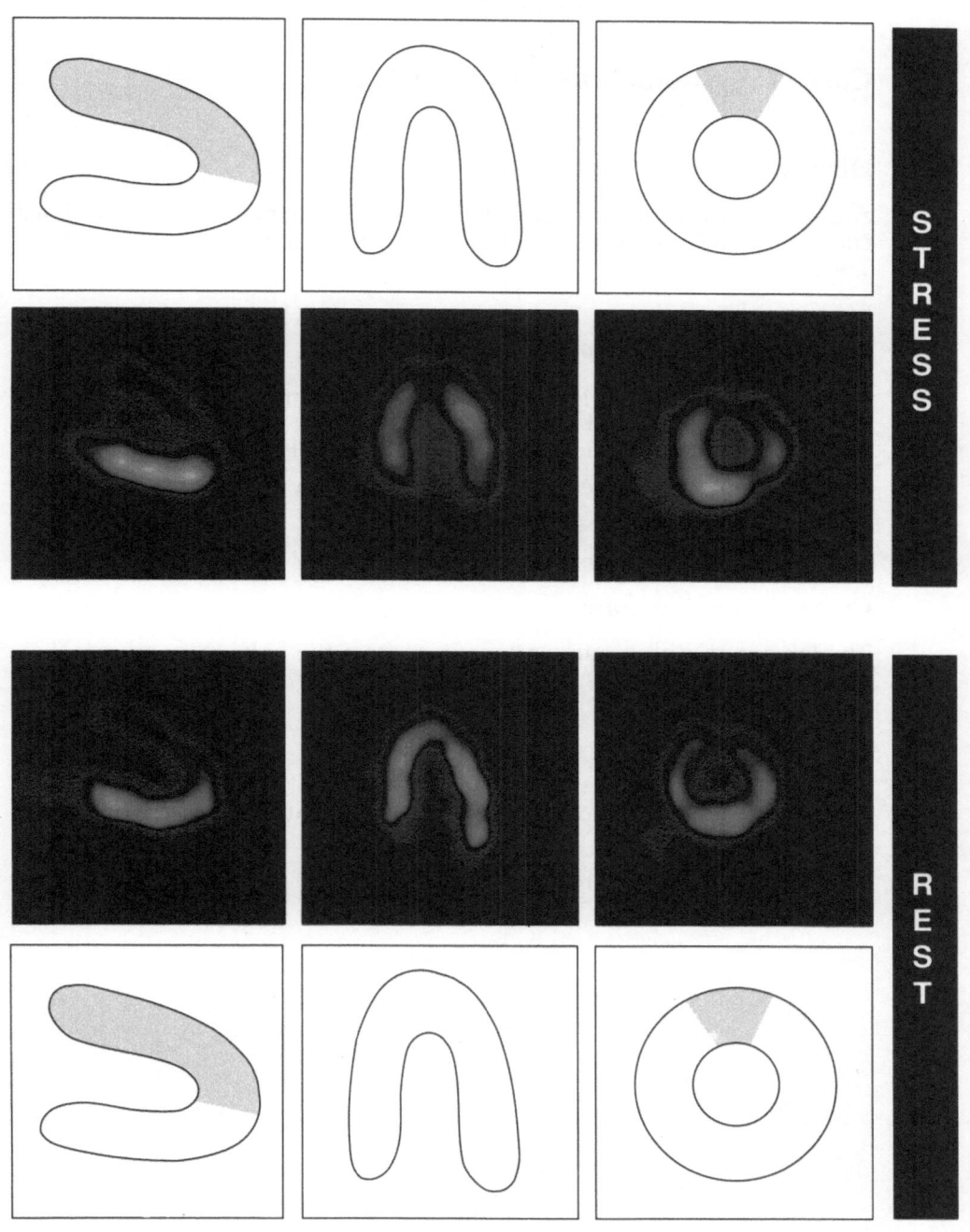

Systemic disease may cause fixed defects of tracer uptake.

Case 66 – Anomalous Origin of LAD

History

A 23-year-old woman was referred for thallium imaging because of exertional chest pain since adolescence. The resting ECG showed inverted anterior T-waves.

Thallium Myocardial Perfusion Tomography

Stress Technique Dipyridamole was infused during bicycle exercise to 75 W. Stress was limited by fatigue without chest pain. At peak stress the blood pressure and the heart rate were 145/90 mmHg and 130/min.

Stress Images There is reduced uptake of tracer in the anterior wall.

Rest Images There is no change.

Coronary Angiography

The left anterior descending artery arose from the pulmonary artery. There was anterior hypokinesis.

Conclusion

Anterior infarction caused by an anomalous left anterior descending artery.

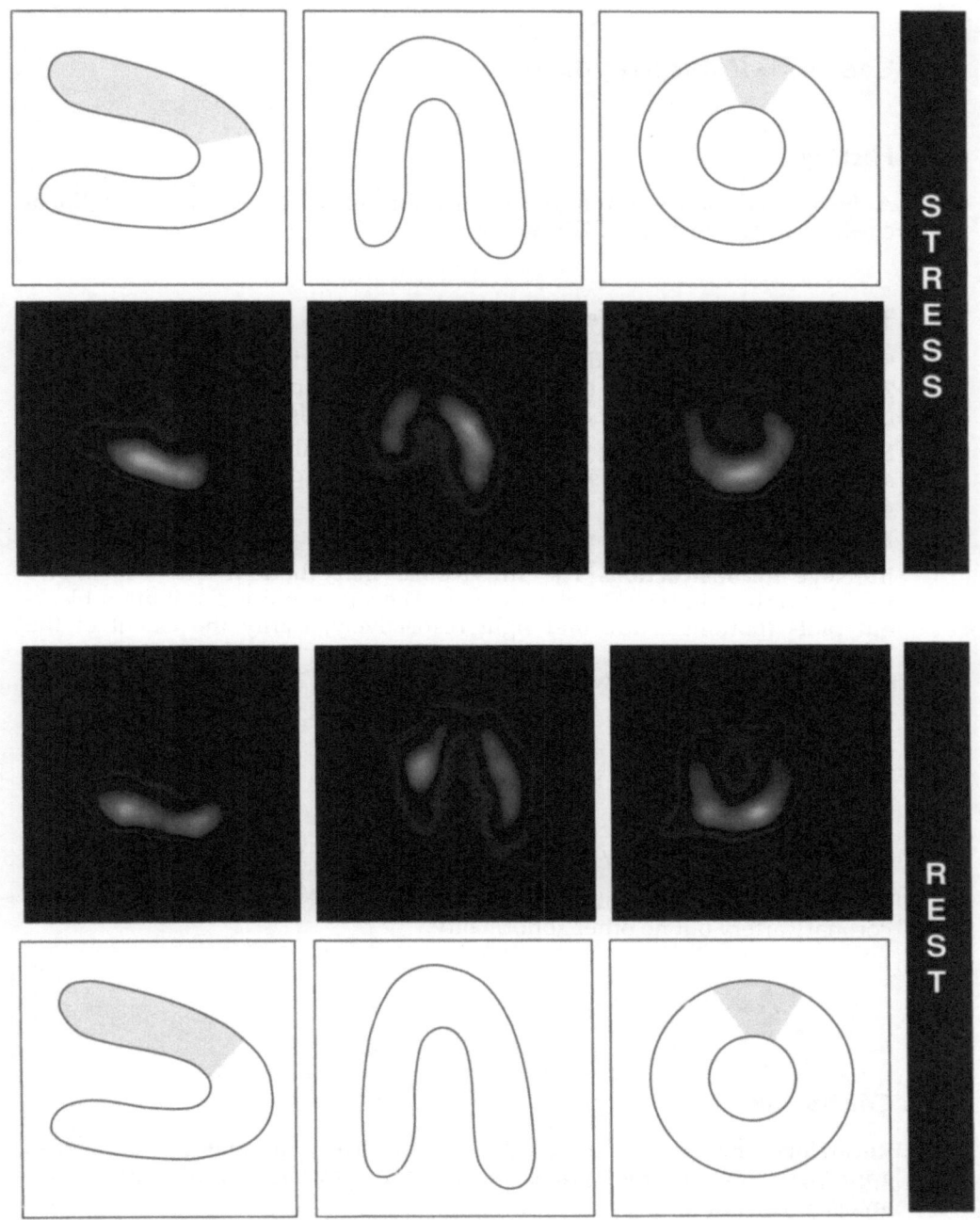

Classical angina in the young may be caused by an anomalous coronary artery.

QUANTIFICATION

Case 67 – Polar Mapping

History

A 59-year-old man was referred for thallium imaging because of exertional chest pain. His resting ECG was normal.

Thallium Myocardial Perfusion Tomography

Stress Technique Dipyridamole was infused during bicycle exercise to 75 W. Stress was limited by fatigue without chest pain. At peak stress the blood pressure and the heart rate were 138/76 mmHg and 110/min.

Stress Images Uptake of tracer in the lateral wall is lower than in the septum. This is the reverse of normal. There is also reduced uptake in the apex.

Rest Images The abnormal areas improve.

Bullseye Reconstructions The stress polar map (bottom left) also shows reduced uptake in the inferolateral wall. The stress and redistribution black-out plots (bottom centre and right respectively) clarify the extent of the abnormality by blacking out pixels with activity that is more than two standard deviations below normal.

Coronary Angiography

There was a stenosis of the left main coronary artery but no other abnormality.

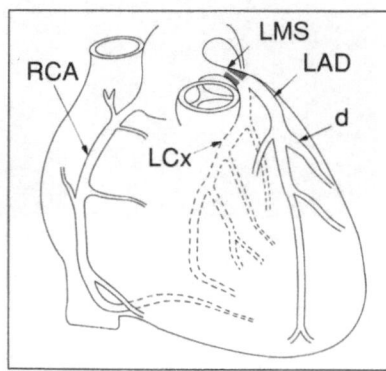

Conclusion

Reversible inferolateral and apical ischaemia. The abnormality is difficult to appreciate from the tomograms but is clearly revealed by the quantitative analysis.

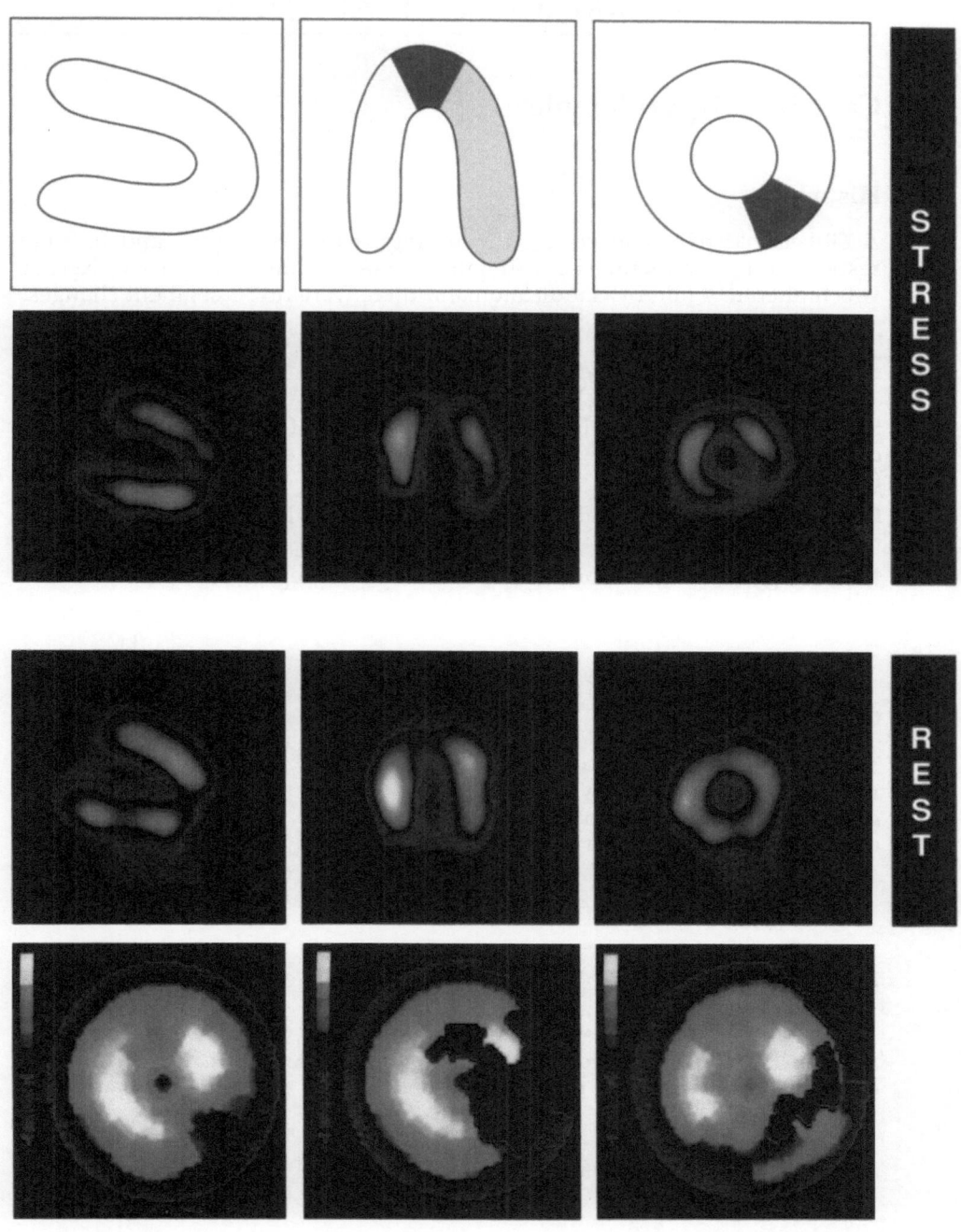

Uptake of tracer in the lateral wall is normally 20% higher than in the septum. Quantitative analysis may reveal an abnormality that is not obvious from the tomograms.

Case 68 – Dipyridamole

History

A 69-year-old man had suffered from angina for six months and had not responded to treatment. The resting ECG showed inferior Q-waves. Exercise was limited to 4 min by claudication and there were no ST segment changes.

Thallium Myocardial Perfusion Tomography

Stress Technique Dipyridamole 0.56 mg/kg was infused intravenously and caused chest pain. Blood pressure and heart rate after infusion were 129/65 mmHg and 77/min.

Stress Images There is reduced uptake of tracer in the anterior wall, septum and apex and also in the inferior wall.

Rest Images There is improvement in all areas except the inferior wall.

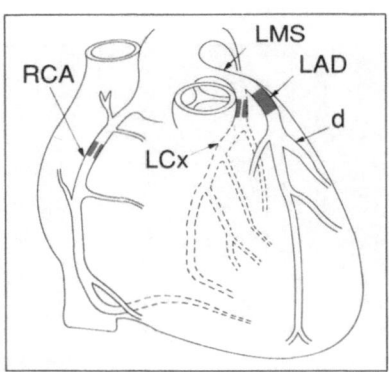

Coronary Angiography

The left anterior descending artery was occluded proximally. There were stenoses of the left circumflex artery and of the right coronary artery.

Conclusion

There is reversible ischaemia of the anterior wall, septum and apex with inferior infarction. This defect is unlikely to have been revealed by dynamic exercise alone because of the claudication.

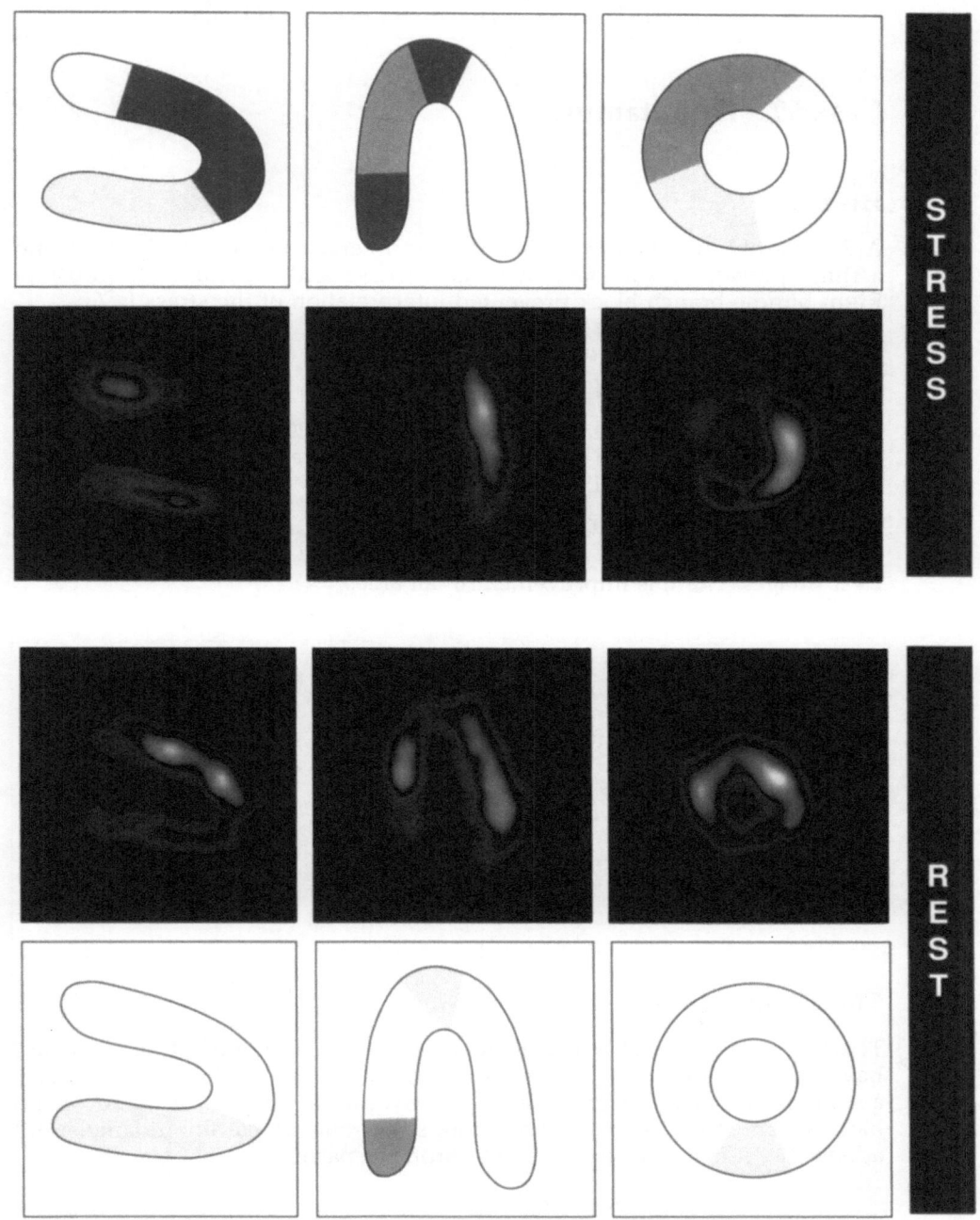

STRESS

REST

Dipyridamole may reveal inequalities of myocardial perfusion and is helpful in patients who cannot exercise. It may also provoke myocardial ischaemia. It is contraindicated in patients with bronchospasm.

Case 69 – Dobutamine

History

A 73-year-old man had exertional chest pain and palpitations. Arthritis and asthma prevented adequate dynamic exercise and dipyridamole infusion. Right bundle branch block prevented interpretation of the stress ECG.

Thallium Myocardial Perfusion Tomography

Stress Technique Dobutamine was infused to 20 µg/kg/min. Stress was limited by chest pain. At peak stress the blood pressure and the heart rate were 164/62 mmHg and 130/min.

Stress Images There is reduced uptake of tracer in the inferior wall and apex.

Rest Images There is improvement in all areas.

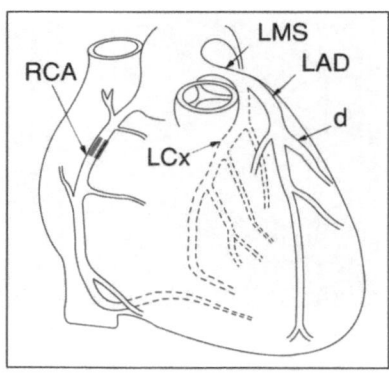

Coronary Angiography

There was a stenosis of the right coronary artery. The other coronary arteries were normal.

Conclusion

There is reversible ischaemia of the inferior wall and apex. This could not have been demonstrated by any other non-invasive technique. The primary action of dobutamine is to increase myocardial oxygen demand. Beta-blockade must be stopped 72 h before stress but, unlike dipyridamole and adenosine, it is safe in patients with bronchospasm.

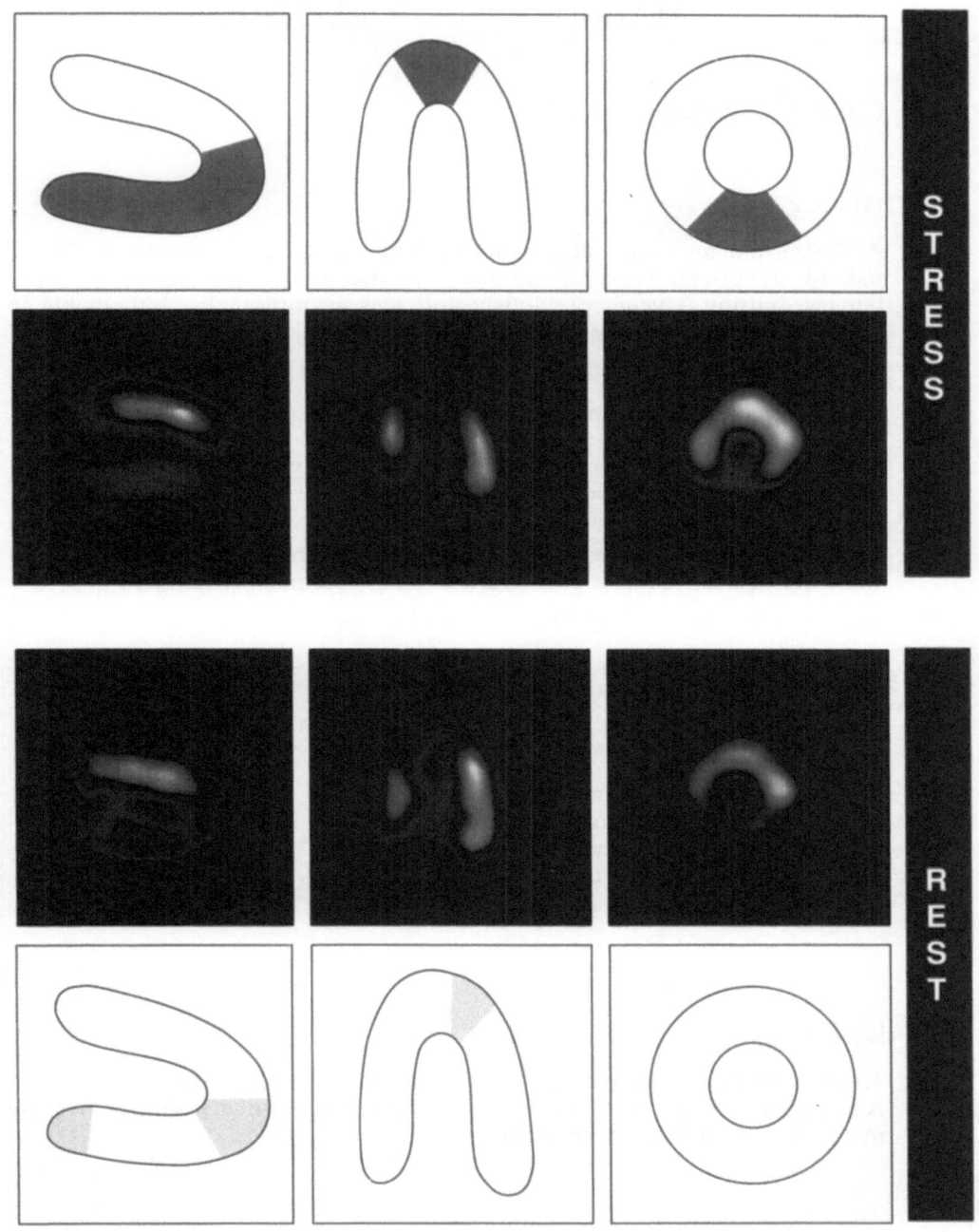

STRESS

REST

In patients who are unable to exercise and who have a history of bronchospasm, dobutamine may be the only simple method of provoking myocardial ischaemia.

Case 70 – Adenosine

History

A 76-year-old man was referred for thallium imaging in order to assess the risk of peripheral vascular surgery. He had undergone coronary artery bypass grafting 3 years previously and was asymptomatic, but unable to exercise freely because of claudication.

Thallium Myocardial Perfusion Tomography

Stress Technique Adenosine was infused at 140 μg/kg/min for 6 min without symptoms. The blood pressure and heart rate following infusion were 120/86 mmHg and 68/min.

Stress Images There is reduced uptake of tracer in the anterior wall, apex, and inferior wall. Uptake in the fundus of the stomach is visible.

Rest Images There is improvement in all areas.

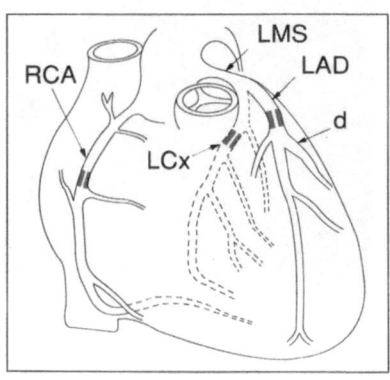

Coronary Angiography

There was disease of all three native coronary arteries and of the grafts to the left anterior descending and right coronary arteries. The circumflex graft was normal.

Conclusion

There is reversible ischaemia of the anterior wall, apex, and inferior wall. Adenosine acts in the same way as dipyridamole but its shorter half-life makes its action more controllable.

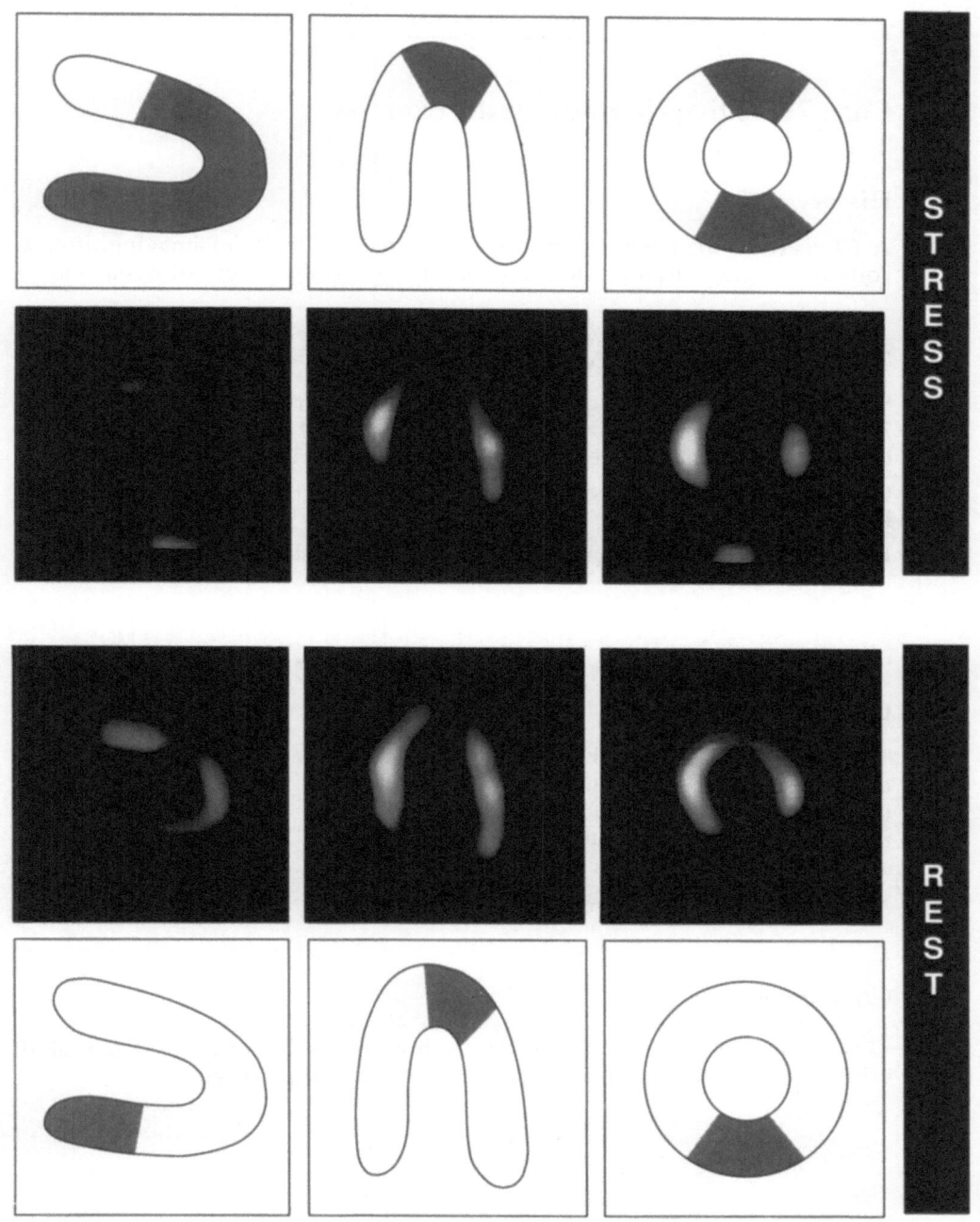

Adenosine is an effective agent for use with myocardial perfusion imaging. Like dipyridamole, it is contraindicated in patients with bronchospasm.

Case 71 – Dipyridamole with Exercise

History

A 60-year-old man with angina was referred for thallium imaging after a coronary angiogram for determination of the site and extent of ischaemia.

Thallium Myocardial Perfusion Tomography

Stress Technique Dipyridamole was infused during bicycle exercise to 75 W. Stress was limited by dyspnoea without chest pain. At peak stress the blood pressure and the heart rate were 140/80 mmHg and 120/min.

Stress Images There is reduced uptake of tracer in the anterior wall extending to the apex.

Rest Images There is improvement in the abnormal areas.

Coronary Angiography

There were stenoses in the left anterior descending and left circumflex arteries of uncertain severity. The right coronary artery could not be intubated.

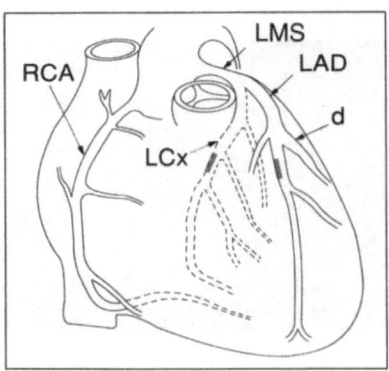

Conclusion

There is reversible ischaemia in the territory of the left anterior descending artery but the right coronary artery territory is well perfused.

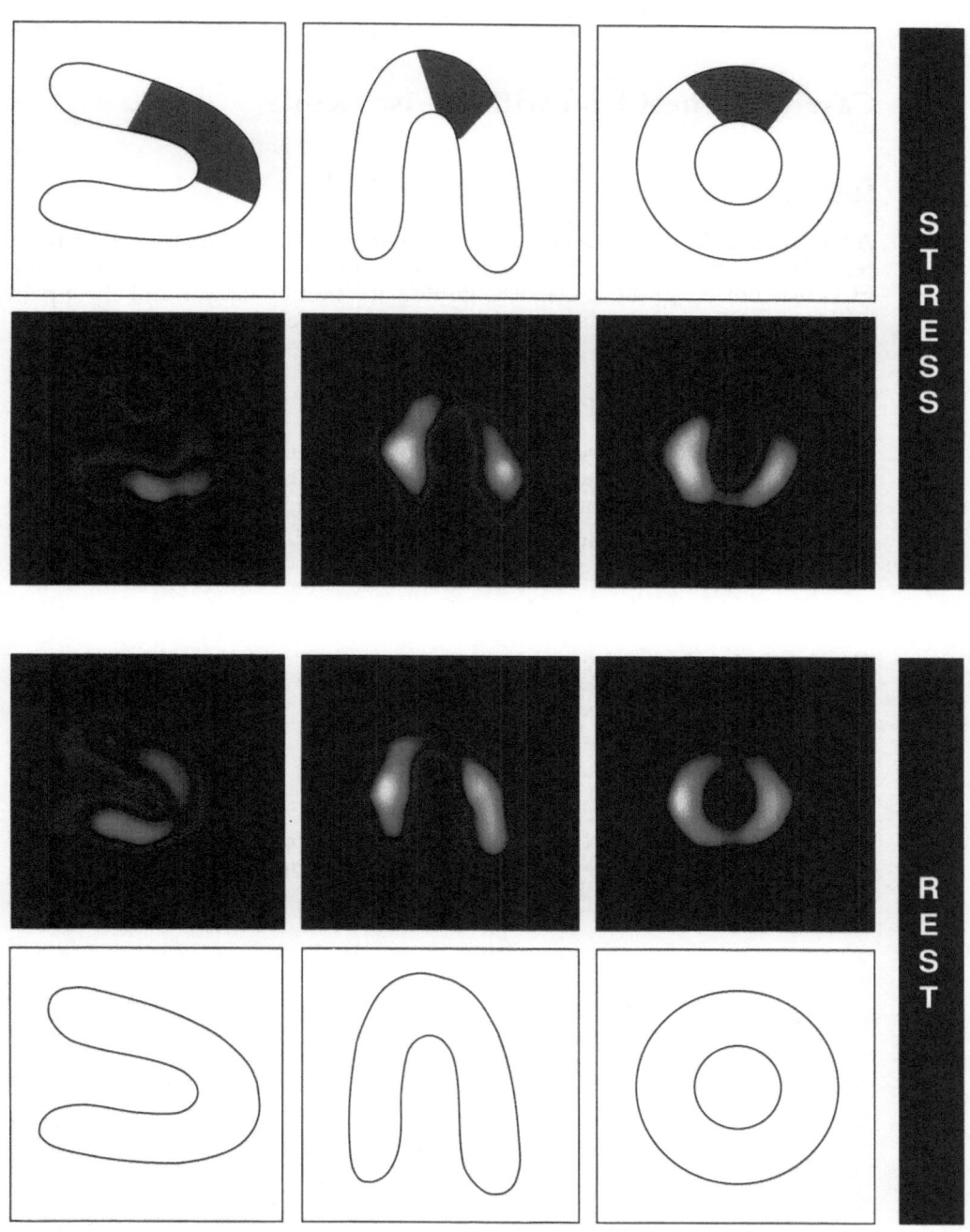

Case 72 – Chest Pain with No Ischaemia

History

A 56-year-old woman had chest pain related to exertion but also occurring at rest. There had been no improvement with medical treatment. Her resting ECG was normal and exercise was limited at 7 min by fatigue and chest pain with 1 mm ST segment depression in the inferior leads.

Thallium Myocardial Perfusion Tomography

Stress Technique Dipyridamole was infused during bicycle exercise to 100 W. Stress was limited by fatigue with chest pain. At peak stress the blood pressure and the heart rate were 180/100 mmHg and 140/min.

Stress Images There is normal uptake of tracer.

Rest Images There is no change.

Coronary Angiography

The coronary arteries were normal.

Conclusion

Normal myocardial perfusion. Ambulatory oesophageal pH monitoring showed the symptoms to be caused by gastro-oesophageal reflux.

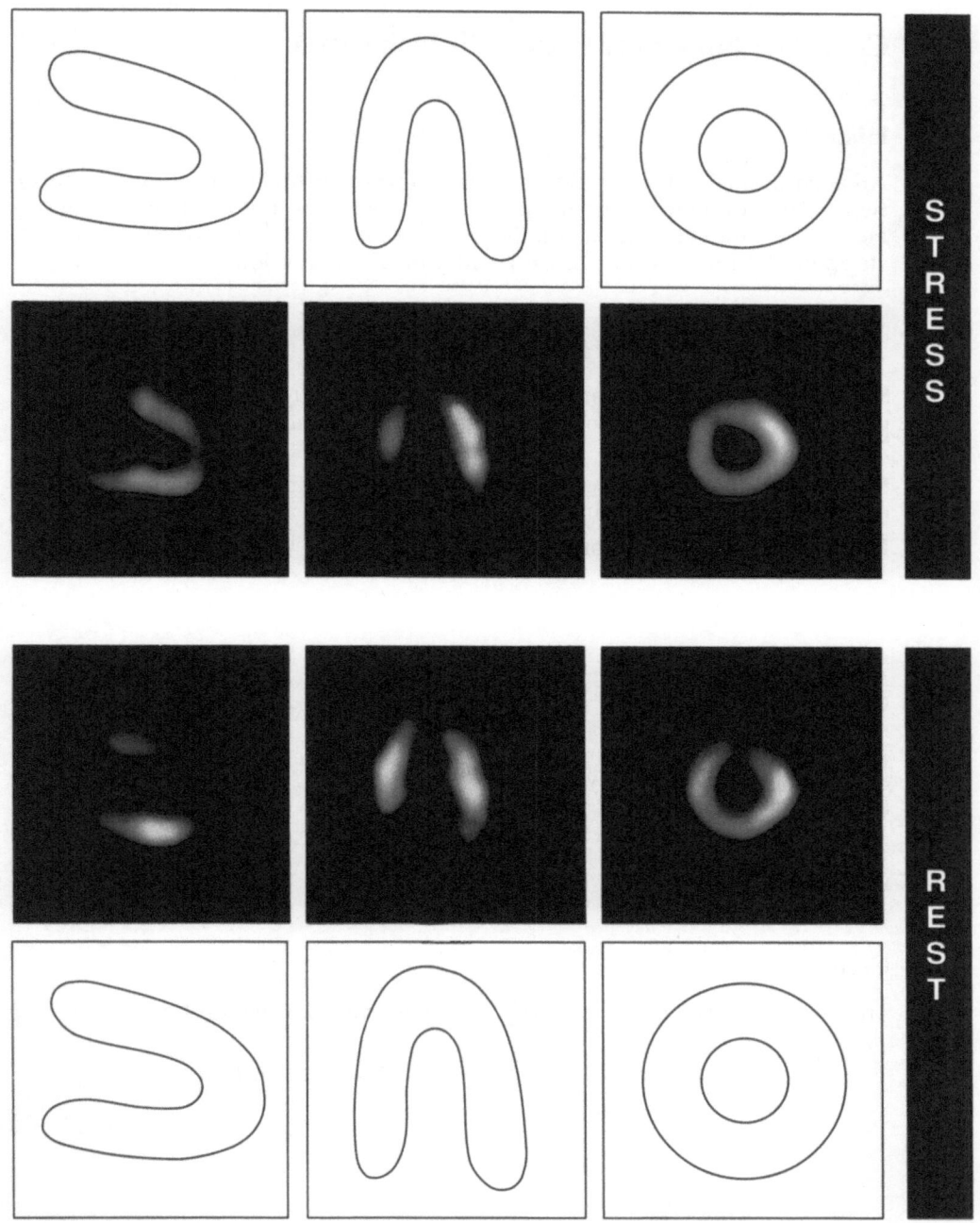

STRESS

REST

Exertional chest pain may not be caused by myocardial ischaemia.

Case 73 – No Chest Pain with Ischaemia

History

An asymptomatic 57-year-old man was referred for thallium imaging because two of his younger brothers had recently died from myocardial infarctions. He was a smoker with a mildly raised cholesterol. An exercise test was stopped at 4 min because of 2 mm inferior ST depression.

Thallium Myocardial Perfusion Tomography

Stress Technique Dobutamine was infused to 20 μg/kg/min without chest pain. At peak stress the blood pressure and the heart rate were 162/76 mmHg and 127/min.

Stress Images There is reduced uptake of tracer in the septum and apex extending to involve the inferior wall.

Rest Images There is improvement in all areas.

Coronary Angiography

There was a stenosis of the proximal left anterior descending artery but the other arteries were normal.

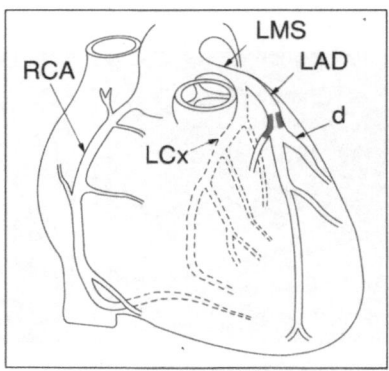

Conclusion

There is ischaemia in the territory of the left anterior descending artery.

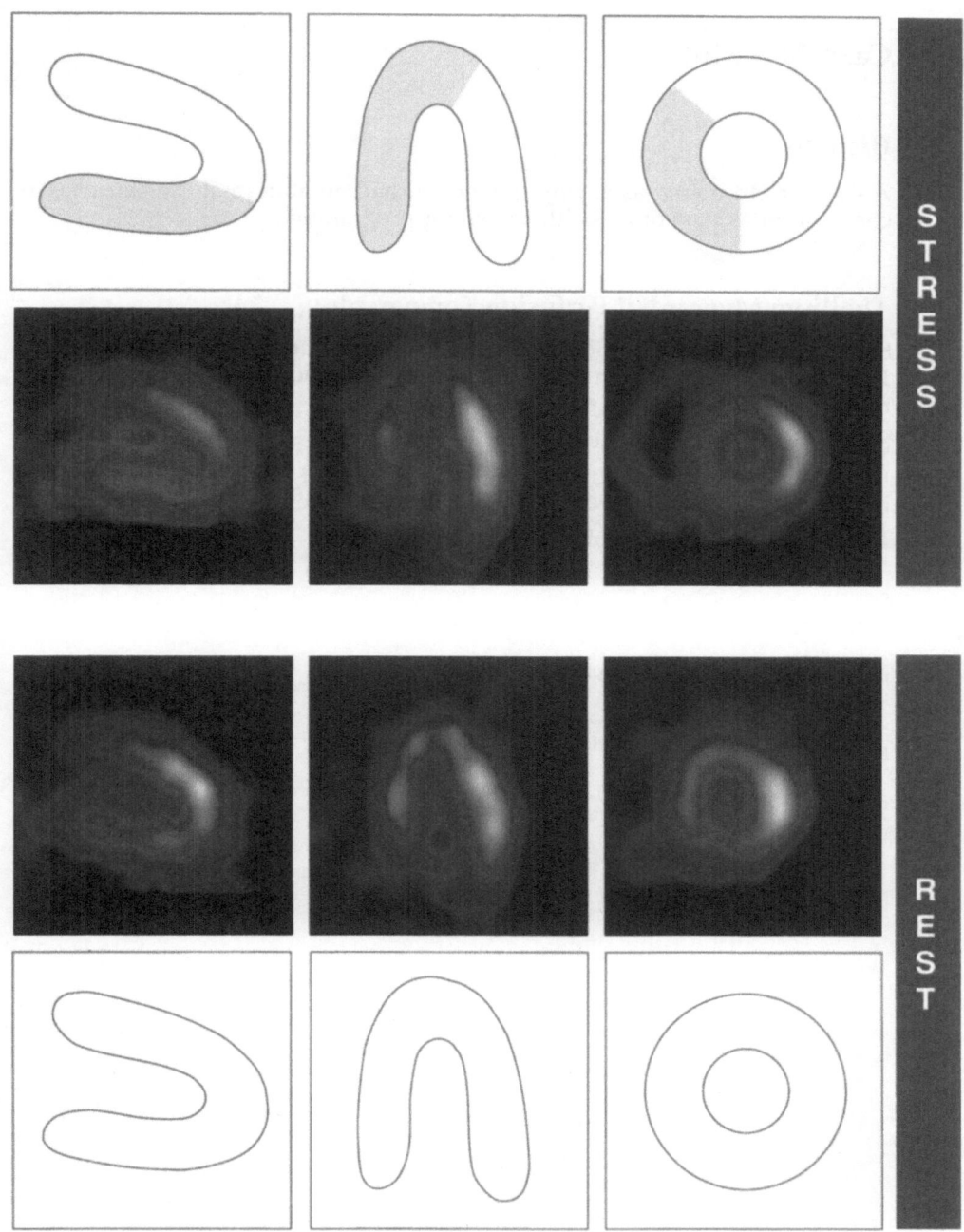

Ischaemia can occur in the absence of symptoms.

Case 74 – Motion

History

A 42-year-old man was asymptomatic but had an abnormal exercise electro-cardiogram as part of a health screening programme.

Thallium Myocardial Perfusion Tomography

Stress Technique Dipyridamole was infused during bicycle exercise to 175 W without chest pain. At peak stress the blood pressure and the heart rate were 190/100 mmHg and 168/min.

Stress Images There is normal uptake in all areas.

Rest Images He moved during the acquisition and there is distortion of the images with apparently reduced uptake in the anterior wall and apex.

Repeat Rest Images The images are now normal.

Conclusion

Normal myocardial perfusion.

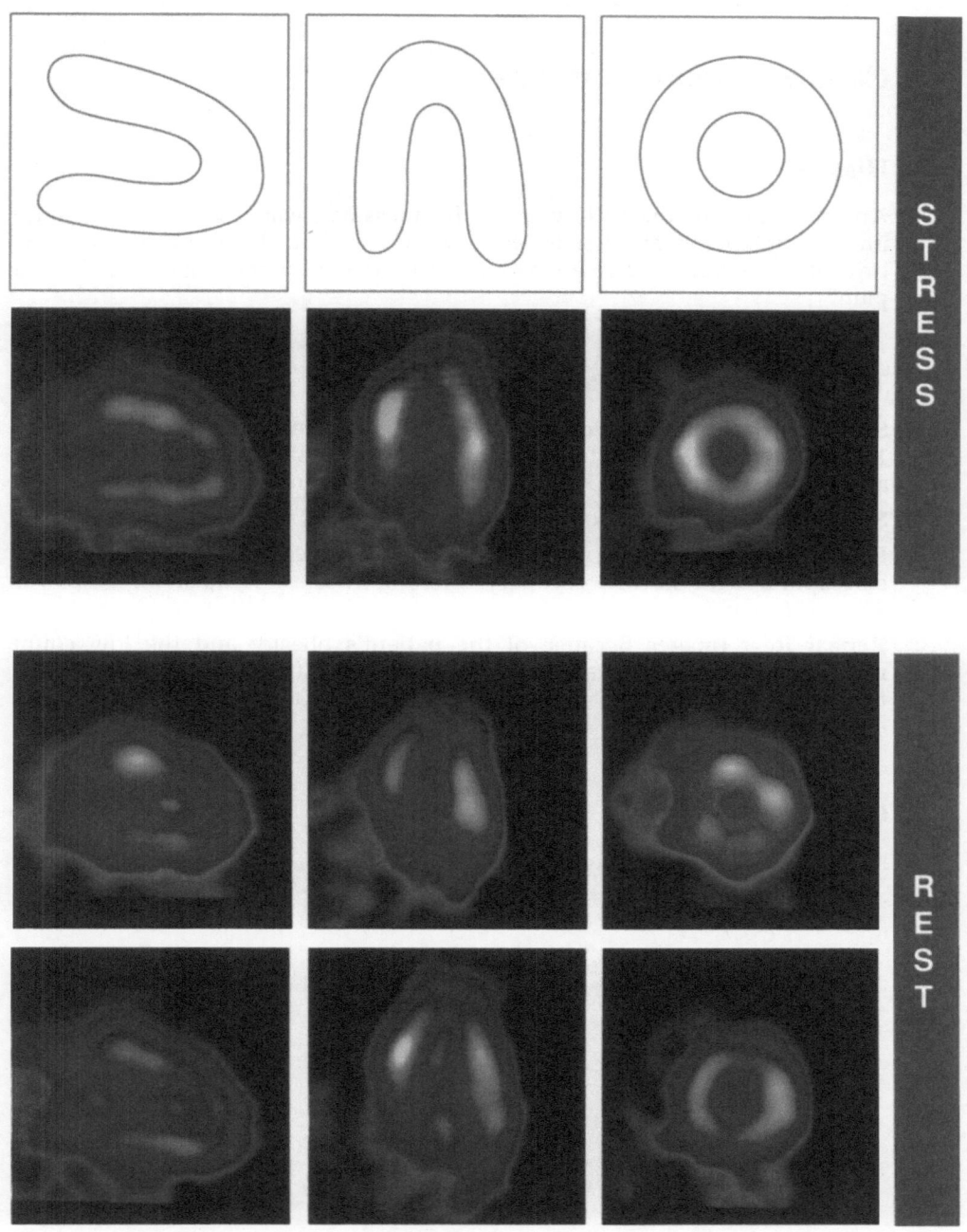

STRESS

REST

Patient motion during acquisition may cause image distortion and simulate abnormal perfusion.

Case 75 – Poor Count Rate

History

An asymptomatic obese 48-year-old businessman was referred for thallium imaging following an exercise ECG which showed 2 mm ST segment depression at 9 min. Exercise was limited by fatigue without associated chest pain.

Thallium Myocardial Perfusion Tomography

Stress Technique Dipyridamole was infused during bicycle exercise to 125 W. Exercise was limited by fatigue. At peak stress the blood pressure and the heart rate were 190/110 mmHg and 168/min.

Stress Images There is normal uptake of tracer.

Rest Images The images are irregular although the apparent defects do not correspond with normal coronary artery territories. Acquisition time was 30 s per frame.

Repeat Rest Images Because of the patient's obesity and the low count rate obtained, imaging was repeated with 45 s per frame. The appearance of the tracer distribution is now homogeneous and normal with some apical attenuation.

Conclusion

Normal myocardial perfusion.

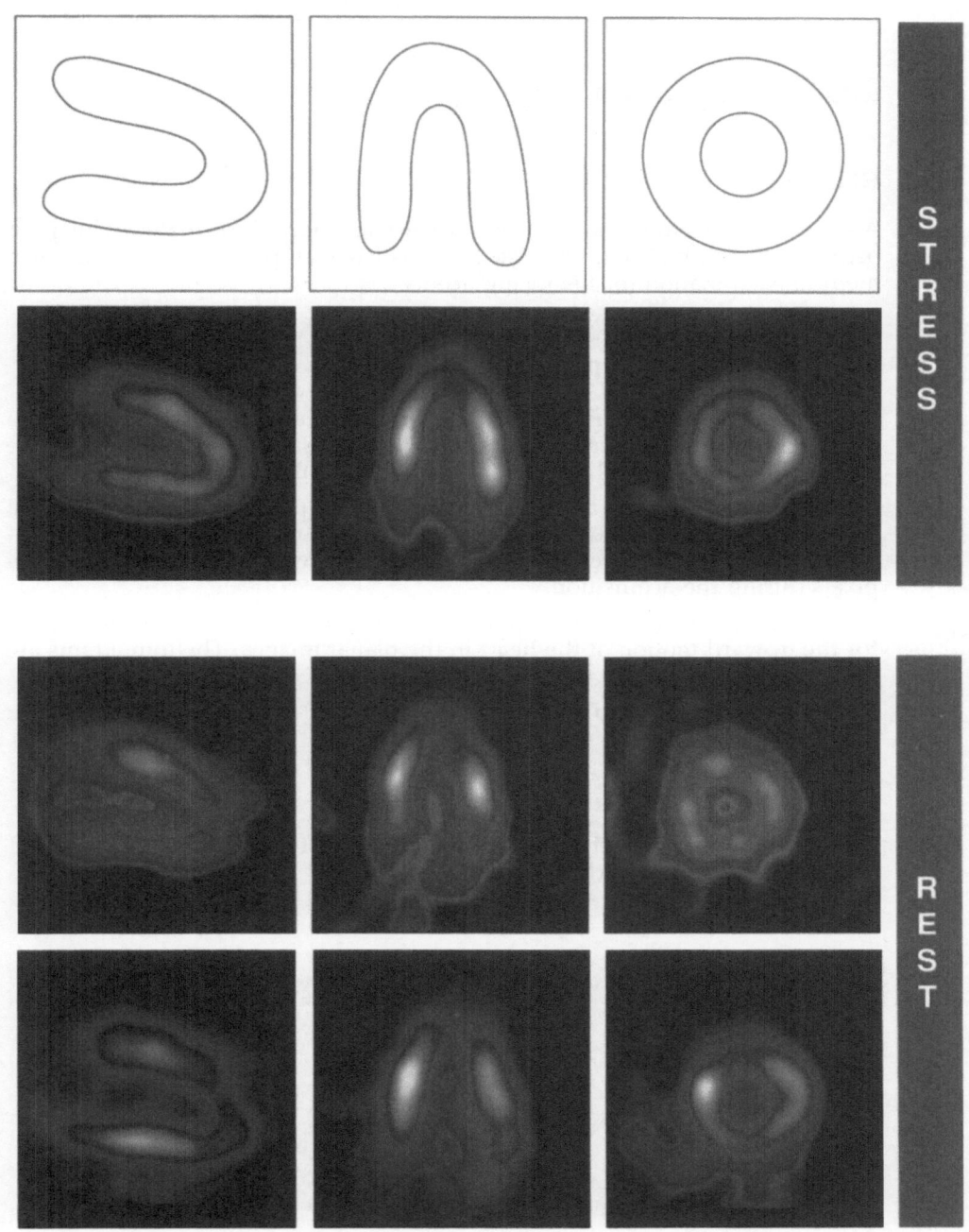

STRESS

REST

Image quality may be degraded in obese patients by a low count rate.
This can be improved by increasing the acquisition time.

Case 76 – Upward Creep

History

A 46-year-old asymptomatic racing driver was referred for thallium imaging because of an abnormal exercise ECG which was performed as part of a medical examination for his racing licence.

Thallium Myocardial Perfusion Tomography

Stress Technique Dipyridamole was infused during bicycle exercise to 150 W. Stress was limited by fatigue without chest pain. At peak stress the blood pressure and the heart rate were 170/80 mmHg and 155/min.

Stress Images There is a focal defect of tracer uptake in the anterior wall with apparent mild reduction in all areas except the lateral wall. Examination of the planar projections showed that the heart moved upwards by 4 pixels during the acquisition.

Corrected Stress Images Computer realignment was performed to correct for the upward motion of the heart in the planar images. The tomograms are now normal.

Rest Images There is no change.

Conclusion

Despite the apparent defect in the uncorrected stress images, the corrected images show normal perfusion.

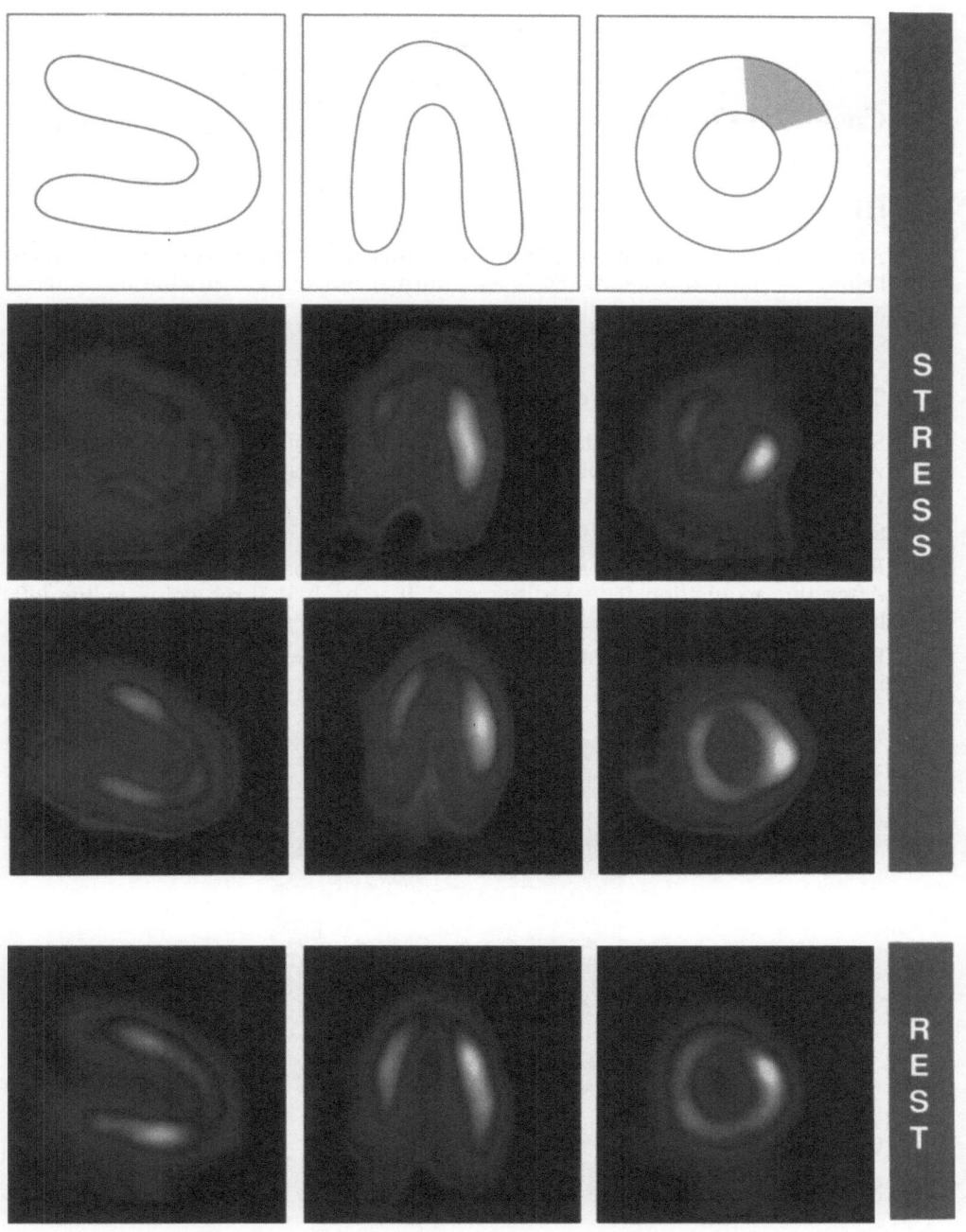

"Upward creep" may cause apparent anterior or inferior defects in images acquired immediately after vigorous exercise. This is the result of excessive lung inflation during exercise which depresses the heart with recovery during imaging.

Case 77 – Objects

History

An obese 50-year-old man had a single episode of chest pain at rest which lasted for 30 min. Resting ECG was normal but he was unable to exercise adequately on the treadmill.

Thallium Myocardial Perfusion Tomography

Stress Technique Dipyridamole was infused during bicycle exercise to 75 W without chest pain. At peak stress the blood pressure and the heart rate were 180/105 mmHg and 130/min.

Stress Images There is normal uptake in all areas.

Rest Images The images are distorted with an apparent defect at the apex. After the acquisition it was discovered that he had three coins in his left breast pocket (see below).

Repeat Rest Images The acquisition was repeated without the coins and the images are again normal.

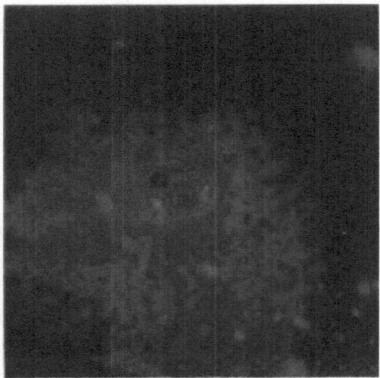

Conclusion

Normal myocardial perfusion with distortion of the images caused by coins.

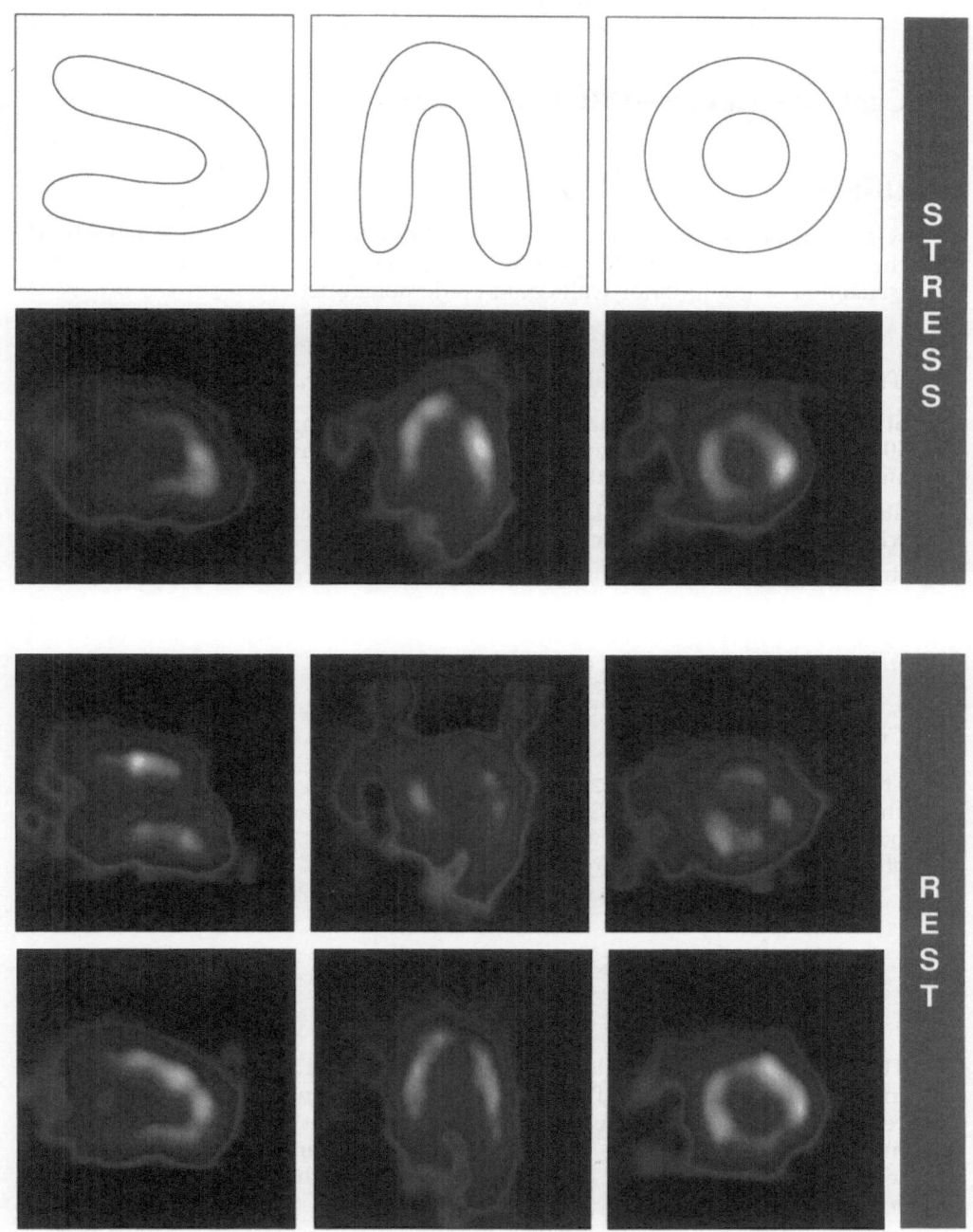

Attenuating objects must be removed from the field of view before imaging.

Case 78 – Reversed Redistribution

History

A 60-year-old woman with angina was known to have a mild stenosis of the left anterior descending artery. Angioplasty was planned if reversible ischaemia of the anterior wall could be demonstrated.

Thallium Myocardial Perfusion Tomography

Stress Technique Dipyridamole was infused during bicycle exercise to 50 W. Stress was limited by chest pain. At peak stress the blood pressure and the heart rate were 190/100 mmHg and 116/min.

Stress Images There is mildly reduced uptake of tracer in the anterior wall with normal uptake in other areas.

Rest Images The defect of the anterior wall is more obvious.

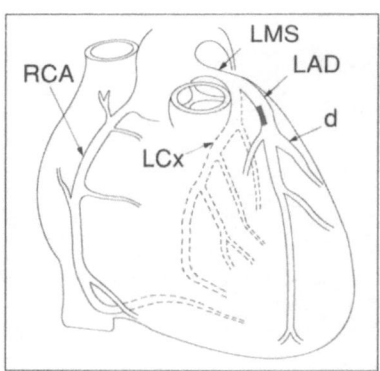

Coronary Angiography

There was a minor stenosis of the left anterior descending artery, of uncertain haemodynamic significance, but the other coronary arteries were normal.

Conclusion

There is a mild anterior defect of the anterior wall which is more marked following redistribution. There is no agreement on the cause of reversed redistribution but it is the result of rapid washout from the affected segment. It is thought to be caused by minor coronary artery disease which leads to subendocardial infarction but where the artery subsequently remains widely patent.

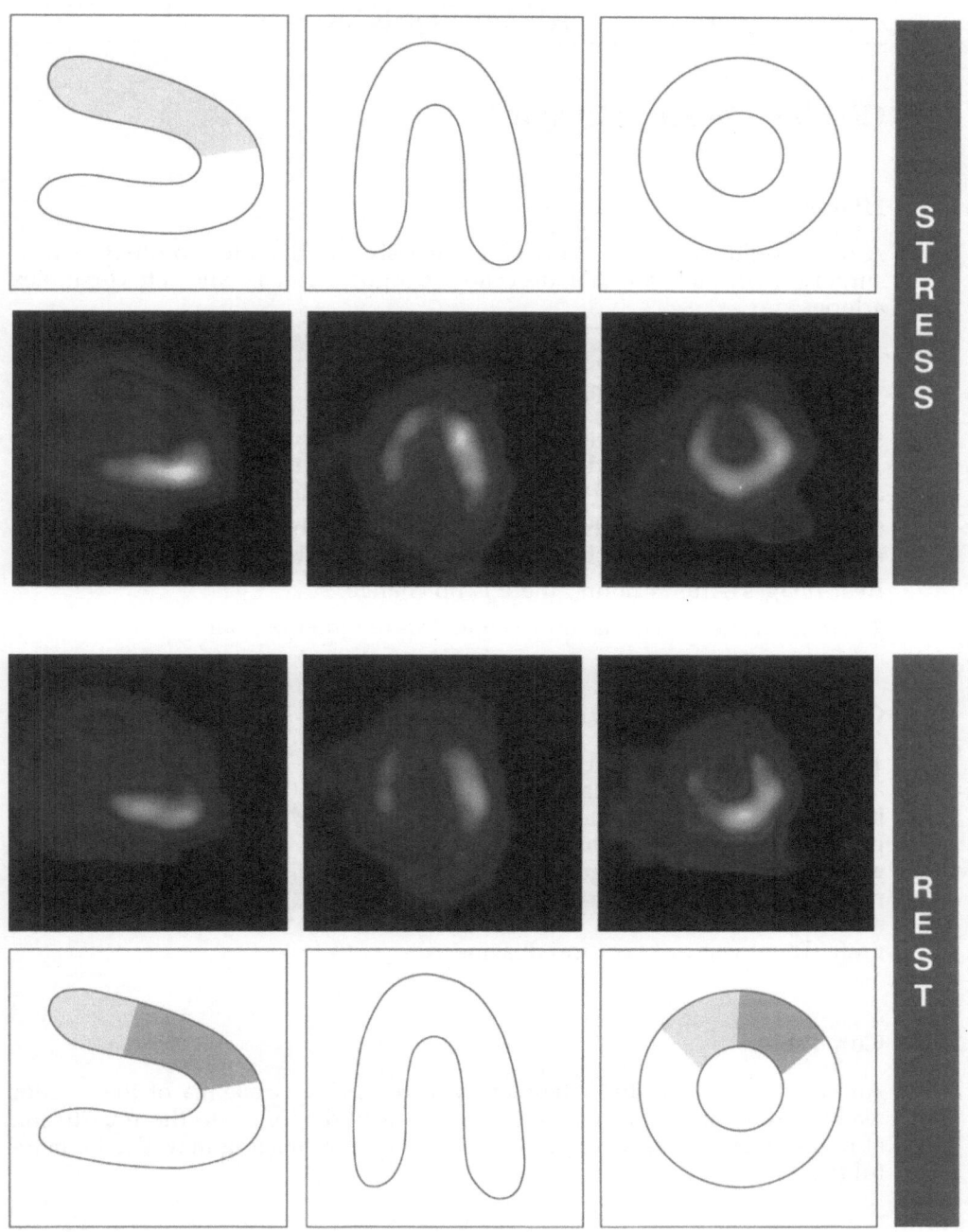

Reversed redistribution may be associated with coronary artery disease although it may also be the result of artefact in the redistribution images.

Case 79 – 24 Hour Imaging

History

A 50-year-old man had recurrent angina six months after coronary bypass surgery to the left anterior descending, right coronary and left circumflex arteries.

Thallium Myocardial Perfusion Tomography

Stress Technique Dipyridamole was infused during bicycle exercise to 125 W. Stress was limited by chest pain. At peak stress the blood pressure and the heart rate were 180/120 mmHg and 116/min.

Stress Images There is absent uptake of tracer in the distal anterior wall and apex, and reduced uptake in the inferior and basal anterior walls.

Rest Images After 4 hours, there is no change.

24 Hour Images There is improvement in the inferior wall.

Coronary Angiography

The native left anterior descending artery had severe proximal stenoses and its graft was patent though with very poor flow. The left circumflex artery graft was patent with good flow. The native right coronary artery was occluded and there was an ostial stenosis of its graft. There was anteroapical dyskinesis.

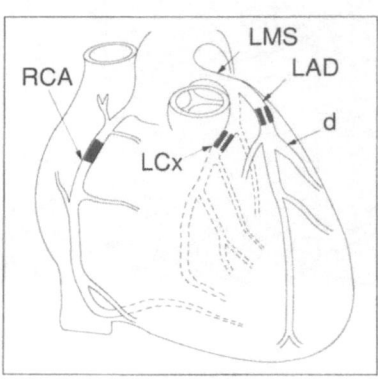

Conclusion

Anteroapical myocardial infarction with reversible ischaemia of the inferior wall. In this case, 24 h imaging was useful to demonstrate the reperfusion although image quality was reduced. Reinjection imaging may also be helpful (see case 80).

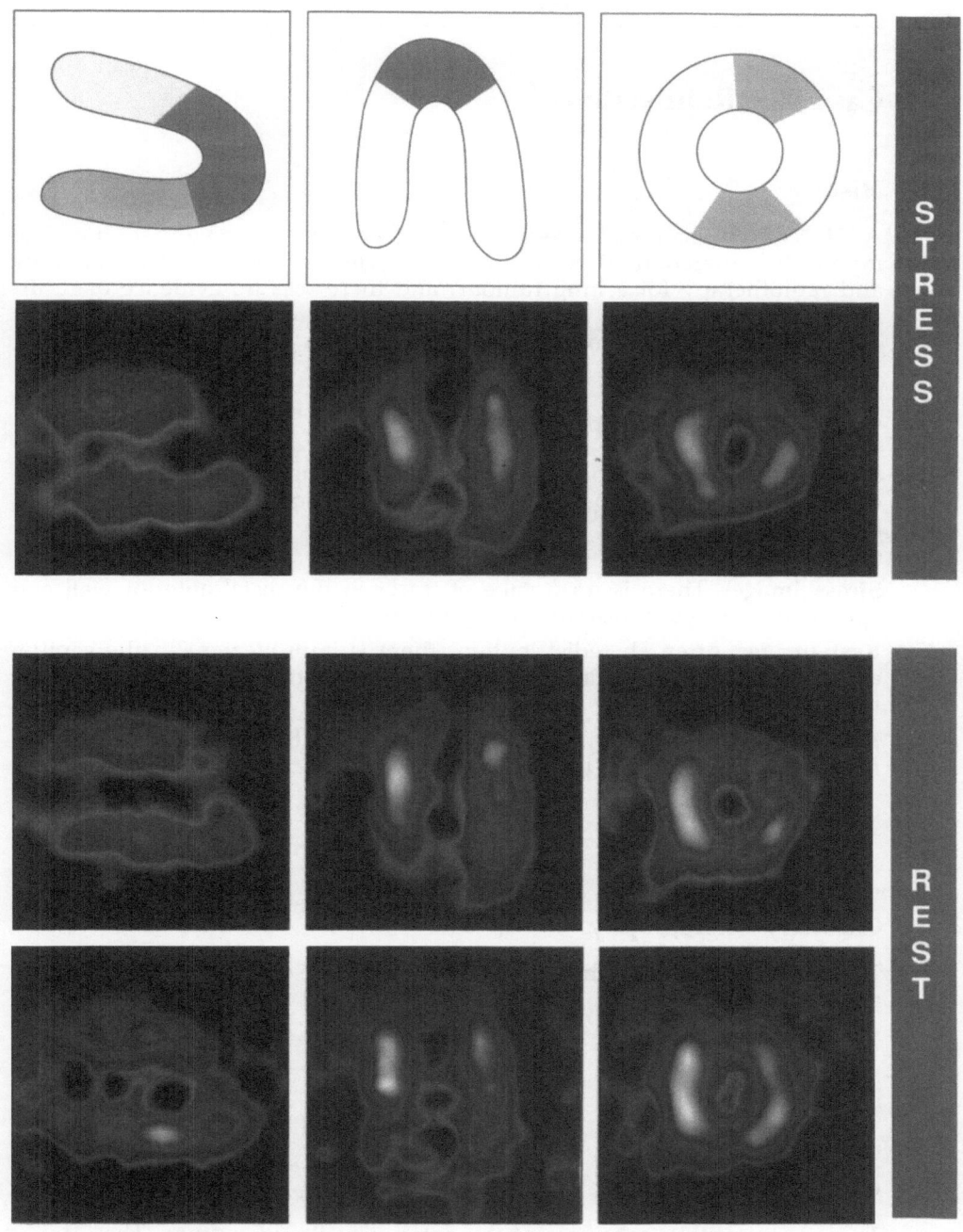

Myocardial viability may be underestimated in the 4 h images because of slow wash-in of thallium to the territory of a severely stenosed artery.

Case 80 – Reinjection

History

A 61-year-old man had exertional chest pain and a history of possible myocardial infarction 10 years previously. He had received chemotherapy and radiotherapy for a lung tumour, and there was no evidence of recurrence. His resting ECG was normal and his exercise ECG was limited at 4 min by dyspnoea without ST segment changes.

Thallium Myocardial Perfusion Tomography

Stress Technique Adenosine was infused at 140 µg/kg/min for 6 min without chest pain or dyspnoea. At peak stress the blood pressure and the heart rate were 106/70 mmHg and 77/min, and there was 2 mm ST segment depression.

Stress Images There is no uptake of tracer in the distal anterior wall and apex with reduced uptake in the septum and the inferior wall.

Rest Images After 4h redistribution, there is improvement in the septum and some improvement in the anterior wall but little change in the inferior wall.

Reinjection Images After resting injection of 37 MBq thallium, there is now marked improvement in the inferior wall and apex.

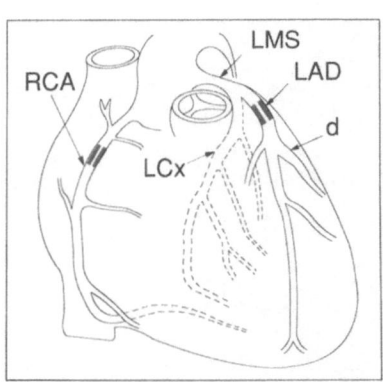

Coronary Angiography

There were stenoses of the proximal left anterior descending and right coronary arteries.

Conclusion

There is reversible ischaemia of the anterior wall and septum. The inferior wall and apex improve following reinjection.

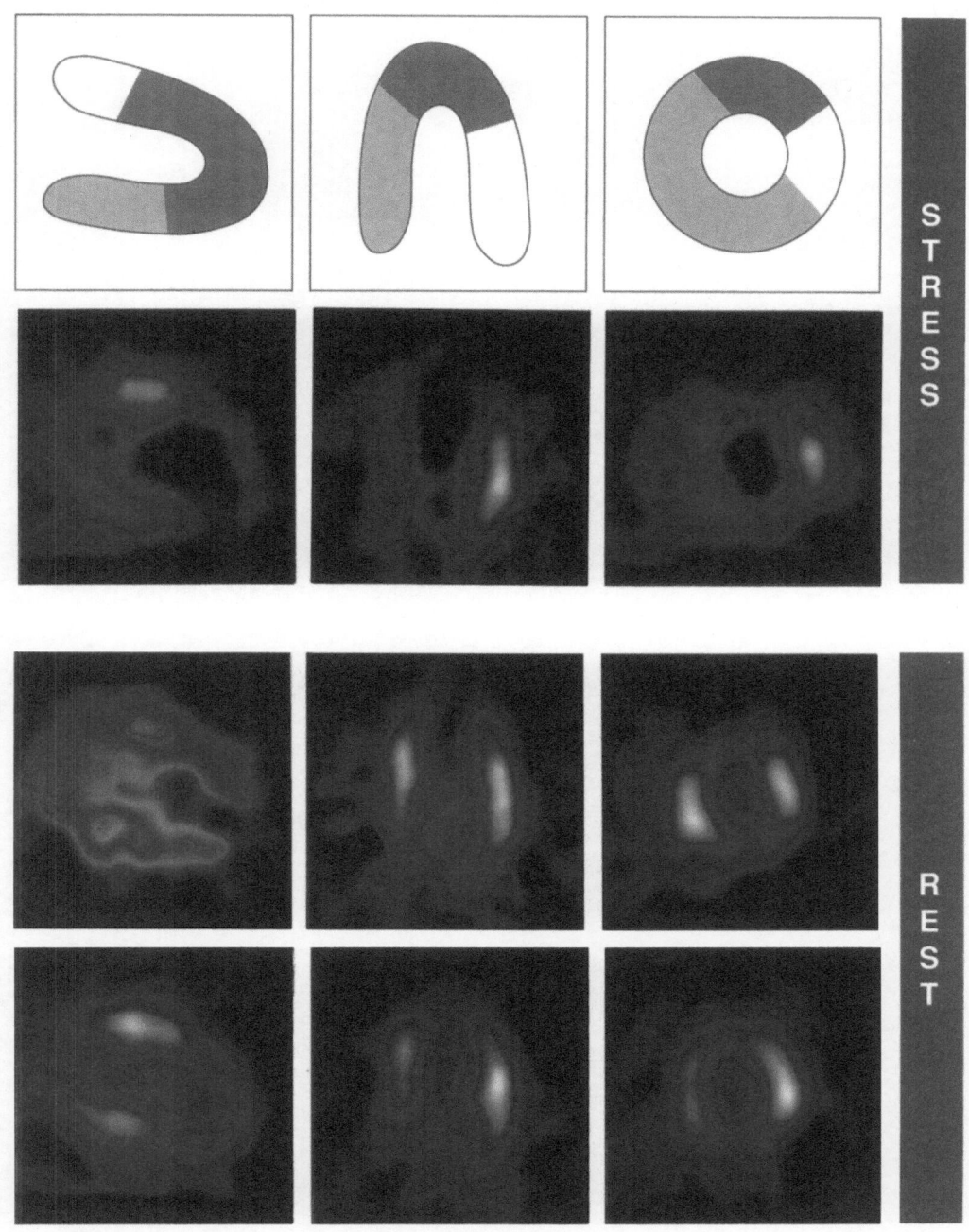

STRESS

REST

Reinjection of thallium may be useful in determining myocardial viability when doubt remains after redistribution imaging.

Chapter 7

Clinical Applications

Detection of Coronary Artery Disease

A range of investigations is normally used in patients with suspected coronary artery disease, the simplest "investigation" being the history. Typical angina is a good indicator of myocardial ischaemia and abolition of symptoms is the primary aim of treatment. Symptoms do not indicate the site or extent of ischaemia, however, and it is helpful to have an objective assessment of myocardial ischaemia in order to guide future management. Myocardial perfusion scintigraphy is the only non-invasive and widely available method of assessing myocardial perfusion. It, therefore, has an obvious role in the detection of perfusion abnormalities caused by coronary artery disease. Many studies have assessed the sensitivity and specificity of the technique for the detection of disease, the coronary arteriogram usually being used as the standard by which the accuracy of scintigraphy is judged. The wisdom of this approach can be debated, but at least the arteriogram provides a universal standard for coronary arterial anatomy even if it is a less good standard by which to judge coronary arterial function. Rozanski and Berman[1] have reviewed 15 such studies involving 1023 patients with disease and 478 without disease. They found that figures varied widely but the overall sensitivity and specificity for the detection of coronary artery disease was 80% and 92% respectively. This was significantly better than exercise electrocardiography where the figures were 64% and 82%.

It is reasonable to ask, therefore, whether thallium scintigraphy should be used in place of exercise electrocardiography in patients with suspected coronary artery disease. Several factors militate against this. The most important is the radiation burden to the patient, but the additional expense and the lower availability of thallium imaging will also influence the decision. The main place of thallium imaging for the diagnosis of coronary artery disease is if the electrocardiogram is uninterpretable because of resting abnormalities (left bundle branch block, pre-excitation, left ventricular hypertrophy, drug effects), or if doubt remains because of equivocal ST segment changes or a normal exercise electrocardiogram despite a high pretest likelihood of disease.

A special case is the asymptomatic individual who requests an exercise test in order to rule out the possibility of coronary artery disease. Sadly, there is a discrepancy between recommended and actual practice. Exercise electrocardiography and exercise thallium scanning should not be performed as screening tests for coronary artery disease in low risk individuals, including those without symptoms.[2] Any test without perfect specificity will produce a higher number of false positive results than true positive results in such a population. Between one-tenth and one-third of asymptomatic men with abnormal exercise electrocardiograms will have normal coronary arteries. Unfortunately in some countries, particularly those with a privatised medical system, exercise testing has become common in asymptomatic individuals. A reasonable role for thallium scintigraphy is then to adjudicate on the presence of disease if the exercise electrocardiogram is equivocal or abnormal.

The position in asymptomatic patients who have a "high risk" of coronary artery disease is more difficult. Although asymptomatic patients with hypertension or hypercholesterolaemia have an increased risk of coronary artery disease, it is not sufficiently high that the post-test likelihood of disease following an abnormal thallium scan exceeds 50%. In other words there will still be more false positives than true positives in this population. Only in patients with established peripheral vascular disease does the pretest likelihood of coronary disease reach a sufficiently high level to warrant exercise testing in patients without cardiac symptoms. The patient with claudication or an abdominal aortic aneurysm may therefore have a thallium scan (with dipyridamole or dobutamine) in order to gauge the risk of vascular surgery.[3,4]

The concept of pretest and post-test likelihood of disease arises from Bayes' theorem which is central to the correct application of any diagnostic test.[5,6] The theorem predicts that the greatest contribution to diagnosis from a test with sensitivity and specificity similar to thallium scintigraphy is made when the pretest likelihood of disease is around 50% (Fig. 7.1). If the pretest

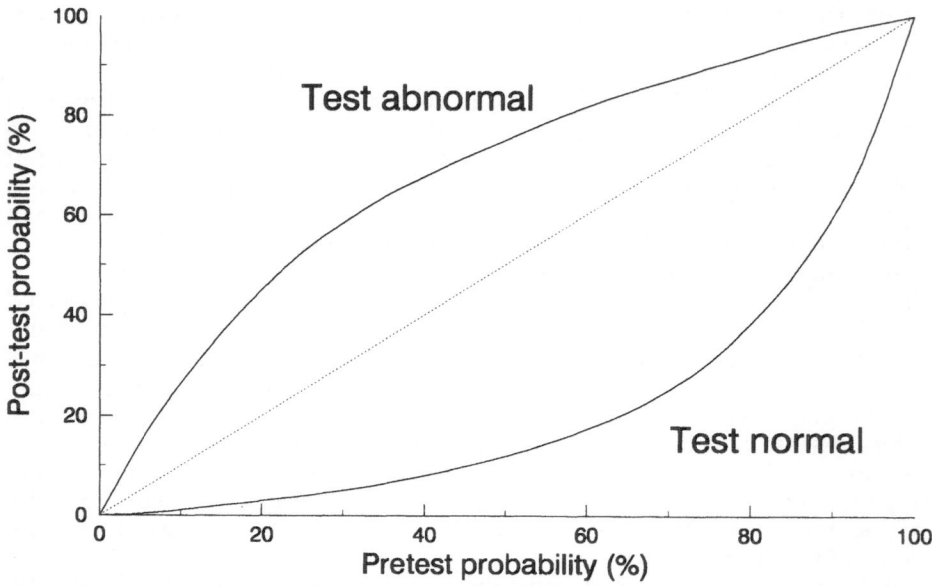

Fig. 7.1. Bayes' theorem relates the pretest probability of disease to the post-test probability. The result of the test makes the largest change in probability of disease if the pretest probability is between 30% and 70%.

likelihood of disease is very low, then even an abnormal test does not increase the likelihood of disease by very much. Conversely, a normal test in a patient with a very high pretest likelihood does not significantly lower the likelihood of disease. It is always worth considering the pretest likelihood of disease before requesting a diagnostic test with less than perfect sensitivity and specificity.

Management of Established Coronary Artery Disease

Stable Angina

As in the diagnosis of coronary artery disease, the presence of typical angina of effort is a reasonable indicator of myocardial ischaemia. It is helpful to have objective confirmation, however, especially since the level of exercise achieved during a formal exercise test can be used to judge the effects of treatment or of progression of disease. The exercise electrocardiogram is the most commonly used objective test. It provides less information than thallium scintigraphy and is less accurate for the detection of ischaemia, but it is simple, cheap and widely available. There are a number of occasions when the electrocardiogram may be unhelpful and in these cases thallium imaging should be used as the primary stress test. Particularly in the light of the later discussion of the assessment of prognosis, it is reasonable for patients with stable angina to have at least one thallium scan but in the patient known to have ST segment changes during myocardial ischaemia, electrocardiography can be used for regular assessment.

The role of thallium scintigraphy in patients with stable angina differs between general and specialist hospitals. Although practice varies between countries, in the United Kingdom the majority of patients with stable angina are referred to general hospitals which may not have the facilities for coronary arteriography. Medical management is directed at abolishing symptoms and if intolerable symptoms remain despite optimal medical treatment, then referral to a specialist centre for possible angioplasty or bypass surgery is required. More commonly, symptoms are improved to tolerable levels by medical treatment and the important question becomes whether the risk of future infarction or death can be improved by mechanical intervention. In these patients, thallium imaging is an ideal prognostic tool allowing the separation of patients into those who can safely continue on medical treatment and those who are at high risk and who may benefit more from intervention. In contrast, the patient with stable angina in a specialist centre has often already been selected to require intervention, and coronary arteriography cannot be avoided. Whilst the coronary arteriogram is not an ideal method of assessing coronary artery function, clinical decisions can often be made from a knowledge of coronary anatomy alone. In such patients, the role of thallium imaging is to act as a baseline for studies after intervention.

Myocardial Infarction

Thallium imaging plays very little role in the immediate management of acute myocardial infarction. In fact, it is an effective tool for the diagnosis of infarction because perfusion defects can be visualised immediately after coronary occlusion and before electrocardiographic changes are apparent. The most important priority in patients with suspected infarction, however, is admission to a coronary care unit. Few hospitals have the facilities for performing portable thallium scans on the coronary care unit.

On recovery from myocardial infarction, management should be very similar to that of patients with stable angina. Persistent reversible ischaemia should be sought, and this is most commonly done from the history and from exercise electrocardiography. Submaximal exercise electrocardiography may be performed before discharge from hospital although maximal exercise at six weeks is common. If the exercise electrocardiogram suggests continuing ischaemia, then thallium imaging is a reasonable next step since it will provide the distinction between ischaemia in a territory unrelated to the infarct and ischaemia in a related territory. Whilst the clinical importance of such a distinction is unclear, many physicians would treat ischaemia in an unrelated territory more aggressively since it is likely to put a larger area of myocardium at risk.

Many patients with acute myocardial infarction will now be given the benefit of thrombolytic treatment in the early hours. It is unusual that all the threatened myocardium is salvaged and more commonly a central region of necrosis is surrounded by an area of salvaged myocardium which continues to be nourished by the recanalised artery. Alternatively, viable and necrotic cells may coexist in a region of partial infarction. It has been debated whether angioplasty of the infarct related lesion might provide any benefit but it is now clear that allowing the lesion to stabilise on medical treatment alone produces the best long-term results. Longer-term management is dictated by whether there is persistent reversible ischaemia, and thallium imaging is the ideal method of assessing such ischaemia since the resting electrocardiogram is unlikely to be normal.

Monitoring the Effects of Intervention

An essential element to any intervention, whether in medicine or in an unrelated field, is to assess the effect of the intervention from studies before and after the procedure. Some cardiologists are accustomed to monitoring patients after angioplasty or bypass surgery from the history and exercise electrocardiography alone. This may be difficult because the pain of myocardial ischaemia can be modified by surgery and because many patients experience different chest pains unrelated to myocardial ischaemia for some time after surgery. Thallium tomography can be particularly helpful because the ability to visualise ischaemia directly and to relate its site to the known coronary anatomy allows the success of intervention to be confirmed, unexpected complications to be detected (patients may suffer silent myocardial infarction early after coronary bypass surgery), and future recurrence of symptoms to be assessed objectively from changes in the pattern of perfusion (cases 43 to 49).

Percutaneous coronary angioplasty has a high primary success rate: the appearance of the coronary arteriogram is improved in four-fifths of patients. In one-third of these, however, the stenosis will recur within six months and further angioplasty may be required. Both exercise electrocardiography and thallium tomography can be used to detect the recurrence (case 46), although the management of recurrent ischaemia in the absence of symptoms is difficult. Symptoms should probably be the guide to the need for further angioplasty since a lesion that has already been dilated is unlikely to be unstable and to present with acute infarction without preceding symptoms.

Prognosis in Coronary Artery Disease

The most valuable contribution that thallium imaging can make to the management of patients with coronary artery disease is in the assessment of the risk of myocardial infarction or death. Prognosis has long been known to depend on the severity of the coronary disease but the problem lies in an objective assessment of severity. Many invasive cardiologists feel most at home if a coronary arteriogram is available. That there is a relationship between the severity of disease assessed in this way and the amount of myocardium in jeopardy is reflected in the better prognosis of patients with left main stem disease and three vessel disease with surgical rather than medical treatment.[7] However, the coronary arteriogram is a crude method of assessing the functional significance of disease. Visual assessment of coronary arteriograms has long been known to have a large intra-observer and interobserver variability[8,9] and a poor association with post mortem anatomy.[10-14] More recently, a poor relationship between luminal narrowing and coronary function has also been demonstrated.[15] Some attempt can be made to improve the assessment using either a coronary artery score[16-18] or digitised tracing of the lesions to combine the effects of luminal narrowing and length and morphology of the stenosis.[19] The exercise is complicated by the fact that coronary arteries are not passive conduits but active organs[20] that control the shear stress along their walls by dilating in response to increases in flow.[21] This normal dilatation is impaired or reversed by atheromatous disease.[22] There can be no doubt therefore that coronary artery function must be assessed by a separate technique and that the main role of coronary arteriography is as an anatomical guide during angioplasty or surgery.

Exercise electrocardiography is the most commonly performed of the tests of coronary function. Several parameters can provide prognostic information including exercise time, ST segment depression and blood pressure response.[23-26] All of these are relatively crude measures of the extent of ischaemia, however. Exercise radionuclide ventriculography provides a more refined assessment because abnormal regional contraction is an early manifestation of reversible ischaemia. Extensive abnormalities impair left ventricular ejection fraction which is an excellent indicator of prognosis.[27-34] Measurements made during exercise are superior to measurements at rest because they reflect the extent of infarction and of reversible ischaemia.

Because it is the extent of jeopardised myocardium that determines risk it is most rational to look at myocardial perfusion directly. The evidence that thallium myocardial perfusion imaging provides prognostic information in stable angina[35-40] and following myocardial infarction[41-45] is overwhelming. Even in asymptomatic patients, the thallium scan can identify those at high risk of future events.[46,47] Two important papers on the subject are from

Ladenheim and colleagues. In 1689 patients with coronary artery disease without prior infarction, it was shown that the extent and severity of the reversible thallium defects were independent predictors of cardiac events at one year.[48] The cardiac event rate varied from 0.4% in patients with normal exercise perfusion, to 78% in patients with both severe and extensive perfusion defects. In a subsequent paper the same group demonstrated the incremental prognostic power of the history, exercise electrocardiography, and myocardial perfusion imaging.[49]

Thus it could be argued that myocardial perfusion imaging should be performed in all patients with coronary artery disease in order to assess prognosis and to select patients who, irrespective of symptoms, deserve intervention in order to prevent future infarction or death. Such a policy assumes that intervention in patients with few or absent symptoms but large areas of reversible ischaemia can improve prognosis. Although this has not been proved there is some supporting evidence. It has been shown, for instance, that coronary angioplasty can be performed safely and with good anatomical results in asymptomatic patients with coronary artery disease, and that five-year prognosis is excellent.[50] Whether it is any better than without intervention remains to be established, but until this evidence is available it is reasonable to assume that abolishing reversible ischaemia is ultimately beneficial.

The powerful prognostic value of myocardial perfusion imaging is difficult to square with the increasing evidence that the degree to which coronary atheroma impairs coronary flow reserve is not necessarily related to the instability of the lesion and hence the risk of coronary thrombosis. Little et al.[51] have shown that only one-third of infarctions occur because of occlusion of the most severe stenosis, and that two-thirds occur at stenoses that were less than 50%. Similar results have been shown by Hackett et al.[52] and by Brosius and Roberts.[53] Thus, there will always be patients who present with myocardial infarction or sudden death without preceding angina and we do not yet have a diagnostic technique that is capable of detecting such early lesions. Presumably the prognostic power of myocardial perfusion imaging arises from the fact that patients with extensive flow-limiting lesions are also likely to have thrombogenic lesions (even if not flow limiting) and so are at high risk of infarction.

References

1. Rozanski A, Berman DS. The efficacy of cardiovascular nuclear medicine exercise studies. Semin Nucl Med 1987;17:104–20.
2. Petch MC. Misleading exercise electrocardiograms. Br Med J 1987;295:620–1.
3. Fletcher JP, Antico VF, Gruenewald S, Kershaw LZ. Dipyridamole–thallium scan for screening of coronary artery disease prior to vascular surgery. J Cardiovasc Surg 1988;29:66.
4. Lette J, Waters D, Lapointe J et al. Usefulness of the severity and extent of reversible perfusion defects during thallium–dipyridamole imaging for cardiac risk assessment before noncardiac surgery. Am J Cardiol 1989;64:276–81.
5. Diamond GA. Reverend Bayes' silent majority. An alternative factor affecting sensitivity and specificity of exercise electrocardiography. Am J Cardiol 1986;57:1175.
6. Detrano R, Leatherman J, Salcedo EE, Yiannikas J, Williams G. Bayesian analysis versus discriminant function analysis: their relative utility in the diagnosis of coronary disease. Circulation 1986;73:970–7.

7. European Coronary Surgery Study Group. Prospective randomised study of coronary artery bypass surgery in stable angina pectoris. Lancet 1980;ii:491–5.
8. Zir LM, Miller SW, Dinsmore RE, Gilbert JP, Harthorne JW. Interobserver variability in coronary angiography. Circulation 1976;53:627–32.
9. Galbraith JE, Murphy ML, Desoyza N. Coronary angiogram interpretation: interobserver variability. JAMA 1981;240:2053–9.
10. Grodin CM, Dyrda I, Pasternac A, Campeau L, Bourassa MG. Discrepancies between cine angiographic and post-mortem findings in patients with coronary artery disease and recent myocardial revascularisation. Circulation 1974;49:703–9.
11. Blankenhorn DH, Curry PJ. The accuracy of arteriography and ultrasound imaging for atherosclerosis measurement: a review. Arch Pathol Lab Med 1982;106:483–90.
12. Isner JM, Kishel J, Kent KM. Accuracy of angiographic determination of left main coronary arterial narrowing. Circulation 1981;63:1056–61.
13. Roberts WC, Jones AA. Quantitation of coronary arterial narrowing at necropsy in sudden coronary death. Am J Cardiol 1979;44:38–44.
14. Vlodaver Z, Frech R, van Tassel RA, Edwards JE. Correlation of the antemortem coronary angiogram and the postmortem specimen. Circulation 1973;47:162–8.
15. White CW, Wright CB, Doty DB et al. Does visual interpretation of the coronary arteriogram predict the physiologic importance of a coronary stenosis? N Engl J Med 1984;310:819–24.
16. Balcon R. Prognostic significance of coronary angiography. Eur Heart J 1984;5:73–5.
17. Balcon R. The relationship between prognosis and angiographic and exercise data. Acta Med Scand 1984;694 (suppl):101–3.
18. Moise A, Clement B, Saltiel J. Clinical and angiographic correlates and prognostic significance of the coronary extent score. Am J Cardiol 1988;61:1255–9.
19. Nissen SE, Gurley JC. Assessment of the functional significance of coronary stenoses. Is digital angiography the answer? Circulation 1990;81:1431–5.
20. Chesebro JH, Fuster V, Webster MWI. Editorial comment. Endothelial injury and coronary vasomotion. J Am Coll Cardiol 1989;14:1191–2.
21. Bing RJ. Editorial comment. Control of shear stress in the epicardial coronary arteries of humans: impairment by atherosclerosis. J Am Coll Cardiol 1989;14:1200–1.
22. Vita JA, Treasure CB, Ganz P, Cox DA, Fish RD, Selwyn AP. Control of shear stress in the epicardial coronary arteries of humans: impairment by atherosclerosis. J Am Coll Cardiol 1989;14:1193–9.
23. Chaitman BR. The changing role of the exercise electrocardiogram as a diagnostic and prognostic test for chronic ischemic heart disease. J Am Coll Cardiol 1986;8:1195–210.
24. Rautaharju PM, Prineas RJ, Eifler WJ et al. Prognostic value of exercise electrocardiogram in men at high risk of future coronary heart disease: multiple risk factor intervention trial experience. J Am Coll Cardiol 1986;8:1–10.
25. Stone PH, Turi ZG, Muller JE et al. Prognostic significance of the treadmill exercise test performance 6 months after myocardial infarction. J Am Coll Cardiol 1986;8:1007–17.
26. Goldschlager N, Sox HC. The diagnostic and prognostic value of the treadmill exercise test in the evaluation of chest pain, in patients with recent myocardial infarction, and in asymptomatic individuals. Am Heart J 1988;116:523–35.
27. Dewhurst NG, Muir AL. Comparative prognostic value of radionuclide ventriculography at rest and during exercise in 100 patients after first myocardial infarction. Br Heart J 1983;49:111–21.
28. Pryor DB, Harrell FE Jr, Lee KL et al. Prognostic indicators from radionuclide angiography in medically treated patients with coronary artery disease. Am J Cardiol 1984;53:18–22.
29. Bonow RO, Kent KM, Rosing DR et al. Exercise-induced ischaemia in mildly symptomatic patients with coronary artery disease, and preserved left ventricular function: identification of subgroups at high risk for death during medical therapy. N Engl J Med 1984;311:1339–45.
30. Fioretti P, Brower RW, Simoons ML et al. Prediction of mortality in hospital survivors of myocardial infarction. Comparison of predischarge exercise testing and radionuclide ventriculography at rest. Br Heart J 1984;52:292–8.
31. Iskandrian AS, Hakki AH, Goel IP, Mundth ED, Kane-Marsch SA, Schenk CL. The use of rest and exercise radionuclide ventriculography in risk stratification in patients with suspected coronary artery disease. Am Heart J 1985;110:864–72.
32. Gillespie JA, Moss AJ. Postinfarction risk profiling: past, present and future considerations. J Am Coll Cardiol 1986;8:50–1.
33. Corne RA. Risk stratification in stable angina pectoris. Am J Cardiol 1987;59:695–7.
34. Abraham RD, Harris PJ, Roubin GS et al. Usefulness of ejection fraction response to

exercise one month after acute myocardial infarction in predicting coronary anatomy and prognosis. Am J Cardiol 1987;60:225–30.

35. Brown KA, Boucher CA, Okada RD et al. Prognostic value of exercise thallium-201 imaging in patients presenting for evaluation of chest pain. J Am Coll Cardiol 1983;1:994–1001.

36. Koss JH, Kobren SM, Grunwald AM, Bodenheimer MM. Role of exercise thallium-201 myocardial perfusion scintigraphy in predicting prognosis in suspected coronary artery disease. Am J Cardiol 1987;59:531–4.

37. Iskandrian AS, Heo J, Decoskey D, Askenase A, Segal BL. Use of exercise thallium-201 imaging for risk stratification of elderly patients with coronary artery disease. Am J Cardiol 1988;61:269–72.

38. Kaul S, Finkelstein DM, Homma S, Leavitt M, Okada RD, Boucher CA. Superiority of quantitative exercise thallium-201 variables in determining long-term prognosis in ambulatory patients with chest pain: a comparison with cardiac catheterization. J Am Coll Cardiol 1988;12:25–34.

39. Bairey CN, Rozanski A, Maddahi J, Resser KJ, Berman DS. Exercise thallium-201 scintigraphy and prognosis in typical angina pectoris and negative exercise electrocardiography. Am J Cardiol 1989;64:282–7.

40. Hendel RC, Layden JJ, Leppo JA. Prognostic value of dipyridamole thallium scintigraphy for evaluation of ischemic heart disease. J Am Coll Cardiol 1990;15:109–16.

41. Gibson RS, Watson DD, Craddock GB et al. Prediction of cardiac events after uncomplicated myocardial infarction: a prospective study comparing predischarge exercise thallium-201 scintigraphy and coronary angiography. Circulation 1983;68:321–36.

42. Leppo JA, O'Brien J, Rothendler JA, Getchell JD, Lee VW. Dipyridamole–thallium-201 scintigraphy in the prediction of future cardiac events after acute myocardial infarction. N Engl J Med 1984;310:1014–18.

43. Wilson WW, Gibson RS, Nygaard TW et al. Acute myocardial infarction associated with single vessel coronary artery disease: an analysis of clinical outcome and the prognostic importance of vessel patency and residual ischemic myocardium. J Am Coll Cardiol 1988;11:223–34.

44. Gimple LW, Hutter AM, Guiney TE, Boucher CA. Prognostic utility of predischarge dipyridamole–thallium imaging compared to predischarge submaximal exercise electrocardiography and maximal exercise thallium imaging after uncomplicated acute myocardial infarction. Am J Cardiol 1989;64:1243–8.

45. Younis LT, Byers S, Shaw L, Barth G, Goodgold H, Chaitman BR. Prognostic value of intravenous dipyridamole thallium scintigraphy after an acute myocardial ischemic event. Am J Cardiol 1989;64:161–6.

46. Younis LT, Byers S, Shaw L, Barth G, Goodgold H, Chaitman BR. Prognostic importance of silent myocardial ischaemia detected by intravenous dipyridamole thallium myocardial perfusion imaging in asymptomatic patients with coronary artery disease. J Am Coll Cardiol 1990;14:1635–41.

47. Fleg JL, Gerstenblith G, Zonderman AB et al. Prevalence and prognostic significance of exercise-induced silent myocardial ischaemia detected by thallium scintigraphy and electrocardiography in asymptomatic volunteers. Circulation 1990;81:428–36.

48. Ladenheim ML, Pollock BH, Rozanski A et al. Extent and severity of myocardial perfusion as predictors of prognosis in patients with suspected coronary artery disease. J Am Coll Cardiol 1986;3:464–71.

49. Ladenheim ML, Kotler TS, Pollock BH, Berman DS, Diamond DA. Incremental prognostic power of clinical history, exercise electrocardiography and myocardial perfusion scintigraphy in suspected coronary artery disease. Am J Cardiol 1987;59:270–7.

50. Anderson HV, Talley JD, Black AJR et al. Usefulness of coronary angioplasty in asymptomatic patients. Am J Cardiol 1990;65:35–9.

51. Little WC, Constantinescu M, Applegate RJ et al. Can coronary angiography predict the site of a subsequent myocardial infarction in patients with mild-to-moderate coronary artery disease? Circulation 1988;78:1157–66.

52. Hackett D, Davies G, Maseri A. Pre-existing coronary stenoses in patients with first myocardial infarction are not necessarily severe. Eur Heart J 1988;9:1317–23.

53. Brosius FC, Roberts WC. Comparison of degree and extent of coronary narrowing by atherosclerotic plaque in anterior and posterior transmural acute myocardial infarction. Circulation 1981;64:715–22.

Chapter 8
The Future

Instrumentation

For many years the single-headed gamma camera has been the standard instrument for almost all nuclear medicine imaging procedures. It is unlikely that we shall see a fundamental change in gamma camera technology but improvements are being made continuously. Advances in the design and stability of the photomultiplier tubes, the uniformity of the detector, and energy and temporal resolution have together halved the intrinsic resolution of the device in the last decade. Coupled with a computer capable of rapid data acquisition, processing, and display, we have an excellent instrument for emission tomography. In the next decade we can expect further improvements. Cameras with multiple heads are already available to increase the speed of data acquisition. Such increases will either be used to decrease imaging time or to reduce the radiation burden to the patient. Whilst the problems of uniformity and precision of orbit increase exponentially with the number of heads, experience and high quality engineering are providing the solution. The characteristics of the collimator are also important and 6–12-fold increases in sensitivity can be obtained by optimising the design. Modern tomographic cameras have a system resolution of 5 mm to 6 mm.

Improvements in computer technology will also be beneficial. Rapid data processing will increase patient throughput. The extraction of functional information from the images will be simplified and three-dimensional displays may become commonplace. The combination of functional nuclear medicine data with anatomical information from other tomographic imaging techniques such as X-ray transmission tomography and magnetic resonance imaging will be possible.

Single photon emission tomography has learned from positron emission tomography and it will continue to do so. The versatility of positron emitting radiopharmaceuticals is unlikely to be matched by single photon emitters but the complexity and expense of positron tomography will always exceed that of single photon tomography. In the next decade, we can expect close comparisons between the two techniques with both industry and the user searching for the most effective method of assessing myocardial perfusion and metabolism. The outcome is uncertain.

Radiopharmaceuticals

We have mainly been concerned with thallium as a tracer of myocardial perfusion and with its clinical role in patients with coronary artery disease. Our extensive experience with thallium means that it is still the standard against which other radiopharmaceuticals must be judged. The cases presented in Chapter 6 provide ample evidence of its value. It is likely, however, that thallium will be replaced by (perhaps a number of) technetium-based perfusion tracers. The most important advantages of technetium are that it is constantly available from a generator and that modern gamma cameras have been optimised to image its 140 keV emission. Technetium-based myocardial perfusion tracers are already available and their cost can be expected to fall. The ideal tracer has not yet been designed but we can expect that the manipulation of myocardial uptake, extraction fraction and residence time within the myocardium will provide us with something closer to the ideal.

At present there is a choice of two commercially available technetium agents (see Chapter 2):

- ^{99m}Tc-MIBI which is almost a pure perfusion agent which does not redistribute, therefore requiring separate injections for stress and rest.
- ^{99m}Tc-teboroxime which has very avid myocardial uptake and rapid washout and is the closest to a pure perfusion agent that we have.

Future agents will build upon the properties of these two. An important variable is the rate of washout from the myocardium. Very rapid washout (of the order of minutes) will allow repeated studies of myocardial perfusion during interventions such as thrombolysis or vasodilation. With cameras capable of rapid tomographic acquisition it will also be possible to investigate the significance of different rates of washout from normal and diseased myocardium. Longer residence times will be less demanding of acquisition technique and will allow us to combine myocardial perfusion studies with wall motion studies by gating the tomograms to the electrocardiogram. An agent with low liver uptake will avoid the problem of imaging the inferior left ventricle and high renal excretion will reduce the radiation exposure to the patient.

An important goal is the assessment of myocardial metabolism as well as perfusion using single photon emitters. At the moment, positron emission tomography is the most versatile method of assessing myocardial metabolism, but we are slowly learning that thallium also gives some metabolic information because redistribution requires viable as well as perfused myocardium. In this respect it is superior to agents that do not redistribute, although it is not yet clear whether ^{99m}Tc-MIBI may provide similar information. The relatively low first pass extraction of this agent means that viable myocardium that is poorly perfused (and may therefore be hibernating) might have the opportunity to extract tracer over the few minutes that the agent remains in the blood in significant concentrations. Given a variety of tracers with different properties, a number of approaches might provide similar information to positron emission tomography. These may be the use of multiple tracers, dual energy acquisition, serial imaging of two different tracers, or the combination of early and late imaging.

The development of other forms of tracer can also be expected. Experience is accumulating with ^{123}I-metaiodobenzylguanidine (^{123}I-MIBG) which demonstrates the adrenergic innervation of the heart,[1,2] ^{123}I-labelled fatty acids which demonstrate fatty acid metabolism[3-7] and ^{111}In-antimyosin antibody which reveals damaged or necrotic myocytes.[8-12] We can also hope for the development of a technetium-labelled analogue of glucose and for other receptor specific agents or labelled drugs that are relevant to the study of the myocardium.

Advances in myocardial perfusion imaging cannot be complete without a brief description of positron emission tomography. Radionuclides which emit positrons include carbon-11, nitrogen-13, oxygen-15 and fluorine-18. Their advantage over gamma-emitting radionuclides is that they are easily incorporated into metabolically active tracers and so allow the study of a range of metabolic pathways. The main disadvantages are their very short half-lives (typically seconds or minutes) so that a cyclotron is required close to the point of dispensing, and the requirement for specialised cameras to image their distribution in the body. Although conventional cameras can be adapted to image the 511 keV gamma rays produced by the annihilation of positrons and electrons, specialised devices that make better use of the properties of the positron rely on the detection of gamma rays emitted simultaneously in opposite directions.

In the heart, the principal applications of positron emission tomography have been the quantitative assessment of regional myocardial perfusion using rubidium-82 or ^{13}N-ammonia and the imaging of myocardial glucose metabolism using [^{18}F]-fluorodeoxyglucose (FDG). The former allows the non-invasive measurement of coronary flow reserve[13] and the latter allows hibernating myocardium to be identified as areas with reduced perfusion in which metabolism has switched from the normal utilisation of fatty acids to glucose.[14,15] The significance of this is that it may be possible to identify patients with ischaemic heart failure who do not have angina but who may benefit from revascularisation by the restoration of myocardial function.

Alternative Imaging Techniques

Nuclear cardiology is only one of several imaging techniques used in the investigation of the cardiac patient and it is important to be aware of the potential of all of them. Echocardiography, magnetic resonance imaging and ultrafast X-ray tomography are the most important techniques because they provide information on ventricular function and they also have the theoretical ability to assess coronary arterial flow and myocardial perfusion. Echocardiography and Doppler ultrasound are mature techniques and they are unlikely to benefit from fundamental advances in our understanding of physical principles. Table 8.1 summarises recent developments in the application of ultrasound and their significance for the practice of nuclear cardiology. Perhaps the most important factor is that echocardiography is widely available and is often performed by the cardiologist rather than by a third person. Familiarity with the technique may often mean that even where the corresponding nuclear technique is superior the echocardiographic equivalent may be used. An example is in stress wall motion studies where

Table 8.1. Recent developments in echocardiography and their significance for the practice of nuclear cardiology

Stress	Echocardiography with dynamic exercise is difficult but pharmacological stress is more successful. Dobutamine is superior to dipyridamole or adenosine for an anatomical technique such as echocardiography. The problem of measuring quantitative information makes stress radionuclide ventriculography preferable when both are available.
Transoesophageal	This approach produces excellent images especially of the deeper structures. It will have little impact on the value of nuclear cardiology which is primarily concerned with function and has never rivalled echocardiography as an anatomical technique.
Intravascular	Imaging of the vascular wall is an important advance for the assessment of atheroma. Direct imaging of the anatomy of atheromatous plaques coupled with an isotopic method of assessing their metabolic activity may become important in the detection and monitoring of disease.
Doppler	Doppler measurements of coronary flow acquired either transoesophageally or intravascularly have been achieved but they cannot rival the direct measurement of myocardial perfusion which is the most important variable for the individual myocyte.
Contrast	Intra-aortic injection of microbubble contrast is able to demonstrate inequalities of myocardial perfusion and of coronary flow reserve. Similar information from venous injection and quantitative measurements of myocardial perfusion are unlikely to be achieved and so the technique will not challenge the use of radioactive tracers.

the quantitative information provided by radionuclide ventriculography is superior to the qualitative information of echocardiography, but the latter may be sufficient for many clinical purposes.

X-ray transmission tomography has not played a large part in the management of the cardiac patient because the relative slowness of the technique means that electrocardiographically triggered information cannot be obtained. The only important contribution of conventional X-ray tomography has been in the assessment of the pericardium and of the aorta. The development of the electronic scanner has reduced acquisition times to between 50 and 100 ms. In this machine there are no moving parts and, instead of an X-ray source and target rotating mechanically around the patient, a beam of electrons is steered magnetically around a semicircular target. This has allowed the acquisition of tomographic images at up to 17 frames per cycle and hence of four-dimensional datasets which show global and regional ventricular function in excellent detail.[16-19] More importantly, it allows a bolus of X-ray contrast to be followed through the myocardium and this may provide an absolute measurement of myocardial perfusion.[20,21] Whilst the technique has been successfully implemented in phantom studies and in patients with intra-aortic injections, quantitative information from a venous injection is more difficult. If such measurements can be achieved, then the combination of myocardial perfusion with a high resolution imaging technique which might allow the distinction between endocardial and epicardial flow could be very important. More sophisticated measurements of myocardial metabolism are unlikely to be achieved and the complexity and expense of the technique mean that it is unlikely to replace radiopharmaceuticals for the routine assessment of myocardial perfusion.

Magnetic resonance imaging provides similar anatomical information to X-ray tomography but ionising radiation and contrast injections are not required.[22] It is, therefore, a serious rival to radionuclide ventriculography particularly since the possibility of imaging during dipyridamole[23] and dobutamine stress[24,25] has been demonstrated. Its greatest strength is that it provides functional and, to some extent, biochemical information and so many aspects of cardiovascular anatomy and function can be studied at a single sitting. Table 8.2 summarises the types of information that can be acquired and their potential impact on the use of radioisotopes. Considerable development will be required before magnetic resonance can rival isotope techniques for the assessment of myocardial perfusion and metabolism.

We believe that no single technique provides all the answers required for the management of the cardiac patient and that the cardiologist must be familiar with all of them if they are to be used appropriately. The newer

Table 8.2. Information provided by magnetic resonance imaging and its potential impact on the value of isotope techniques

Anatomy	Excellent three-dimensional anatomical information provided by spin echo imaging.
Ventricular function	Cine imaging gives accurate measurements of ventricular volumes, wall motion and wall thickening.[26] This is more accurate than radionuclide ventriculography and can be performed during pharmacological stress.[23,24] Availability of scanners, expertise and imaging time will determine whether radionuclide ventriculography is replaced.
Valve function	Accurate measurements of regurgitation can be made from ventricular volumes[27] and pressure gradients across stenoses can be measured by cine velocity mapping.[28] Radionuclides have had a small role to play but the magnetic resonance measurement of regurgitant fraction is more accurate than the radionuclide measurement.
Flow measurements	Cine velocity mapping provides accurate measurements of flow in the heart and vessels.[29,30] Isotopes cannot provide similar measurements but Doppler ultrasound can.
Tissue perfusion	Perfusion and diffusion can be measured by velocity-sensitive techniques in static organs such as the brain but not in the heart. Myocardial perfusion may be measured by real-time imaging by following boluses of magnetic resonance contrast.[31] As with ultrafast X-ray tomography, reliable measurements may be difficult from an intravenous injection and isotope techniques will not be replaced.
Tissue metabolism	Relaxation measurements give some indication of biochemical state but the parameters that determine relaxation·times are too far removed from biochemical parameters to be of value. Magnetic resonance spectroscopy provides more sophisticated biochemical information but poor sensitivity limits its applicability.[32] The translation of research spectroscopy into clinical practice may never be practical. Radionuclides will not be replaced in clinical practice but important information will be provided in research laboratories.
Chemical shift imaging	The separation of water and fat images has allowed the assessment of the composition of atheroma.[33] The relative value of magnetic resonance, intravascular ultrasound and isotope techniques has yet to be established but imaging of the vessel wall is our best hope for the early detection of atheromatous disease.

imaging techniques are able to measure ventricular volumes and wall motion just as well as radionuclide ventriculography and so this aspect of nuclear cardiology may become less important. The newer techniques are, however, either more complex or more invasive and so the simpler and less costly techniques of echocardiography and nuclear medicine will not be replaced. On the other hand, none of the new techniques provides as simple and as reliable a method of assessing myocardial perfusion as thallium tomography. In this book we have tried to demonstrate the wealth of information that can be provided and how it may be used to make important management decisions. Given that a cardiologist's familiarity with a technique is the most important factor in making it of value to him or her, we believe that we have provided a means by which thallium tomography may continue to benefit the patient with cardiovascular disease.

References

1. Henderson EB, Kahn JK, Corbett JR et al. Abnormal I-123 metaiodobenzylguanidine myocardial washout and distribution may reflect myocardial adrenergic derangement in patients with congestive cardiomyopathy. Circulation 1988;78:1192–9.
2. Schofer J, Spielmann R, Schuchert A, Weber K, Schluter M. Iodine-123 metaiodobenzyl-guanidine scintigraphy: a noninvasive method to demonstrate myocardial adrenergic nervous system disintegrity in patients with idiopathic dilated cardiomyopathy. J Am Coll Cardiol 1988;12:1252–8.
3. van der Wall EE. Myocardial imaging with radiolabeled free fatty acids: applications and limitations. Eur J Nucl Med 1986;12:S12–S15.
4. Visser FC, van Eenige MJ, Duwel CMB, Roos JP. Radioiodinated free fatty acids: can we measure myocardial metabolism? Eur J Nucl Med 1986;12:S20–S23.
5. Demaison L, Dubois F, Apparu M et al. Myocardial metabolism of radioiodinated methyl-branched fatty acids. J Nucl Med 1988;29:1230–6.
6. Ugolini V, Hansen CL, Kulkarni PV, Jansen DE, Akers MS, Corbett JR. Abnormal myocardial fatty acid metabolism in dilated cardiomyopathy detected by iodine-123 phenyl-pentadecanoic acid and tomographic imaging. Am J Cardiol 1988;62:923–8.
7. Vyska K, Machulla HJ, Stremmel W et al. Regional myocardial free fatty acid extraction in normal and ischemic myocardium. Circulation 1988;78:1218–33.
8. Khaw BA, Strauss HW, Moore R et al. Myocardial damage delineated by indium-111 antimyosin Fab and technetium-99m pyrophosphate. J Nucl Med 1987;28:76–82.
9. Braat SH, de Zwaan C, Teule J, Heidendal G, Wellens HJJ. Value of Indium-111 monoclonal antimyosin antibody for imaging in acute myocardial infarction. Am J Cardiol 1987;60: 725–6.
10. Yasuda T, Palacios IF, Dec GW et al. Indium 111-monoclonal antimyosin antibody imaging in the diagnosis of acute myocarditis. Circulation 1987;76:306–11.
11. Carrio I, Berna L, Ballester M et al. Indium-111 antimyosin scintigraphy to assess myocardial damage in patients with suspected myocarditis and cardiac rejection. J Nucl Med 1988;29:1893–900.
12. Tamaki N, Yamada T, Matsumori A et al. Indium-111 antimyosin antibody imaging for detecting different stages of myocardial infarction: comparison with technetium-99m pyrophosphate imaging. J Nucl Med 1990;31:136–42.
13. Gould KL, Goldstein RA, Mullani NA et al. Noninvasive assessment of coronary stenosis by myocardial perfusion imaging during pharmacologic coronary vasodilation. VIII. Clinical feasibility of positron cardiac imaging without a cyclotron using a generator-produced rubidium-82. J Am Coll Cardiol 1986;7:775–89.
14. Brunken R, Tillisch J, Schwaiger M et al. Regional perfusion, glucose metabolism and wall motion in chronic electrocardiographic Q-wave infarctions: evidence for persistence of viable tissue in some infarct regions by positron emission tomography. Circulation 1986;73: 951–63.

15. Tillisch J, Brunken R, Marshall R et al. Reversibility of cardiac wall motion abnormalities predicted by using positron tomography. N Engl J Med 1986;314:884–8.
16. Lipton MJ. Cine computerized tomography. Int J Card Imaging 1987;2:209–21.
17. Lanzer P, Garrett J, Lipton MJ et al. Quantitation of regional myocardial perfusion by cine computed tomography: pharmacologic changes in wall thickness. J Am Coll Cardiol 1986; 8:682–92.
18. Roig E, Chomka EV, Castaner A et al. Exercise ultrafast computed tomography for the detection of coronary artery disease. J Am Coll Cardiol 1989;13:1073–81.
19. Tanenbaum SR, Kondos GT, Veselik KE, Prendergast MR, Brundage BH, Chomka EV. Detection of calcific deposits in coronary arteries by ultrafast computed tomography and correlation with angiography. Am J Cardiol 1989;63:870–2.
20. Feiring AJ, Lipton MJ, Higgins CB et al. Measurement of myocardial perfusion by ultrafast CT. J Am Coll Cardiol 1985;5:500.
21. Wolfkiel CJ, Ferguson JL, Chomka EV et al. Measurement of myocardial blood flow by ultrafast computed tomography. Circulation 1987;76:1262–73.
22. Underwood SR, Firmin DN. Magnetic resonance of the cardiovascular system. Oxford: Blackwell's Scientific Publications, 1990.
23. Pennell DJ, Underwood SR, Ell PJ, Swanton RH, Walker JM, Longmore DB. Dipyridamole magnetic resonance imaging: a comparison with thallium-201 emission tomography. Br Heart J 1990;64:362–9.
24. Pennell DJ, Underwood SR, Swanton RH, Walker JM, Ell PJ. Dobutamine thallium-201 myocardial perfusion tomography. J Am Coll Cardiol 1991 (in press).
25. Pennell DJ, Underwood SR, Manzara CC et al. Magnetic resonance imaging of reversible myocardial ischaemia during dobutamine stress. Proceedings of the Ninth Annual Meeting. Berkeley: Society of Magnetic Resonance in Medicine 1990;116 (abstract).
26. Longmore DB, Klipstein RH, Underwood SR et al. Dimensional accuracy of magnetic resonance in studies of the heart. Lancet 1985;i:1360–2.
27. Underwood SR, Klipstein RH, Firmin DN et al. Magnetic resonance assessment of aortic and mitral regurgitation. Br Heart J 1986;56:455–62.
28. Kilner PJ, Firmin DN, Rees RSO et al. Valve and great vessel stenosis: assessment with magnetic resonance jet velocity mapping. Radiology 1991;178:229–35.
29. Underwood SR, Firmin DN, Klipstein RH, Rees RSO, Longmore DB. Magnetic resonance velocity mapping: clinical application of a new technique. Br Heart J 1987;57:404–12.
30. Rees RSO, Firmin DN, Mohiaddin RH, Underwood SR, Longmore DB. Application of flow measurements by magnetic resonance velocity mapping to congenital heart disease. Am J Cardiol 1989;64:953–6.
31. Wilke N, Engels G, Stehling M et al. Myocardial perfusion study with serial ultrafast MR imaging at rest and during dipyridamole induced stress (abstract). J Mag Reson Imag 1991;1:205.
32. Conway MA, Bristow JD, Blackledge MY, Rajagopalan B, Radda GK. Cardiac metabolism during exercise in healthy volunteers measured by ^{31}P magnetic resonance spectroscopy. Br Heart J 1991;65:25–30.
33. Mohiaddin RH, Firmin DN, Underwood SR et al. Chemical shift magnetic resonance imaging of human atheroma. Br Heart J 1989;62:81–9.

Subject Index

Abnormal appearances 33–6
  classification 34
Adenosine 17, 18
  (Case 70) 184
Aminophylline 17
Amyloidosis 35
  (Case 40) 124
Angina 18, 19, 209
Angiogram, correlations
  abnormal angiogram, normal thallium
    (Case 57) 158
  normal angiogram, left bundle branch block
    (Case 56) 156
  normal angiogram, Syndrome X (Case 55)
    154
Angiography, prognosis before and after. *See*
    Prognosis
Angioplasty
  after angioplasty study (Case 45) 134
  before angioplasty study (Case 44) 132
  recurrence of stenosis (Case 46) 136
  two-vessel disease, culprit lesion (Case 43)
    130
Anterior attenuation 33
  (Case 3) 50
Aortic stenosis 19
Apical attenuation 33
  (Case 5) 54
Artefacts
  low count rate (Case 75) 194
  motion (Case 74) 192
  objects (Case 77) 198
  upward creep (Case 76) 196
Artificial intelligence 37
Atherosclerosis, post heart transplant 36
  (Case 62) 168
Atrioventricular block 18
Attenuation correction 28

Bayes' theorem 208
Beta-blockers 15, 19
Breasts, strapping 26, 33
  (Case 3) 50
Bronchospasm 17
"Bullseye" image 37, 39
  (Case 67) 178

Bypass grafting
  postoperative study (Case 48) 140
  preoperative study (Case 47) 138
  recurrent ischaemia (Case 49) 142

Caffeine 17
Carbon-11 217
Cardiomyopathy
  dilated 35
    (Case 58) 160
  hypertrophic 35
    (Case 60) 164
  ischaemic 35
    (Case 59) 162
Chest pain 17, 18
  no chest pain with ischaemia (Case 73) 190
  normal scan (Case 35) 114
  with no ischaemia (Case 72) 188
  see also Prognosis before angiography
Circumferential profile analysis 39
Cocoa 17
Coffee 17
Colour scale 31, 32, 37
Connective tissue disorders 35
Coronary arterial anatomy 36
  (Case 64) 172
Coronary artery disease 16, 17, 19, 35, 36, 41
  detection of 207–9
  management of 209–11
  prognosis 211–12
    (Cases 34–42) 112–28
Coronary muscle bridge 35
  (Case 61) 166
Count distribution 31, 37, 38
Count rate (Case 75) 194

Data acquisition 26–7
Data processing 27–9
Diabetes 35, 36
Diagonal LAD
  (Case 11) 66
  (Case 17) 78
Diastolic coronary flow 35
Dilation of left ventricle 33
  (Case 41) 126
  (Case 42) 128

Dipyridamole 16–18, 20
  (Case 68) 180
  with exercise (Case 71) 186
Distal LAD
  (Case 12) 68
  (Case 18) 80
Dobutamine 18–19
  (Case 69) 182
Drug treatment 13–14
Dynamic exercise 15–16, 19

ECG
  left bundle branch block 35
    (Case 53) 150
  left ventricular hypertrophy 35
    (Case 54) 152
  marked changes with minor ischaemia (Case 51) 146
  marked changes with no ischaemia (Case 50) 144
  Wolff-Parkinson-White syndrome 35
    (Case 52) 148
Echocardiography, recent developments 218
Electrocardiogram gated blood pool emission tomography 24
Emission tomography 23–5
Exercise electrocardiography 211

[^{18}F]-fluorodeoxyglucose (FDG) 217
Fatty acid metabolism 217
Fluorine-18 217

Gamma camera 23, 215
Grading perfusion defects 34

Horizontal long axis (HLA) 29
Hypertension 35
Hypertrophic cardiomyopathy 33, 35
  (Case 60) 164

^{123}I-labelled fatty acids 217
^{123}I-metaiodobenzylguanidine (^{123}I-MIBG) 217
Image interpretation 31–43
  computer-aided 37
Image quality 26
Image reconstruction 27
Imaging techniques 23–9
  alternative 217–20
^{111}In-antimyosin antibody 217
Inferior attenuation (Case 4) 52
Instrumentation, future 215
Intrinsic correction 28
Ischaemia 34

LAD, anomalous origin of (Case 66) 176
LAD infarction/LCx ischaemia (Case 30) 104
LAD infarction/RCA ischaemia (Case 31) 106
LAD/LCx
  infarction (Case 25) 94
  ischaemia (Case 21) 86

LAD/LCx/RCA
  infarction (Case 27) 98
  ischaemia (Case 26) 96
LAD/RCA
  infarction (Case 24) 92
  ischaemia (Case 20) 84
LCx
  infarction (Case 14) 72
  ischaemia (Case 8) 60
LCx Infarction/LAD Ischaemia (Case 33) 110
LCx Infarction/RCA Ischaemia (Case 32) 108
Left bundle branch block 35, 36
  (Case 53) 150
  (Case 56) 156
Left main coronary artery (Case 22) 88
Left ventricle 34
  dilated after infarction (Case 42) 128
  dilated on exercise (Case 41) 126
Left ventricular hypertrophy 33, 35
  (Case 54) 152
Lung uptake, of thallium 37
  (Case 40) 124

Magnetic resonance imaging 215, 219
2–methoxy-isobutyl-isonitrile (MIBI) 9
Mixed reversible ischaemia and infarction
  LAD infarction/LCx ischaemia (Case 30) 104
  LAD infarction/RCA ischaemia (Case 31) 106
  LCx infarction/LAD ischaemia (Case 33) 110
  LCx infarction/RCA ischaemia (Case 32) 108
  RCA infarction/LAD ischaemia (Case 28) 100
  RCA infarction/LCx ischaemia (Case 29) 102
Monitoring effects of intervention 210
Motion (Case 74) 192
Myocardial damage following acute anaphylaxis (Case 65) 174
Myocardial distribution of thallium 37–40
Myocardial glucose 217
Myocardial hypertrophy 35, 36
  (Case 54) 152
Myocardial infarction 18, 209–10
Myocardial perfusion 1
Myocardial perfusion tracers 5
Myocardium
  hibernating 35, 217
    (Cases 79, 80) 202–4
  stunned 35, 217
  viability 35, 217
    (Cases 79, 80) 202–4

^{13}N-ammonia 217
Nitrogen-13 217
Normal appearance 31–3
  common variations in 33
Normal heart
  normal horizontal heart (Case 2) 48
  normal vertical heart (Case 1) 46
Normal variants
  anterior attenuation (Case 3) 50
  apical attenuation (Case 5) 54

inferior attenuation (Case 4) 52
  papillary muscle (Case 6) 56
Nuclear medicine 1

Objects (Case 77) 198
Orthotopic cardiac transplantation 36
  (Case 62) 168
Oxygen-15 217

Pacemaker 26
Papillary muscle (Case 6) 56
Partial redistribution 34
Patient preparation 25–6
PDA
  (Case 9) 62
  (Case 15) 74
Percutaneous coronary angioplasty 210
  (Cases 43–46) 130–6
Pharmacological stress 16–19
  adenosine (Case 70) 184
  dipyridamole (Case 68) 180
  dipyridamole with exercise (Case 71) 186
  dobutamine (Case 69) 182
Polar maps
  (Case 67) 178
  distribution of myocardial counts in 39
  reconstruction 39
Positron emission tomography 35, 215, 217
Postreconstruction correction 28
Prereconstruction correction 28
Prognosis 211–12
  adverse prognostic signs
    dilated left ventricle after infarction (Case
      42) 128
    dilated left ventricle on exercise (Case 41)
      126
    high lung uptake (Case 40) 124
  after angiography
    controlled chest pain, three vessel
      disease, major ischaemia (Case
      39) 122
    controlled chest pain, three vessel
      disease, minor ischaemia (Case
      38) 120
  before angiography
    chest pain, normal scan (Case 35) 114
    controlled chest pain
      major ischaemia (Case 37) 118
      minor ischaemia (Case 36) 116
    no chest pain, normal scan (Case 34) 112
Projectional imaging 24
Proximal LAD
  (Case 10) 64
  (Case 16) 76

Quality control 31
Quantification 36–41
  (Case 67) 178

Radioactive tracers 1, 6
Radiopharmaceuticals 5–11
  development 5

future 216
RCA
  (Case 7) 58
  (Case 13) 70
RCA infarction/LAD ischaemia (Case 28) 100
RCA infarction/LCx ischaemia (Case 29) 102
RCA/LCx
  infarction (Case 23) 90
  ischaemic (Case 19) 82
Redistribution imaging 26, 34
Reinjection
  (Case 80) 204
  imaging 34
Reperfusion
  reinjection (Case 80) 204
  reversed redistribution (Case 78) 200
  24 hour imaging (Case 79) 202
Reverse redistribution 35
  (Case 78) 200
Reversible ischaemia 33, 35
Reversible right ventricular ischaemia (Case
  63) 170
Right ventricle 34
Rubidium-82 217

Sarcoidosis 35
Short axis planes (SA) 28, 29
Single vessel myocardial infarction
  diagonal LAD (Case 17) 78
  distal LAD (Case 18) 80
  LCx (Case 14) 72
  PDA (Case 15) 74
  proximal LAD (Case 16) 76
  RCA (Case 13) 70
Single vessel reversible ischaemia
  diagonal LAD (Case 11) 66
  distal LAD (Case 12) 68
  LCx (Case 8) 60
  PDA (Case 9) 62
  proximal LAD (Case 10) 64
  RCA (Case 7) 58
Stenosis, recurrence (Case 46) 136
Stress images 26–7
Stress techniques 13–22
  choice of 19–20
Syndrome X 35
  (Case 55) 154

^{99m}Tc-MIBI 9–10, 216
^{99m}Tc-teboroxime 10, 216
Tea 17
Technetium-based myocardial perfusion
  tracers 216
Thallium-201 6–8
  development 5
  emission tomography 24
  imaging, and tomography 2
  injection 25
  limitations 8
  lung uptake of 37
  myocardial distribution of 37–40
  problems with 1–2

role in cardiac imaging 1
  scintigraphy 1
Three vessel disease
  infarction (Case 27) 98
  ischaemia (Case 26) 96
  prognosis (Cases 38–39) 120–2
Tomography versus planar imaging 2
Tracer delivery inequalities 35
Tracer uptake defects 35
24–hour imaging (Case 79) 202
Two vessel disease, culprit lesion (Case 43)
    130
Two vessel myocardial infarction
  LAD/LCx (Case 25) 94
  LAD/RCA (Case 24) 92
  RCA/LCx (Case 23) 90
Two vessel reversible ischaemia

LAD/LCx (Case 21) 86
LAD/RCA (Case 20) 84
left main coronary artery (Case 22) 88
RCA/LCx (Case 19) 82

Upward creep 31
  (Case 76) 196

Ventricle size and shape 33
Ventricular fibrillation 18
Vertical long axis (VLA) 28, 29

Washout analysis 41
Wolff–Parkinson–White syndrome (Case 52)
    148

X-ray transmission tomography 215, 217, 218